A Christian Worldview & Mental Health

A Seventh-day Adventist Perspective

A Christian Worldview & Mental Health

A Seventh-day Adventist Perspective

Edited by:

Carlos Fayard
Barbara Couden Hernandez
Bruce Anderson
George T. Harding IV

Andrews University Press
Berrien Springs, Michigan

Andrews University Press
Sutherland House
8360 W. Campus Circle Dr.
Berrien Springs, MI 49104–1700
Telephone: 269-471-6134
Fax: 269-471-6224
Email: aupo@andrews.edu
Website: http://universitypress.andrews.edu

ISBN 978-1-883925-68-0

Printed in the United States of America
15 14 13 12 11 1 2 3 4 5

Library of Congress Cataloging-in-Publication Data

A Christian worldview and mental health : Adventist perspectives / Carlos Fayard ... [et al.], editors.
p. cm.
Includes bibliographical references and index.
ISBN 978-1-883925-68-0 (pbk. : alk. paper) 1. Mental health--Religious aspects--Seventh-Day Adventists--Congresses. 2. Psychiatry and religion--Congresses. 3. Psychology and religion--Congresses. I. Fayard, Carlos, 1954–

BT732.4.C37 2011
261.5'15--dc23

2011012751

Project Director	Ronald Alan Knott
Project Editor	Deborah L. Everhart
Copy Editor	Deborah L. Everhart
Indexer	Carol J. Schoun
Cover Designer	Tiago Baltazar
Text Designer	Tiago Baltazar
Typesetters	Tiago Baltazar, Deborah L. Everhart

Typeset: 11/15 Minion Pro

While numerous articles and books have been written about the theoretical and philosophical foundations of mental health, mental illness, research, and treatment, comparatively few have been published on the interrelationship of spirituality, religion, and psychiatry. This volume, while discussing a wide variety of topics, is held together by writers who share a common biblically-based worldview. I believe that many mental health professionals, academics, and others will find *A Christian Worldview and Mental Health* stimulating, challenging, and rewarding. My hope would be that it inspire a new generation of interest, research, and clinical applications in this important area.

Richard K. Harding, M.D., Chair and Professor
Department of Neuropsychiatry and Behavioral Science
University of South Carolina School of Medicine
Past president, American Psychiatric Association

This volume provides timely new information that provides a foundation that can usher in a new era in which we thoughtfully and comprehensively confront the challenge of mental health and mental illness in the church and society. The collection of essays provide an in-depth look, not only at a biblically-informed, nuanced, conceptual perspective on mental health but also a practical guide for scholars, mental health professionals, and clergy. It will be an indispensable handbook for many.

David R. Williams, Ph.D
Florence and Laura Norman Professor of Public Health
and of African and African American Studies
Harvard University

This volume is simultaneously comprehensive and useful. It builds on the historic commitment of Seventh-day Adventists to wholistic health by drawing on empirical research, clinical practice, and the Bible.…Some parts present a Seventh-day Adventist perspective, such as the chapter on the Sabbath as a resource for marriage enrichment, while others draw on concepts shared by people in many faith traditions. It concludes with a section on the education and supervision of mental health practitioners. As such, it will be of value to students and educators in the social/behavioral and health sciences, as well as those in religion and theology.

Lisa M. Beardsley, Ph.D, Director of Education
General Conference of Seventh-day Adventists

The book's major contributions lie with its intentionality to apply a Christian worldview to various clinical practices and institutional cultures. In this sense it moves from the theoretical to the applied in creative and suggestive ways. It provides a reasoned integrative path of how mental health clinicians and educators alike can confidently claim a faith that seeks understanding without it being sacrificed on the table of humanistic philosophy. And yet, it challenges those who hold Christian worldviews to make their claims credible through empirical evidence.

Edwin I. Hernandez, Ph.D
Research Fellow at the Center for the Study of Latino Religion
University of Notre Dame

Through scientific and careful analysis, the authors explore some of the factors that impact the state of human mental wellness and healing. Any therapeutic recommendations harmonize with their worldview of God's restorative intention. The primacy of mental health in the way we adapt and adjust to physical disability underscores the importance of a unified biblical worldview. To face physical adversity with an equanimity of spirit is bolstered by belief in an eternal God Who moves to ensure the ultimate best.

Allan R. Handysides, Ch.B., Director, Department of Health Ministries
General Conference of Seventh-day Adventists

TABLE OF CONTENTS

SECTION 4: CLINICAL APPLICATIONS

SECTION 5: EDUCATION AND TRAINING

PREFACE AND ACKNOWLEDGEMENTS

Akumal is a beautiful location on the Mexican Caribbean where the initial steps were taken for the formulation of what has come to be known as Positive Psychology. Coincidentally, Akumal is the place where the initial idea for the development of a symposium on mental health issues informed by Seventh-day Adventist ideas and practices was born.

Edward Zinke, president of the Foundation for Adventist Education, provided the initial impetus and financial support, along with Humberto Rasi, executive director of the Foundation for Adventist Education and Special Projects Coordinator for the Department of Education, General Conference of Seventh-day Adventists. The Department of Psychiatry at Loma Linda University School of Medicine and its chair William Murdoch gave crucial financial and logistical guidance.

George T. Harding IV had a profound influence on the organization of the symposium. As a leader in the American Psychiatric Association, and having served as the president of its Section on Religion and Psychiatry, Dr. Harding made available his wisdom, wide network of connections with Seventh-day Adventist professionals, and access to funds from the Harding-Evans Foundation and Versafund.

Meaningful organizational and financial support was provided by Carla Gober, Director of the Center for Wholeness and Spiritual Life at Loma Linda University, and, through her efforts, the Office of the President at Loma Linda University. Henry Lamberton, Associate Dean for Student Affairs at Loma Linda University School of Medicine, and Barbara Hernandez, Associate Professor of Counseling and Family Science at Loma Linda University, contributed their time, talents, and vast experience to the successful organization of the symposium. To each one of them I offer my deepest gratitude.

Rancho Palos Verdes, California, the location for this symposium, is far from Akumal, and very likely the impact of our symposium is far from the revolutionary change in the behavioral sciences brought about by Positive Psychology. There are a number of powerful reasons for Seventh-day Adventists to reflect together on the impact of our spiritual heritage on how we think about and practice the mental health professions. This volume, which consists of the presentations made at the symposium, is offered to the reader with the hope of explicating the unique perspectives and contributions of Seventh-day Adventism on mental health practice, programming, and education.

–Carlos Fayard

ABBREVIATIONS FOR BIBLE VERSIONS

AMP	Amplified Bible
ASV	American Standard Version
CEV	Contemporary English Version
ERV	English Revised Version
ESV	English Standard Version
GW	GOD'S WORD Translation
HCSB	Holman Christian Standard Bible
KJV	King James Version
LB	Living Bible
MSG Bible	*The Message*
NASB	New American Standard Bible
NIV	New International Version
NKJV	New King James Version
NRSV	New Revised Standard Version
YLT Bible	Young's Literal Translation

Section 1

Seventh-day Adventists and Mental Health

A Christian Worldview and Mental Health: An Introduction and Background to the Symposium

Carlos Fayard

WORLDVIEWS AND MENTAL HEALTH

As in any realm of scientific and professional endeavor, once religious claims of some sort are made, there is a host of implications that follow. How do science and religion relate? Which set of ideas has control over the other? Do religion's assumptions about the nature of reality, history, and the role of revelation inform and shape the interpretation and use of scientific data? What is a believing scientist to do when a faith-based paradigm is unacceptable by the scientific community, and yet, to be relevant, some kind of common ground is necessary?

More precisely, for the mental health field, do Adventist ideas about the role of the Word of God in human life, health, and healing make a difference on constructs ranging from notions of human nature and ethics to the role of spirituality in clinical interventions? Does a wholistic paradigm make a difference? If it makes a difference, is it visible in our teaching, research, and practice? Should it be?

I will briefly expand on the rationale for choosing the terms that guided the organization of this symposium. It might be ironic for a gathering of believers to call on Ludwig Wittgenstein to help us define the notion of a worldview. He tells us that a worldview is part of the riverbed that channels one's thinking. Theologian N.T. Wright (1992) affirms that worldviews "form the grids through which humans, both individually and in groupings, perceive all of reality" (p. 32). Closer to home for mental health professionals, Sigmund Freud (1933) defined worldview as "an intellectual construction which solves all the problems of our existence in virtue of a comprehensive hypothesis" (p. 1). The omnipresence and relevance of worldviews are perhaps more apparent in the behavioral sciences than in many other areas of scientific and applied knowledge, as worldviews answer basic questions about who we are, or what it means to be human. In the words of Bevan and Kessel, "Worldviews are like sand at a picnic; they get into everything" (Bevan & Kessel, 1994, as cited by Bufford, 2007, p. 293).

Don Browning (2000), at the University of Chicago, has been a leader in identifying some of the assumptions that are embedded in the theories of psychotherapy, whether or not they are explicitly recognized. For instance, judgments about notions of ultimate reality such as the existence of God and the value of religion, and notions about human nature such as theories of motivation and the role of spirituality in human development, are routinely promoted. Theories of psychotherapy have implicit ethical theories and clear notions about human flourishing and derailment.

Should Adventist Christians simply throw the proverbial baby out with the bath water because of the philosophical and spiritual entanglement found in psychotherapeutic theory? Do we as committed Adventists—who take the Bible as the Word of God and have embraced the mission of our church—reach different conclusions about human nature, ethics, the nature of reality, and what constitutes a life worth living from the ones found in psychological theory? If we have a different worldview, does it make a difference in the way we do research, train students, and carry out clinical work? In other words, if we develop and apply a worldview anchored in Scripture that is shaped by the Christian experience of the Seventh-day Adventist community, what difference will it make in the crucial areas of clinical practice, education and training, theory development, and research?

A BRIEF HISTORY OF PSYCHOTHERAPEUTIC THEORY AS A WORLDVIEW

Mental health professionals reflect, to some extent, the worldview of their founding fathers, who frequently were hostile to religion in general, and to Christianity in particular. For instance, Sigmund Freud

(1933) said the following when addressing the question of the impact of psychoanalytic understanding on a worldview:

> Of the three forces which can dispute the position of science [art, philosophy, and religion], religion alone is a really serious enemy.... If one wishes to form a true estimate of the full grandeur of religion, one must keep in mind what it undertakes to do for men. It gives them information about the source and origin of the universe, it assures them of protection and final happiness amid the changing vicissitudes of life, and it guides their thoughts and actions by means of precepts which are backed by the whole force of its authority. It fulfills, therefore, three functions. In the first place, it satisfies man's desire for knowledge; it is here doing the same thing that science attempts to accomplish by its own methods, and here, therefore, enters into rivalry with it. It is to the second function that it performs that religion no doubt owes the greater part of its influence. In so far as religion brushes away men's fear of the dangers and vicissitudes of life, in so far as it assures them of a happy ending, and comforts them in their misfortunes, science cannot compete with it" (p. 3).

Freud's extraordinary recognition is truly a lamentation. His personal negative views on religion have been well documented (see Nicholi, 2003) and are quite apparent in his copious theorizing, as in his books *The Future of an Illusion* and *Totem and Taboo,* among others. Freud's influence on generations of mental health practitioners cannot be minimized. Christian psychoanalyst Randall Lehman Sorenson (2004) examined references to spirituality or religion in psychoanalytic journals and assessed Freud's impact on his followers: "The proportion of wholesale pathologizing of religion in psychoanalytic journals decreased significantly following Freud's death, compared to more nuanced and balanced accounts of religion that have appeared in the years since" (p. 34).

Carl Jung has been thought to be a friend of religion. One of his quotations has been heard many times in sermons, indicating the superiority of religion over any kind of psychological theory or therapy:

"Among all my patients in the second half of life...there has not been one whose problem in the last resort was not that of finding a religious outlook on life...none of them has been really healed who did not regain his religious outlook" (1933, p. 229). However, Jung also wrote this: "the Christian church has failed to stand the baptism by fire, that is the test of reality" (1933, p. 100). He claimed that figures, such as Christ, "do not exist outside the psyche" (quoted in Foster, 1994, p. 111). It is fair to say that Jung did have an influence in the field of religion and mental health as his views paved the way for Eastern-based (immanent) spiritualities into psychotherapeutic theory and practice (Clarke, 1994).

Carl Rogers who himself trained at a seminary came to this conclusion: "Neither the Bible, nor the prophets—neither Freud nor research—neither the revelations of God nor man—can take precedence over my own direct experience" (1961, p. 89). Certainly this worldview has clear correlations to Roger's implicit ethical system and approach to psychotherapy (Browning, 2000) and the questionable value he gives to religious ideas. But no one has been as vitriolic in his language as Albert Ellis (1980), the founder of Rational Emotive Therapy: "Devout and orthodox religiosity is in many respects equivalent to irrational thinking and emotional disturbance...the elegant therapeutic solution to emotional problems is to be quite unreligious..." (p. 636).

The hostility of the founding fathers of psychotherapy is no longer as strong. The book written by Christian psychoanalyst Randall Sorenson (2004) quoted above was edited by a popular analytic publisher. Even Albert Ellis co-edited a volume on the application of Rational Emotive Therapy to Christian populations (Nielsen, Johnson, & Ellis, 2001). The American Psychological Association has published a series of volumes that reflects this shift. However, when surveys are conducted, clinicians tend to describe themselves as "spiritual but not religious," which according to Pargament's research reflects a negative view for organized religion (Zinnebauer & Pargament, 2005).

The decrease in hostility has resulted in a more ecumenical environment of tolerance towards what is deemed to be spiritual.

However, these two most powerful paradigms emerging in the world of psychotherapy theory and practice—namely evolutionary psychology and Buddhist psychology—have no room for the fundamental Christian assumption that God is real and active in human affairs.

Evolutionary psychology is frequently utilized as an overarching theoretical context to explain behavior and basic human motivation (e.g., Buss, 2007). I am not suggesting that scientific psychology should incorporate explicit Christian beliefs, but different assumptions about human nature result in different explanatory models. A case in point is the interpretation of altruistic behavior, and the implications derived in the field of moral psychology, where evolution is construed to shape even selfless behaviors out of selfish motives. A second very influential paradigm in the field of psychotherapy comes from Buddhist philosophies. Mindfulness interventions teach individuals how to become detached by focusing in the present and decreasing judgment; "befriending the problem" as attachment is thought to cause suffering. Through mindfulness Buddhists explore "the richness of pure experience"—those brief moments when the mind is not involved in the construction of meaning. By contrast, a Christian's informed approach may seek to facilitate detachment from negative aspects in one's life by developing a closer walk with Christ and finding a richness of experience in the abiding of the Holy Spirit.

Some could argue that just as Christians have come to appreciate aspects of psychoanalytic theory, discarding the elements that conflict with a Christian perspective, the same may happen with Evolutionary Psychology and Buddhist-inspired interventions. The purpose of this symposium, however, is not necessarily to seek points of contact with existing theories, nor to develop an apologetic against these or other theories. It is to nurture the development of an affirmative perspective that is grounded in the Bible as the Word of God, and find that in embracing the mission of our church we may reach different conclusions about human nature, ethics, the nature of reality, and what constitutes a life worth living. And if we do this, we must articulate it affirmatively in the way we do research, train students, and carry out clinical work.

WORLDVIEWS HAVE PRACTICAL IMPLICATIONS: A BRIEF CLINICAL EXAMPLE

Let me insert a brief clinical example to illustrate this point. I once saw a single young person who reported to have had a physical relationship with two individuals who were married. The disclosure of molestation through the age of nine provided a possible way to understand a behavior that puzzled and distressed my patient. "I am not like that! I was not raised that way!" was repeated several times while sobbing. What worldview would be appropriate to understand this person's predicament? A worldview that drives self-reproach and judgment into hopelessness (this model would exclude psychological, emotional, and developmental factors)? A worldview that highlights unconscious relational patterns in which traumatic experience is mastered by turning active that which was suffered passively (a worldview that would diminish moral responsibility)? Yet another worldview would question the patient's self-condemnation as an expression of a moral reaction that is itself the cause for the distress, and therefore the target of treatment (a worldview model that sees religion as immoral). Will the worldview of the therapist have a crucial impact on the assessment of the problem and the direction of treatment? Unavoidably so!

I suggest that in the clinical example given above, a biblical-Christian worldview would confidently affirm (explicitly if the patient is a believer, implicitly if the patient is not) my patient's worth in God's eyes regardless of the condition that brought this person to my office. A wholistic view of human nature would neither be hesitant about the appropriate use of medications if needed nor of engaging the patient's spirituality as aides to treatment. It would use both as needed and appropriate. Although a clear ethical breach would be recognized, it would not lead to condemnation (John 8:11). In summary, human flourishing and derailment as applied to this case would be informed by a wholistic view of human nature—a notion of ultimate reality that welcomes God as integral to personal well-being and which is not devoid of personal ethical expectations. The conceptual result would lead to clinical interventions that may use elements from other paradigms—addressing the impact of trauma on development, for example. Interventions informed by an evolutionary psychology worldview or a Buddhist worldview would result in some areas of substantial difference.

BACKGROUND TO THE SYMPOSIUM

Why, then, should we as a community of believers care about these issues? The Seventh-day Adventist church operates a large chain of hospitals and clinics where mental health services are delivered as well as a large educational system literally covering the planet where students are trained to enter mental health related professions or are taught about the behavioral sciences. Unlike other Christian organizations, the Seventh-day Adventist church has a distinctive element of its identity that has been referred to as the "Health Message." Perhaps unique to the Christian body, Adventists see health concerns as a matter of doctrinal truth as reflected in fundamental belief 22—*Christian behavior*. To us, matters of health are not just conduits for outreach and compassionate service. Our bodies, including the brain, mediate the quality of our spiritual lives. Health concerns are at the center of our theology, our self-understanding as a church, and our mission.

Some fear that we may not have lived up to the privilege that our church founders passed on to the present generation as they developed such an incredible organization and community. Here are some concerns: Can we say that the ideals of wholeness found in our theology have been clearly assimilated in health and mental health settings? Can we claim that each patient who enters a Seventh-day Adventist facility encounters an organizational culture and health care delivery parameters that reflect a wholistic approach?

What about the educational system? Seventh-day Adventist universities currently educate and train mental health professionals in every conceivable branch of practice. Do the curricula offered reflect something beyond competent education and training comparable to that found in reputable organizations down the road? Do we have faculty who are identified with a spiritually sensitive approach? Do our students call for it? Do they want it? Those of us in the trenches of the Adventist educational and health care systems and who care about the answers to these questions know that the response is mixed.

Finally, can we say that Adventist health organizations provide the critical context for the clinical education and training necessary to realize the vision of whole-person care? There is no other link in the educational process in mental health as crucial as this one. Educators know that the answer to this question is not as encouraging as it ought to be. There is a lot of work to do.

CHALLENGES AND CONCERNS

I will now turn to briefly discuss current challenges and concerns in graduate education, academic scholarship, and clinical training and education in the Seventh-day Adventist system.

GRADUATE EDUCATION

Perhaps a way to approximate an assessment of the state of current affairs in this regard is to ask a few more questions. In 1977, the Education Department of the General Conference published a series of papers by behavioral scientists, mental health practitioners, and theologians called "Adventist Concepts in Psychology." Although naturally dated by now, the richness of these contributions did not seem to move beyond the important step of legitimizing mental health training and mental health treatment in the Adventist church. Sadly, the conceptual aspects of this effort did not seem to fare quite as well. This is perhaps most apparent when the transcripts from graduate students of Seventh-day Adventist programs are compared to those of programs self identified as Christian. The differences are significant in quantity and quality, and not in our favor.

Let me hasten to indicate that meaningful effort is underway to be more intentional and modify the current state of affairs. The papers prepared by Dr. Murdoch and his collaborators, and by Dr. Hernandez give us reasons to hope. Now, could I be more personal here? As someone who came to the United States hoping that I would be educated in this manner several years ago, I am amazed at the incredible untapped resources Adventists have to realize this vision. The Christian programs that provide more depth and substance in the training of their students participate in an integrated health system where the richness of clinical training opportunities are simply unparalleled. We could only dream of such opportunity! This point was recently brought home as I drove around Loma Linda with a well-respected researcher who works at one of these programs.

A clear and present danger is the perception that some students and trainees have that we "talk the talk, but don't walk the walk." That is, we claim to train and provide whole-person care, when the content of our teaching and practice is often basically comparable to secular organizations. In my view, there is no deeper injury in the formation process than the one that comes from the belief that hypocrisy and apathy carry the day.

ACADEMIC SCHOLARSHIP

Some Adventist scholars are doing cutting-edge work in mental health, and some participated in the symposium. However, to my knowledge, Adventists are not known as leaders in the field that relates mental health and Christianity. Some are conducting excellent research and should be recognized by the rest of us for their contributions, and be encouraged to continue. But when it comes to articulating various aspects of a Christian worldview in the mental health literature, we are yet to produce noticeable scholarship. Perhaps Adventist pragmatism and service orientation may not have inspired us to contribute in this arena.

The result nevertheless is that if explicitly relating faith and practice in mental health is not a prominent area of scholarship and investment, the curricula and training are bound to reflect primarily a professional focus.

Some argue that a "Christian environment" is the differential element in the formation process. After several years of involvement in an "Adventist Christian environment," I would say: *good, but not good enough*. The cautious side of this argument would say that if we don't have much to say, we better not say much as it would hurt our credibility. It was the hope of the organizers of this symposium that this trend may be changed with the contributions of the papers presented. My personal assessment is that this is an area with varying levels of progress as reflected by the papers read during the symposium, and that much work remains.

CLINICAL EDUCATION AND TRAINING

The reputation of Adventist hospitals and clinics is just as diverse as that found in any other organization. However, are these facilities widely recognized for providing spiritually informed care? Do people who value a wholistic philosophy of medical care flock to them? Perhaps they do, but if so, it is a well kept secret. Some argue, for example, that a Christian endocrinologist of similar competency to a non-Christian but caring physician would make a difference in the quality of care delivered. It might not be by much, but it should as I will elaborate below. Now, when it comes to mental health, a whole-person Christian approach should make a critical difference.

If the parent health organizations and administrations either fail to value this differential element or if they do not nurture its implementation as it demands expertise and resources they may not possess, the promise of Adventist health care facilities becoming a model for intentional and integrated whole-person care will not be realized. Paradoxically, in this age, given the mounting support for comprehensive systems of care, ignoring spiritual, nutritional, and psychological components may even fail to meet regulatory expectations (see Deane Wolcott's paper in this volume for a review of the issues). It goes without saying that if the health care facility is not providing whole-person care, little integrative clinical training is likely to take place either. Students and trainees may encounter these experiences in a haphazard way when they stumble upon such a teacher or clinician, but it would be very difficult to incorporate it into a trainee's professional identity.

CHRISTIAN WORLDVIEW AND MODELS OF INTEGRATION

The debates on the proper role and relationship between religion and science have not been particularly prominent in the mental health field, perhaps because of the influence of the founding fathers as discussed. The behavioral sciences have held a conceptual control on religion. That is, they have attempted to explain religion as a set of behaviors, cognitions, and social forces. Christian psychologists have been an exception (see Stevenson, Eck, & Hill, 2007, for a detailed account of various approaches to this task). For the purposes of the symposium, I will summarize three dominant models of relating faith and science in the mental health field: the *levels of explanation model*, the *integration model*, and the *fermentation model*. As the reader goes through the papers compiled in this volume, aspects of these approaches can be discerned.

The *levels of explanation model* basically posits that humans are best understood in terms of the hierarchy of disciplines of relative complexity which study different aspects of human experience, and that should not be confused. For example, theology belongs in one place, psychology in another, biology in another, chemistry in another, and so on. Theological understanding and ideas cannot be used to guide research in chemistry or interpret data in biology. Psychology should not be treated differently. This model operates under a scientific worldview and tends to produce more rigorous research as shown in fields such as the psychology of religion, or the health benefits of religious practices.

The *integration model* assumes that there are areas in which there is an overlap between religion and mental health, and therefore Christian theology is a partner in the exploration process. Some of the most helpful results from this model come from studies on forgiveness, among other subjects. Integrationists, as they call themselves, have been most active in the education of psychologists for clinical service, with the doctoral programs at Fuller Theological Seminary and Biola University being outstanding examples. A focus of endeavor has been how to facilitate access to spiritual resources in the clinician's office to help those in emotional pain. For instance, an integrationist may adopt a Cognitive-Behavioral Therapy approach to the treatment of depression appropriating Christian cognitions to counter the negative cognitions that contribute to the depression.

Early on, Integrationists utilized a "filter" methodology, in which basically psychological theory is controlled by, or goes through the filter of, Christian theology. Whatever is deemed compatible is kept and whatever is deemed to be in conflict with the Christian faith is discarded.

The *integration model*—and its variant, the "filter" methodology—is by its very nature in a state of constant tension, definition, and re-definition. Thus the worldview emerging from this paradigm is less coherent than the *levels of explanation* model. In an honest attempt to establish and maintain a dialogue with relevant psychological theory and practice, the integrationist sometimes becomes enamored with the ideas coming from psychological theory, which in fact become the controlling worldview. Christianity is then domesticated in some fashion. The result is that psychological theory becomes a sort of filter for Christian ideas.

Finally, the *fermentation model* argues that the place from which the conversation between psychology and Christianity starts is a Christian understanding of reality. The agenda of this model is to develop a distinctive Christian psychology shaped primarily by Scripture and the writings of prominent Christian authors such as Augustine and others. This is one of the newest efforts in the field. Among other contributions, Christian psychology is legitimizing the use of the Bible as a primary source for forming psychological theory. A good example is the work of Roberts (2007) on moral emotions and virtues. Like the *levels of explanation* model, this approach has a more integrated worldview, but has yet to grapple with the implications of diversity within the Christian community (for a discussion on this topic, see Murphy, 2005).

When we adopt a Christian worldview as informed by a Seventh-day Adventist perspective, should we select one of the models summarized above? I have my own bias in this regard, which I believe is revealed in fairly explicit ways. But in a more general context, I agree with Johnson and Jones (2005) who argue that a Christian worldview of mental health will not necessarily differ in every respect from modern or postmodern psychology except when the mental health feature under consideration is worldview dependent. What areas of mental health are *not* so worldview dependent? Mostly those associated with basic science such as biological mechanisms (genetics, neurobiology, and basic motivational components). Also psychological mechanisms, like learning and memory; cognitive processes; and social processes, such as cybernetics, social influence, group dynamics, and social skills. In my view, worldview issues are present in the basic sciences in regards to the kinds of questions asked, the preferred methodology utilized, and how the interpretation of findings is connected to a larger body of knowledge or theoretical corpus.

How do we identify areas of mental health that *are* worldview dependent? These are most often subject to social and cultural influence, the ones that are most complex, most existential, and the understanding of which is the most value-laden. These would include areas through which "the riverbed of one's thinking flows" (Wittgenstein, p. 97), such as epistemology, philosophical anthropology (notions of human nature), areas of moral ethics or values, the definitions of what it means to be healthy, to be mature, to flourish or derail during the lifespan, and finally, definitions of healing or the nature of interventions. All of these have a direct impact on what one would consider adequate education and training.

SEVENTH-DAY ADVENTIST PERSPECTIVES

When we talk about Seventh-day Adventist perspectives, what are we talking about? As a lay person who is also privileged through my profession to hear about what *really* is going on in Adventism from across the world, because Loma Linda attracts folks from all over the United States and around the Adventist world, I have witnessed an assortment of astonishing developments in the last quarter of a century. As documented by the wave of the Valuegenesis studies (Gillespie, 2002), a grace orientation has become more the norm rather than the exception. The personally devastating remnants of "last generation theology" have loosened their grip on the Adventist soul. Along with this development, which I have found psychologically healthy, has been a polarization in the body politic (by the way, I do not believe that the shift to a grace orientation contributes to the fragmentation seen in our community). Very few doctrines have continued to function as a point of theological contact for most within our community of faith, and even fewer seem to be compelling in the lives of younger Adventists. One perhaps unintended and negative effect has been the de-legitimization of many religious practices and beliefs. When de-legitimization is coupled with a weakened sense of belonging to a community as demonstrated by the graying present in many Anglo congregations, the real question is: if we talk Adventist perspectives, would anyone listen?

Thus, when we approach the topic of Seventh-day Adventist perspectives, can we identify ideas that could be both compelling (i.e., perceived as "legitimate") and central to Seventh-day Adventist experience? Here is my own decidedly limited and humble effort circumscribed to the purposes of this symposium and the edited book that resulted from it. Here is the question that some of the symposium organizers hoped to have participants focus in on: *What could we mean by an affirmative Adventist spiritual identity relevant to mental health theory and practice*?

I would like to offer a couple of rudimentary proposals to answer this question. One has to do with the attitude that should guide our methodology. The second has to do with what I think Adventists from different persuasions may find spiritually compelling. Because Adventists have vigorously sought to provide an intelligent foundation for our faith, we have as a community engaged in a variety of activities, from medicine to archaeology, which we have believed can only strengthen both faith and science. These emphases should result in a humble epistemology as we approach topics in mental health using a biblical-Christian worldview.

The second consideration has to do with what one might identify as Adventist spirituality at its best. I realize that as I bring up the topic of spirituality I am already walking on thin ice for some, so let me explain. I simply mean, by spirituality, the experience of faith: how our faith is lived out, not just what the twenty-eight doctrines stipulate. I nominate compassionate service as the primary candidate. Other Christians seem perplexed by what they perceive as our timid Christianity. Adventists tend to keep matters of the Spirit to themselves or in their heads, and less evident in their day-to-day social practices. Prayer and prayerful, Spirit-led Bible study are kept to the sanctity of our personal chambers, and seldom become apparent during corporate activities. But compassionate service is not. We all grew up with mission stories of self-denial and daring for God. Generation after generation of Seventh-day Adventists has trained in the health professions to serve their communities and the world. The disproportionate size of the health and educational Adventist system relative to the membership is a testimony to the noble power of compassionate service.

More precisely, when we talk about health care delivery as "the right arm of the Gospel" (White, 1903), the image is one of action as opposed to one of contemplation. Ellen White's guidance in this regard is priceless: healing *is* ministry. Thus, Seventh-day Adventist spirituality in mental health is very likely one that invites reflection, but would be somewhat restless until it finds pragmatic ways of expressing itself. It might perceive theoretical constructs as having relative significance insofar as they may facilitate compassionate action and engagement in the hospital ward, the consulting room, the supervisory discussion, the classroom, and perhaps in mostly applied research. I think it less likely that Adventists may sit around just talking about these issues without keeping an eye on their application.

In summary, Seventh-day Adventist perspectives need to have a humble epistemology simply because as we seek to understand God, there is much we just cannot know (Isa. 55:8–9); science, on the other hand, presents both limitations and challenges that result in a necessarily constantly precarious status. Because Seventh-day Adventists see compassionate service as a natural outflowing of their spirituality, there may be more emphasis on contributions that have a predominantly applied context and that lead toward a full restoration of health, rather than being concerned as to how to make Christian assumptions explicit along the way.

OVERVIEW OF THE BOOK

The contents of this volume demonstrate a diverse use of the notion of a worldview in mental health. In part, that is due to the multidisciplinary nature of this book; the organizers intentionally invited academics in theology, philosophy, and ethics to dialogue with sociologists, historians, psychologists, psychiatrists, social workers, and marriage and family therapists. Furthermore, the mental health field is not very familiar with the concept of a worldview and its impact on both the providers and the recipients of clinical services (Josephson & Peteet, 2004); thus, this is a conceptual tool that contributors to this volume use in various ways. Sometimes, the notion of a worldview is explicitly utilized, and at other times it is implicit in the writing. Finally, the diverse angles from which the contributors proceed mirror the observations made by Mathisen (2003) as to how academics engage the integration of faith and learning in their respective disciplines. Some describe an explicit Christian worldview as the foundation for their ideas. Others apply components of the scientific worldview to their research or clinical application as it interacts with the worldview of Christians. Yet others think critically about a Christian worldview relying on competing worldviews.

Understanding where we come from as a community is essential to the development of a healthy perspective on the Christian worldview we hold as Seventh-day Adventists. In this first section of the book, George Harding takes the reader into a fascinating and very personal history as to where Adventists have contributed on mental health issues and where we are today. Ellen White's ideas and experience are foundational to almost everything Adventist. In the second section, Merlin Burt sheds light on the historical context that informed her writings on mental health, and on Ellen White's own interaction with emotional suffering. I can only wish his article would have been available when I was starting my career as her statements were frequently used as a hammer, and I, a young psychology student, was the nail upon which it was used.

Essential to the task of thinking Christianly about mental health issues are the challenges present in the conversation between faith and science. Mental health practitioners rarely stop to consider how their scientific knowledge is developed or how philosophical assumptions about human nature shape clinical theory. Edward Zinke provides a helpful historical overview on the tension between the worldview of faith and the emergence of the worldview of science, which has shaped the philosophical assumptions underlying the behavioral sciences. Miroslav Kiš illuminates the ways in which a Christian worldview can inform the epistemological process as applied to mental health disciplines. Richard Rice opens a powerful vista from which mental health professionals can think biblically about what it means to be human. He applies it to specific areas that contribute to mental health, followed by further applications by Bruce Anderson. Finally, Gerald Winslow weaves epistemological and ethical considerations to offer a critical appraisal of the inherent limits of the scientific endeavor when applied to human beings. The notion of human freedom defies the boundaries of the scientific method and worldview.

The third section of this book focuses on research findings. David Williams skillfully points to the benefits associated with a spiritual walk, and warns against uncritical assertions about the power of religion on human emotional well-being. The articles by Jana Boyd, and by Barbara Couden Hernandez and Jamie Aten, illustrate how ideas important to Adventists can guide research and inform the religious experience of Seventh-day Adventists.

The fourth section of this volume attempts to exemplify how Seventh-day Adventists grapple with different aspects of a Christian worldview in their clinical activity. Carlos Fayard examines how Adventist ideas about being human can inform the manner in which psychotherapy is practiced. Henry Lamberton and Antonia Ciovica focus on the most important topic of forgiveness. David Mee-Lee and Bruce Anderson share their considerable expertise on how the most successful treatment of addictions is suffused with ideas that can be traced to a Christian view of personal redemption. The article by Kendal Boyd appropriates current approaches in psychotherapy and applies them with a Christian worldview in mind. Finally, Deane Wolcott and Carlos Fayard bring the reader to the reality and challenge of applying a Christian worldview into a clinical context. The good news is that it not only works, but it also makes financial sense.

The final section of this book deals with the most important subject of how a Christian worldview can be passed on to the next generation of mental health clinicians. Barbara Couden Hernandez not only articulates a model to help trainees integrate spiritual considerations in clinical delivery through supervision, but she challenges the supervisor to be a spiritual mentor to the supervisee. William Murdoch, Antonia Ciovica, and Carlos Fayard review the development of a curriculum for mental health professionals that embraces a Christian worldview. They remind us that a trainee needs to develop the intellectual tools, interpersonal skills, attitude, and knowledge base to be competent in dealing with spiritual issues in clinical practice. They argue that having a clinical context in which these skills can be applied under supervision is essential, without forgetting that fostering the spiritual development of the trainee completes the formation cycle.

It is the hope of the editors of this volume that this collection of articles may be only the beginning of a discussion that will contribute to a renewal in Adventist education and training. If so, the outcome will have eternal significance for those we serve: students, trainees, and clients.

SUMMARY AND RECOMMENDATIONS

I am primarily a clinician and a clinical educator, and as such I cannot help but end in the manner I end my clinical reports—with a brief summary of the evaluation and a list of suggestions. As Seventh-day Adventists in the mental health field, we are blessed by a number of opportunities. First, we have a theology that values health and that sees mental health as indivisible from physical or spiritual well-being. Second, we have an educational and health care network committed to whole-person learning and service delivery. Third, we have graduate and post-graduate training programs in every mental health discipline, with ready access to excellent theological resources on the one hand, and clinical training locations supportive of whole-person approaches on the other.

In my opinion, such vast richness remains largely untapped. This is due in part to our own sub-cultural idiosyncrasies, but primarily because we have not sought to develop and articulate core ideas in a systematic way, and across contexts of learning and service delivery. The collection of papers gathered for the symposium seeks to make a humble contribution to remedy the situation. But even if the quality of these papers were to be revolutionary, in addition to good ideas, it would be necessary to have a confluence of the following:

- Mental health clinicians who prayerfully and humbly value the guidance of the Word of God and the presence of the Holy Spirit in their work.

- Teachers and trainers who see themselves as ministers, with as much concern for the spiritual formation of their students and trainees as for their education and competence.
- Administrators who see the fulfillment of this mission as the guiding principle in setting institutional priorities.

As is clear from the training outcome research from graduate psychology Christian programs, the integration of faith and practice in mental health is more "caught than taught" (Sorenson, VandeKemp, & Staton, 1998). The development of human resources that may transfer an Adventist spiritual identity in mental health must be a priority. However, without equally supportive contexts for clinical education, the best efforts will be insufficient. This is the promise of the "Adventist advantage." It is now up to us, the beneficiaries of the vision of our forefathers, to fulfill the mission God has called us to live out.

REFERENCES

Bevan, W., & Kessel, F. (1994). Plain truths and home cooking: Thoughts on the making and remaking of psychology. *American Psychologist, 49,* 505–509.

Browning, D. (2000). *Religious thought and the modern psychologies.* Minneapolis, MN: Augsburg Fortress Publishers.

Bufford, R. K. (2007). Philosophical foundations for clinical supervision within a Christian worldview. *Journal of Psychology and Christianity, 26,* 293–297.

Buss, D. (2007). *Evolutionary psychology: The new science of the mind.* Boston: Allyn & Bacon.

Clarke, J. (1994). *Jung and Eastern thought.* London: Routledge.

Ellis, A. (1980). Psychotherapy and atheistic values: A response to A. E. Bergin's "Psychotherapy and human values." *Journal of Consulting and Clinical Psychology, 48,* 635–639.

Foster, R. (1994). *Prayers from the Heart.* San Francisco: Harper.

Freud, S. (1933). *New introductory lectures on psychoanalysis.* London: Hogarth Press.

Fuller, A. (1994). *Psychology and religion: Eight points of view.* New York: Littlefield Adams.

Gillespie, B. (2002). Adventist schools DO make a difference. *Journal of*

Adventist Education, 65, 12–16.

Johnson, E., & Jones, S. (2005). Finding one truth in four views. In E. Johnson & S. Jones (Eds.), *Psychology and Christianity: Four views.* Downers Grove, IL: InterVarsity Press.

Josephson, A., & Peteet, J. (2004). *Handbook of spirituality and worldview in clinical practice.* Washington, D.C.: American Psychiatric Publishing.

Jung, C. (1933). *Modern man in search of a soul.* London: Harvest Books.

Mathisen, J. (2003). Integrating world views with social roles: Supplying a missing piece of the discussion on faith-learning integration. *Journal of Psychology and Christianity, 22,* 230–240.

Murphy, N. (2005). Integration from a radical-reformation perspective. In A. Duek & C. Lee (Eds.), *Why psychology needs theology.* New York: Eerdmans.

Nicholi, A. (2003). *The question of God: C. S. Lewis and Sigmund Freud debate God, sex, and the meaning of life.* New York: Free Press.

Nicholi, A. (2004). Introduction: Definition and significance of a worldview. In Josephson, A., and Peteet, J. (Eds.), *Handbook of spirituality and worldview in clinical practice.* Washington, D.C.: American Psychiatric Publishing.

Nielsen, S., Johnson, B., & Ellis, A. (2001). *Counseling and psychotherapy with religious persons: A rational emotive behavior therapy approach.* New York: Lawrence Erlbaum.

Roberts, R. (2007). *Spiritual emotions: A psychology of Christian virtues.* Grand Rapids: Eerdmans.

Rogers, C. (1961). *On becoming a person.* London: Constable.

Sorenson, R. (2004). *Minding spirituality.* New York: Analytic Press.

Sorenson, R., VandeKemp, H., & Staton, R. (1998). How students learn integration: Replication of the Sorenson (1997a). model. *Journal of Psychology & Theology, 26,* 340–350.

Stevenson, D., Eck, B., & Hill, P. (2007). *Psychology & Christianity integration: Seminal works that shaped the movement.* Batavia: Christian Association of Psychological Studies.

White, E. G. (1903). *Ministry of healing.* Mountain View, CA: Pacific Press.

Wittgenstein, L. (1969). *On Certainty.* Oxford: Oxford University Press.

Wright, N. (1992). *The New Testament and the people of God.* Minneapolis, MN: Augsburg Fortress Publishers.

Zinnebauer, B., & Pargament, K. (2005). Religiousness and spirituality. *Handbook of the psychology of religion and spirituality.* New York: Guilford Press.

Adventists and Mental Health: Remembering Who We Are

George T. Harding IV

Just six days before Adventism's great disappointment of October 22, 1844, an event took place that would have historic importance for American psychiatry. Superintendents from thirteen of the twenty-four insane asylums in the country met in Philadelphia. They included the author of a treatise on medical jurisprudence of insanity and the founder of the *American Journal of Insanity.* They established an association now known as the American Psychiatric Association.

Thus, we find our denomination's predecessors struggling to bring hope and meaning out of the despair of the great disappointment while American psychiatry was consolidating its professional efforts to deal more effectively with emotional suffering. Evolving slowly, psychiatry spent most of the nineteenth century caring for the institutionalized mentally ill. Professional meetings often focused on the heating and plumbing of asylums and census trends of inmates. The word "psychiatry" did not even appear until two years after the 1844 meeting in Philadelphia. In 1890 the word "psychiatry" was first noted in an American dictionary (Harding IV, 1987).

Through much of the nineteenth century, the term "medical-psychologist" was used, to be followed from 1880 to 1920 by the term "alienists," a word borrowed from the French (Harding IV, 1987, p. 228). It is clear that psychiatry and psychology have considerable overlap; in many cases, knowledge generated in one field is shared and absorbed into the ensuing theoretical development of the other discipline. Hence, concepts from psychology and psychiatry will be used here interchangeably.

How did it happen that Seventh-day Adventists—who grew out of the spiritual revival of the early 1800s and whose purpose was "to prepare a people for the soon coming of the Lord"—should have developed an extraordinary emphasis on health care, calling it "the right arm of the message"? How did Seventh-day Adventists, unlike most other conservative church bodies, choose, as did Quakers, to become a major sponsoring organization of health care institutions, giving major emphasis to mental health and the treatment of mental illness (Blazer, 1998)?

From earliest times, religion and science, including medicine, were interchangeable ideologies; religious orders and organizations often devoted themselves to the care of the sick. In fact, religious beliefs and rituals have had a central role in the lives of humankind, frequently providing the structural framework from which social, cultural, and moral norms develop. Almost all world religions believe in a Supreme Being or group of beings who are in some way interested in human welfare and development. Furthermore, throughout most of known history, it was the religious leaders, whether priest or shaman, who were considered healers (a tradition which continues today in less westernized cultures). Indeed, prior to the 1800s, what scant treatment existed for mental illness was provided by the church.

When the same person exercises both religious and healing functions, we have the possibility of positive coordination and integration between the two domains. Reformers, such as Philippe Pinel (1745 to 1826) in France, began to see the mentally ill as sick rather than sinful or wicked. The Quaker William Tuke (1732 to 1822) opened the York Retreat in England in 1792, and other Quakers were early leaders in the care and treatment of the mentally ill. In the United States, the first hospital to accept psychiatric patients was the Pennsylvania Hospital founded (1752) by the father of American psychiatry, Benjamin Rush, and his friend, Benjamin Franklin. The first public mental hospital in the United States (1775) was the Eastern Virginia Hospital in Williamsburg. Pious Quakers developed psychiatric hospitals along the eastern seaboard; by 1844 there were twenty-four state mental hospitals in the then thirty-four states of the Union (Harding IV, 2001).

But how did Seventh-day Adventists, a conservative religious body, become involved in psychiatric care? After beginnings in upper New

York State in the 1830s, the followers of William Miller crisscrossed the land, urging listeners to prepare for the Advent day. As the predicted date (October 22, 1844) came and went without incident, the disappointed Millerites sought reasons for the failure of their expectations. One Millerite seeking answers was Ellen Gould Harmon, who had experienced her own physical pain in childhood. Following her marriage to James White in 1846, she developed a powerful preaching style which was combined with prophetic visions and a gift for writing and publication. In 1855, a group of Adventists in Battle Creek, Michigan, invited the Whites to move to their town, which offered a tolerant home for them. The church flourished in Battle Creek; by the 1860s, several hundred Seventh-day Adventists were in the area. There Ellen White received visions related to health care and diet reform. In 1863 she was shown the wisdom of healthful living. On June 6, 1863, at the Hilliard Farm in Otsego, Michigan, she later wrote in a document still preserved: "I saw that it was a sacred duty to attend to our health and arouse others to their duty.... We have a duty to speak, to come out against intemperance of every kind—intemperance in working, in eating, in drinking, in drugging—and then point them to God's great medicine: water..." (White, 1863). Two years later, she and her ailing husband, James, visited Dr. James Caleb Jackson's health cure spa in Dansville, New York, which espoused many health reform ideas, including an emphasis on sunshine, rest, and hydrotherapy, or the water cure. On their way home from Dansville, the Whites were visiting friends on Christmas Day in 1865 when Ellen White received instruction about establishing a water cure and vegetarian institution pursuing a balanced, God-fearing course of treatment not only for Adventists but also for the public (Robinson, 1943).

It is quite clear that a major reason why Seventh-day Adventists embraced psychiatry and mental health care, rather than rejecting it, was due to Ellen White, a co-founder of the church. She was a visionary of wholistic health and health care service. Her voluminous writings included numerous articles on health which she termed health reform; mental health principles and the treatment of mental illness were included. Her interest likely was increased by her own childhood illness. After being struck in the face by a rock, she was incapable of attending school on a regular basis and was limited in other activities. Later, her husband, James White, was incapacitated by depression. This was the reason for their visit to Dr. Caleb Jackson's center. James White regained his health in Dansville (Schwarz, 2000). While James and Ellen were uncomfortable with portions of the regime which they considered frivolous, Ellen White envisioned what enlightened health care could mean to sickly people and a hurting world. She maintained her active interest in and advocacy of healthful living throughout her long career. Early supporters of her advocacy for a health reform facility were John and Ann Kellogg, parents of the fourteen-year-old future doctor John Harvey Kellogg and his younger brother, William Keith Kellogg. Nine months later, in 1866, Ellen White's vision was realized as the Western Health Reform Institute opened in a small two-story farmhouse. The staff consisted of one doctor and a number of willing but untrained assistants.

The institute offered health reforms designed to heal the whole person by caring for the mind, body, and spirit. The Adventist belief in abstinence from alcohol and tobacco, as well as moderation in diet, physical work, and the use of pharmaceutical drugs, were integral to the program. Patients were taught the use of natural cures, including water, sunshine, exercise, rest, and proper diet. This was immediately following the bloodletting of the late eighteenth and first half of the nineteenth centuries and certainly was a novel approach. At that time, medicine frequently practiced purging, leeches, alcohol-based patent remedies, and crude surgical practices with high mortality rates. Many "doctors" and "nurses" had no formal training, relying instead on reading books and apprenticeship training. The institute's first nurses were Adventist volunteer farm women who did everything from chopping wood to administering massage.

Recognizing the need for a more thoroughly trained staff and seeing leadership potential in teenaged John Harvey Kellogg, the

Whites partially subsidized his medical education at the University of Michigan and the Bellevue Hospital Medical College in New York City. In 1875, Dr. Kellogg returned to Battle Creek, joining the Western Health Reform Institute staff. Immediately offered the position of medical director, Kellogg declined, saying he preferred to devote his career to writing and research. The next year he reluctantly agreed to serve for one year. That year stretched out to sixty-seven, as Dr. Kellogg remained medical director until his death on December 14, 1943, at the age of ninety-one (Robinson, 1943).

The dynamic twenty-four-year-old doctor immediately launched a series of innovations. First, he replaced the traditional term "sanatorium" with the new name "sanitarium." The Battle Creek Medical and Surgical Sanitarium was to be a "sanitary place where people learned to stay well" (Schwarz, 1970). He assumed editorial control of the monthly publication, which he renamed *Good Health,* refined and improved the water therapy treatments, added more scientifically-based treatments, revised the diet of the patients, introduced surgery, and hired a professionally trained staff. Ten years later, in 1877, "the San" was erecting a four-story expansion. By 1885, the San had become the "largest institution of its kind in the world" and, as a sanitarium pamphlet pointed out, "at this time there existed no other institution which combined the comforts of the home and the hotel with the medical advantages of a hospital and the added facilities and equipment requisite for the administration of baths of every description, electricity in its different forms, medical gymnastics and other rational agencies, with careful regulation of diet" (Heritage Battle Creek, 2009). When fire destroyed the main building and hospital in February 1902, Dr. Kellogg immediately vowed to rebuild an even larger sanitarium. Despite Ellen White's advice to keep the new structure small and simple, Dr. Kellogg persisted with elaborate plans, laying the cornerstone three months later. The six-story, fireproof brick building was dedicated in May 1903, only fifteen months after the conflagration (Butler, Thornton, & Stolz, 1994).

Over the next several years, there were increasing areas of disagreement between church leaders and the sanitarium administration. By 1907, both parties considered the problems irreconcilable. Dr. John Harvey Kellogg and his brother, William Keith Kellogg, were disfellowshipped and the administration of the sanitarium was no longer under church auspices. Although formally separated from the church, both Kellogg brothers continued to live by Adventist principles, and the sanitarium continued to observe the Sabbath and to promote Adventist health ideas (Schwarz, 2006).

The treatment offered at the sanitarium, the success rate in difficult surgical and medical cases, and its laboratory research continued to enhance the institution's worldwide reputation. Guests like the industrialist John D. Rockefeller Jr. came for several weeks at a time "to get advice and a general looking over" (Heritage Battle Creek, 2009). By 1927, even more space was necessary and a three-million-dollar addition was completed the next year. The fifteen-story towers addition contained over six hundred patient rooms and suites, banquet rooms, and medical offices. The crash of the booming economy early in the next decade reduced the patronage; occupancy dropped over 75 percent and financial difficulties threatened the very existence of the institution. Going into receivership in 1933, the San continued to operate on a reduced basis. Finally, in 1942, it was necessary to sell the building complex to the United States Army and move to smaller quarters. Without the charismatic leadership of Dr. Kellogg, the institution gradually declined in importance as American tastes in health care changed.

In 1957 a group of Seventh-day Adventist doctors purchased "the San" and by 1974 the Battle Creek Sanitarium and Hospital returned to church ownership and control. During the next decade, the hospital changed its emphasis to psychiatric and substance abuse treatment. In 1993, the facility merged with two other local hospitals, becoming part of the Battle Creek Health System (Butler et al., 1994).

The impact of the Battle Creek Sanitarium on American medicine cannot be overemphasized. It was the dominant health care facility of that era. Will and Charles Mayo, founders of the Mayo Clinic, spoke on many occasions of modeling the Mayo Clinic after the Battle Creek Sanitarium. Karl Menninger said that his father, C. F. Menninger, was inspired to develop a group practice and clinic which became the Menninger Clinic after a visit to Rochester, Minnesota, and discussions with brothers Charles and Will Mayo (Menninger, personal communication, 1981).

John Harvey Kellogg was a surgeon, not a psychiatrist, and the Battle Creek Sanitarium and the sanitariums and hospitals it spawned were medical/surgical, not psychiatric, hospitals. Adventist medical leaders who were contemporaries of John Harvey Kellogg, such as Daniel and Loretta Kress, David Paulson, George Thomason, and Harry Miller, were general physicians sometimes giving special attention to surgery, internal medicine, or other specialties. In fact, before the age of specialization, all physicians were generalists, although some had expertise in a special area. A second factor that contributed to Adventism's embracing of psychiatry and mental health care was the earlier acceptance of physicians and medical treatment. With Ellen White's vision, advocacy, and encouragement, Dr. John Harvey Kellogg and those associated with him demonstrated in actual practice a program with specific application to clinical treatment and developed equipment which people could understand and use to treat themselves. Physicians were educated in the affiliated American Medical Missionary College, and nurses, treatment assistants, dietitians, and others were trained. Graduates were encouraged not only to practice in the Battle Creek Sanitarium but to spread out. Sanitariums, clinics, and treatment rooms were soon planted from Melrose, Massachusetts, to St. Helena, Glendale, and Paradise Valley in California, and from Hinsdale, Illinois, to Orlando, Florida. That psychiatry and mental health treatment was medically based, sharing many tenets and practices of medical care, and also contributed to its acceptance.

One of John Harvey Kellogg's contemporaries was my grandfather, George T. Harding II, who is considered by many to have been the first Seventh-day Adventist psychiatrist. George II was a devout Seventh-day Adventist and sufficiently pious, often referred to as "Deac" or "Deacon." He was the younger son of George T. and Phoebe Dickerson Harding, both country physicians. Phoebe was one of the first women doctors in post-Civil War Ohio. She also was the first Harding convert to Adventism and a strong influence on all her children. Her oldest son, Warren Gamaliel, became the 29th president of the United States; her daughter, Mary, taught in the Ohio School for the Blind; and her daughter Carolyn, with her husband Heber Votaw, in 1905 became the first Seventh-day Adventist missionaries to Burma, now Myanmar. The younger son, George II, attended Battle Creek College from 1894 to 1896 with plans to attend the American Medical Missionary College. Recognized for his outstanding academic ability and spiritual dedication, George II was asked by church leaders to attend an established school of medicine to demonstrate that graduates of Battle Creek College could perform in medical school as well as students from other colleges and universities, even prestigious ones such as Rush, University of Michigan, Jefferson, Harvard, and Yale. He attended the University of Michigan. But his plans to join his parents in their country practice in Ohio were dramatically altered when he was found to have rheumatic heart disease with mitral stenosis, the sequelae of childhood rheumatic fever. In those days, people with rheumatic heart disease were plagued with atrial fibrillation and congestive heart failure and rarely lived into their thirties. With this dire prognosis, George II was advised to pursue a "less strenuous" practice, such as the care of persons with tuberculosis or mental illness. Upon graduation in 1900 (the same year that Freud's *Interpretation of Dreams* was published), he joined the staff of the Columbus (Ohio) State Hospital, where he became interested in sickness of the mind as well as of the body. For five years he gained experience in the "moral treatment" that was in vogue in public mental hospitals at the turn of the century. He found some similarities between the needs of the mental patients and those treated at the Battle Creek Sanitarium and suggested trying treatment approaches that had been found effective at Battle Creek.

Anticipating his older brother's move from Ohio to Washington, D.C. (Warren G. Harding would not become president of the United States until 1921), George II served from 1905 to 1907 as superintendent of the original Washington Sanitarium. Seventh-day Adventists made an auspicious entrance into the nation's capitol by installing a sanitarium in General Ulysses S. Grant's magnificent Victorian mansion on Iowa Circle (the mansion dominates what is now called Logan Circle, which is still circled by original Victorian homes). Returning to Columbus, George II opened an office across from the state capitol. Initially, he practiced as a general physician and became a Fellow of the American College of Physicians. With "talk therapy" as part of his method of treatment long before it was commonly called psychotherapy, he gradually came to specialize in the treatment of the mentally ill. Patients treated included the severely ill, such as those with schizophrenia and manic depression (now called bipolar), and those whose illnesses resulted from vitamin deficiency and central nervous system syphilis. These mental health illnesses were the focus of psychiatry throughout the nineteenth century, but he also treated people with depression, anxiety, and adjustment reactions, as well as those less severely incapacitated.

George II was a member of the American Psychiatric Association, where he became acquainted with Adolf Meyer (the father of American psychiatric education), William Alanson White, Harry Stack Sullivan, and other leaders in American psychiatry. His practice strongly reflected his Adventist heritage. His Columbus office included a Battle Creek style treatment room; throughout his career he stressed the importance of hydrotherapy, including the calming effect of warm "neutral baths" on those suffering with insomnia. With his willingness to listen and reputation for being truthful with his patients, his practice grew. But 100 years ago, community hospitals expected psychiatric patients to be cared for in state mental hospitals, and known psychiatric patients were barred from admission. Places were needed to treat psychiatric patients. Although he was chronically ill and on the edge of congestive heart failure most of his adult life, George II had vision, ambition, and a strong wife who was able to manage a household of three children, do the physical work that her husband could not do, and still be actively involved in church and community activities. Recognizing the need, she agreed to accept one, two, or sometimes three patients into their Columbus home for care.

In 1915, two events occurred that changed this "in house home care" arrangement. On July 16, Ellen White died. Throughout her lifetime she had adamantly declined positions on institutional boards, with one exception—the self-supporting Madison (Tennessee) Sanitarium and College. Following her death, Elder A. G. Daniells, the president of the General Conference, recommended that George II take her seat on the Madison board (Daniells, personal communication, 1930). George II felt deeply honored. He soon was impressed with the self-supporting work that Drs. E. A. Sutherland and Percy T. Magan were doing at Madison. Perhaps a self-supporting psychiatric hospital in Columbus might answer a major need. And secondly, when the Harding's fourth child, Charles Weaver, was born in December 1915, Elsie put her foot down on patients in the home, saying, "If you want to have a psychiatric hospital, then open one."

After earnest prayer, George II, with his wife Elsie, opened the Indianola Rest Home as an outreach of the local Adventist church. It was located in rented quarters on Indianola Avenue in the Ohio State University District. Serving women only, the Indianola Rest Home admitted eight patients who suffered primarily from depression. He was seeking to establish an ideal self-supporting medical center where the capable, mature, consecrated Christian physician would find his sole delight in working until the close of time. Dr. Stella Howser, a Seventh-day Adventist physician with some experience in psychiatric hospitals, initially shared the medical leadership. Four years later, when the institution was moved to the countryside south of Columbus and became the Columbus Rural Rest Home, George II recruited physicians, nurses, physical therapists, and others to join the endeavor. Several of the physicians in addition to Stella Howser were women; Dr. Anna Laird, an ex-missionary, arrived with no previous psychiatric training but stayed to become an important member of the staff. After graduating from the University of Colorado School of Medicine, Drs. Mary and Fred Weber joined the staff. Dr. Fred Weber was especially effective in working with alcoholics and made their care and treatment a special ministry.

In 1919, a fifty-acre estate in Worthington, Ohio, was purchased to which George II moved the institution. He and his associates carried on the traditional program of Battle Creek. Dr. Mary Weber's regimen for patients in the "women's cottage" was an early morning glass of fruit juice, followed by a cold mitten friction, a healthy breakfast, a brisk walk, and hydrotherapy. Lunch preceded a period of rest and activities in the craft shop. Appointments with a physician were held throughout the day. A vegetarian diet was provided with care that it be the best.

After supper came an educational activity, then a massage and hot cereal beverage. For those with insomnia, the day's activities ended with a wet sheet pack, a fomentation, or a neutral bath. Other aspects of the Battle Creek program included evening educational programs called "Parlor Talks" and a question box in which patients submitted questions (Harding II, 1919). Once a week George II or an associate would respond. Spiritual issues often arose in these sessions.

During the 1920s, a pharmacist with severe depression—including nihilistic delusions, helplessness, and hopelessness—told his doctor, George II, that his condition was hopeless. Indeed, he felt he was dying and by nightfall would be ready for burial. My grandfather responded that if he were going to die, he might as well accomplish something worthwhile before he departed this life. Thereupon he was directed to take a rake and hoe to remove weeds from the flower beds in front of the patient cottage. Despite the patient's protestations of his terminal state, my grandfather firmly told him to begin his work, which he finally did. By nightfall the patient was much improved. A prescription of a non-gratifying task helped the patient both relieve guilt by doing penance and externalize his internally directed rage and sublimate it through constructive work.

George II realized that clinics like Mayo's, Menninger's, and Harding's needed highly trained medical personnel and shrewd management. In 1920, the year he moved the Columbus Rural Rest Home to its Worthington location, he wrote to Dr. Alfred B. Olsen, superintendent of the Adventist Caterham Sanitarium in England: "If you are interested in teaching and preaching health, you will help a lot in our plans. It is a work I could easily kill myself at because it appeals to me more strongly the older I get, the more I learn and the more I realize the needs of the work in its closing days" (Harding II, personal communication, 1920). Olsen came.

George II also insisted on hiring a competent business manager "who would demonstrate what an advantage it would be to have a real manager, one who knows what good business demands and a recognition of the principles of justice that no one department can ignore the interests of the other." When Olsen resisted bringing a non-physician into the management, George II insisted on the value of specialization and division of labor:

> There will be so much legitimate work for us doctors to do that we ought not to have time to try to do what a really worthwhile businessman can do better. Our place will stand out above others if we provide proper medical supervision by the personal physicians who know the victorious life and have time to make friends with our patients. (Harding II, personal communication, 1920)

Just as John Harvey Kellogg and the Battle Creek Sanitarium were instruments to develop the health message and contribute to its acceptance among Seventh-day Adventists, so George Harding II and the Harding Sanitarium were used to contribute to the acceptance of psychiatry and to develop the mental health message. As A. G. Daniells, president of the General Conference, 1901 to 1922, said to George III:

> In addition to Sister White's vision of the importance of mental health in total health and the church's acceptance of the health message,

> George Harding was a trusted, involved fellow worker and a wise councilor. We church leaders did not understand all of psychiatry's theory and methods but we knew and trusted George Harding and his psychiatry. (Daniells, personal communication, 1931)

George II was a devout Seventh-day Adventist and committed to the church's health message. He believed that sunshine, fresh air, adequate rest, exercise, a proper diet, and faith in God contributed to a healthful life. His practice incorporated Ellen White's instructions on the relationship between mind and body, the power of God, hindrances to the recovery of the sick who center their attention on themselves instead of thinking and caring for others, and the importance of prayer (White, 1903). The following statement from *Ministry of Healing* was hung on the parlor wall of the Columbus Rural Rest Home: "It is a positive duty to resist melancholy, discontented thoughts and feelings, as much a duty as it is to pray" (White, 1903, p. 251). George II embraced Ellen White's assertion that "to deal with minds is the greatest work given to man" (White, 1886, p. 209) and believed that the true principles of psychology are found in the Holy Scriptures (White, 1903, p. 121). As he read the writings of Freud and other psychiatric leaders, he kept in mind the dangers in psychology, wrongly used (White, 1884, Vol. 1, pp. 290–302). His practice tended to confirm Ellen White's statement that nine out of ten diseases originate in the mind (White, 1844, Vol. 5, p. 444).

In 1934, at the age of fifty-five, George Tryon Harding II died following a stroke. During his lifetime, he had steadfastly refused to name the institution after himself, but soon after his burial it became the Harding Sanitarium and, after World War II, the Harding Hospital.

George T. Harding III, who graduated in 1928 from the College of Medical Evangelists, now Loma Linda University, felt that psychiatry had been minimized at Loma Linda, and indicated that the faculty were fearful of teaching it since they felt that psychiatry was largely hypnotism and therefore a thing of the devil. But by observing the psychiatric treatment regime provided in the Harding's self-supporting Worthington (Ohio) facility and reading Karl Menninger's *The Human Mind,* a pioneering self-help book, he became increasingly enthusiastic about psychiatry.

At the age of twenty-nine, George III succeeded his father as medical director in 1934. He proved to be a master at brief evaluations and effective clinical interventions. He continued his clinical practice until the age of eighty, and maintained his interest in psychiatry until his death in November 1985. In 1929, he began teaching psychiatry at the Ohio State University College of Medicine. He also developed one of the first approved psychiatric residency programs at Harding Sanitarium. His appointment and tenure as president of the College of Medical Evangelists from 1948 to 1951 was a symbol of the growing Adventist acceptance of psychiatry.

Harrison S. Evans, also a graduate of the College of Medical Evangelists, came to the Harding Sanitarium in 1936 as its first resident. He received additional training in neurology with the College of Medical Evangelists' world renowned neuropathologist, Cyril Courville. He had additional studies in psychiatry at the Menninger Clinic and the New York Psychiatric Institute, and a personal analysis with Maurice Levine. He became director of residency training in 1939 and, after serving with the CME 47th General Hospital in New Guinea during World War II, medical director of the Harding Hospital. Drs. Harding and Evans innovatively developed a creative psychiatric treatment approach that integrated the spiritual from an Adventist perspective, with the growing scientific knowledge about mental illness and treatment.

As George Harding III and Harrison Evans became professional colleagues and personal friends with Karl and William Menninger of the Menninger Clinic, they saw many similarities in the Harding and Menninger treatment programs. In addition to psychodynamic psychotherapy, both programs had an activity program of physical work, exercise, creative activities, and educational opportunities; these were provided by skilled people trained to be therapeutic. "Milieu therapy," as it is now called, had its beginnings with Ernst Simmell at the Tegel Sanitarium in Berlin. However, it was at Menninger's that it was developed and flowered. William Menninger's brilliant "Guide to the Order Sheet" made it possible for the entire staff to be involved in treatment. However, they noted that one area missing in the Menninger Program was a recognition of, and attention to, the spiritual needs of patients. Although the Menninger brothers' mother was a devoutly spiritual person, the Menninger Program, as in most psychiatric hospitals of that time, included few if any spiritual opportunities. Drs. George III and Evans pointed this out to the Menningers. Later in 1954, when L. Harold Caviness, an Adventist psychiatrist educated at Loma Linda and trained in psychiatry at Harding Hospital, joined the Menninger Clinic staff, he suggested a weekly worship service for patients. This was instituted and continued in the Menninger program for many years.

At the Harding Hospital, the Menninger Guide to the Order Sheet (1982) was modified and expanded to include spiritual/religious concerns (Shafer, 1959). Patients were informed that the spiritual/religious program was available and were encouraged to participate. However, it was not mandatory and patients could choose to participate at whatever level they wished. A weekly worship service, a Saturday morning Bible class led by a psychiatrist, a faith and life discussion group co-led by a chaplain and a clinical professional, and a weekly evening lecture with opportunity for questions and discussion attracted the interest of patients and many attended. Letting patients know that spiritual/religious concerns could be brought to their individual psychotherapy session opened the door to meaningful discussion and personal growth.

In his book, *The Future of an Illusion,* Freud opined that faith is based on the illusion that an idealized father (God) can replace the lost real father who has proven fallible to the child and is no longer a comfort and source of security. Freud's solution to his depiction of this infantile response on the part of individuals to create a mythological God was for them to develop a realistic view of the reality that there is no God. "Man cannot remain a child forever. He must venture at last into the hostile world. This may be called 'education to reality'" (Freud, 1935, p. 86). Although the idea that God is a projected illusion did not originate with Freud, his declaration that religious belief is an infantile projective fantasy cast a long shadow over subsequent practitioners' theories about the relationship between religious belief and mental health. This contributed to many decades in which psychiatry generally viewed religious belief with skepticism and apathy.

Psychologists and psychiatrists who integrated religion with their psychological theories include such notables as Carl Jung (1875–1961), Erich Fromm (1900–1980), and Viktor Frankl (1905–1997). The broadest incorporation of the spiritual with the psychiatric is found in Jung, a Swiss psychiatrist, son of a Protestant clergyman and contemporary of Freud. In stark contrast to Freud, Jung's liberal premise that all psychic products, including visions, dreams, and hallucinations, are facts and should be considered as having the same basis in reality as other physical facts, opens wide the door to religious belief and behavior in psychic functioning that Freud had firmly attempted to close. Furthermore, according to Jung, it is not the business of psychology or psychiatry to prove or disprove the existence of God; it can only address the psychic effects of the God image and its mythic antecedents on human behavior (Harding IV, 2001).

Psychoanalyst Erich Fromm recognized the value of religion in providing healthy feelings of stability and security for individuals. In his book, *Psychoanalysis and Religion,* he stated that "man is not free to choose between having or not having ideals, but he is free to choose between different kinds of ideals, between being devoted to the worship of power and destruction and being devoted to reason and love" (Fromm, 1950, p. 25). Fromm further advocated a surrendering of one's individual goals and identity in favor of living selflessly in community with others, a not uncommon ideal of both Judaic and Christian tradition. Finally, Victor Frankl, the Holocaust survivor and psychiatrist, who wrote *Man's Search for Meaning,* articulated in his book the premise that all humans are on an unmitigated quest for meaning, even in the midst of horror and despair. Frankl clearly credited his spiritual belief as sustaining his mental health throughout his imprisonment. He contrasted his experience to that of other prisoners who lost faith and subsequently their will to live, succumbing to illness and death. Of the three highlighted theorists who have acknowledged the positive merits of religious belief on mental health, Frankl's testimony is the most graphic and recent representation of the positive outcome of melding the two.

The potential benefit of intertwining psychiatry and religious belief has also been addressed by a number of theologians, religious philosophers, and clergy who have debated the merits of incorporating religious beliefs into the best scientific practices in mental health. An early proponent of such an integration was Anton Boisen (1876–1965), a Protestant clergyman who had once experienced a psychotic illness and subsequently had been institutionalized in the mental hospital he later served at as chaplain. Finding a religious renewal during his hospitalization, he believed that other patients could have similar experiences if the psychiatric community were sufficiently sensitive to the meaning of such experiences.

Another theologian, Paul Tillich, asserted that when psychiatry makes either negative or positive judgments about the reality of religious ideas and symbols, it has moved out of the realm of science and into the realm of metaphysics (Tillich, 1957).

Philosopher of religion Paul Recoeur (1913–2005) has countered Freud's view that religion is basically a public expression of obsessive/compulsive neurosis. Recoeur says that humans grow when confronted by sacred figures who challenge them to become more than they are (Harding IV, 2001).

More than fifty years of writing on the positive interaction between religion and psychological health passed before the field of psychiatry officially re-examined its Freudian views on religious belief. In 1956, R. Finley Gayle Jr., the incoming president of the American Psychiatric Association, devoted his entire presidential address entitled, *Conflict and Cooperation Between Psychiatry and Religion* (Stevens, 2010). In that speech, Dr. Gayle called for the formation of a committee on psychiatry and religion (which I chaired from 1995 to 2001) and suggested that mental health chaplains be invited to participate in the venture. Although the next several decades indicated some gains in psychiatric acceptance of religion as non-pathological, diagnoses as late as those found in 1987 (*Diagnostic and Statistical Manual of Mental Disorders* – Third Edition [DSM III]) indicated religious belief as a factor in poorer mental health (Larson & Greenwald, 1997). However, the 1990 guidelines indicated that "patient's religious beliefs were being professionally recognized" as not only acceptable but important treatment factors (Larson & Greenwald, 1997, p. 22).

With the demonstration that psychiatric treatment was not anti-religious but could contribute to more effective treatment, Adventist health care hospitals across the country began to seek Adventist psychiatrists to develop psychiatric programs. They turned to Adventist psychiatrists trained at Harding Hospital. In 1937, an estate given to the Southern New England Conference became the site for the Fuller Memorial Sanitarium, a psychiatric hospital founded and directed by Laurence Senseman, M.D. The Washington Sanitarium and Hospital appointed Henry Andren to introduce psychiatry to that important medical center. Dr. Andren also gave leadership to the Cedarcroft Sanitarium in nearby Maryland. William Brunie, Walter Hofmann, and Vernon Shafer, Ph.D., gave leadership to the Glendale Sanitarium and Hospital, and Charles and Bruce Anderson developed the psychiatric program at the Hinsdale Sanitarium and Hospital. Denis and David Mee-Lee led out in developing the psychiatric program at the New England Sanitarium and Hospital, as L. Harold Caviness did in the reopened Battle Creek Sanitarium. In 1963, Harrison Evans and Clarence Carnahan developed the clinical and educational psychiatric program at Loma Linda University Medical Center, and Stanley Sturges and Charles Bensonhaver developed the Kettering Medical Center Psychiatric Program. It took strong psychiatric leadership to maintain a therapeutic program focused on the patient's needs and the importance of the relationship between doctor and patient, mentoring leading to a corrective emotional experience and psychotherapy and psychoeducation to new ways of relating and living. This was done often in the face of strong hospital administrators' efforts to increase revenues by fully utilizing efficiency of size, the rapidly developing psychopharmacology, in addition to the cost-cutting edicts of managed care.

Another major emphasis of the Adventist church was education, both formal education of students and continuing education of the public. The Battle Creek Sanitarium developed educational programs for nurses, physical therapists, and physicians. The American Medical Missionary College (AMMC) in a short time (1895–1910) educated and graduated a remarkable group of physicians, many of whom were the founding faculty of the College of Medical Evangelists, now Loma Linda University (Knight, 1983). When asked whether the AMMC, which lasted only a dozen years, was worth the effort, Dr. Kellogg cited Dr. Charles Stewart and said, "If we had produced only one Charles Stewart, it would have been worth all of our efforts" (Kellogg, personal communication, 1931). The psychiatric residency program at Harding Hospital also produced a remarkable group of more than 100 psychiatrists who have given leadership to psychiatric programs in Adventist hospitals across North America, chaired departments of psychiatry in four different medical schools, and served patients in hospitals, mental health centers, and private offices.

In 1962, Dr. Evans became chairman of the Department of Psychiatry at the Loma Linda University School of Medicine. He developed a modern psychiatric program and, two years later, approval was granted by the Council on Medical Education for the Department of Psychiatry to offer a psychiatric residency program at Loma Linda. Loma Linda University today is a psychiatric educational center sought after by graduates of Loma Linda University and other medical schools who wish to train in a Christian setting where there is encouragement rather than opposition to integrating spiritual beliefs and scientific psychiatry. The Loma Linda University Department of Psychiatry is the only psychiatry department promoting the integration of Christian spirituality into the theoretical and clinical curriculum of psychiatric medical school and residency education.

Nevertheless, the trend in psychiatry to emphasize the biological (pharmacological) has influenced the Loma Linda University Department of Psychiatry, along with all other departments of psychiatry. To find the proper balance between the biological, psychological, social, and spiritual has been the challenge (Engel, 1980). Recently, Loma Linda Department of Psychiatry leaders have given renewed emphasis to psychotherapy, utilizing not only traditional supportive, psychodynamic, and cognitive behavioral psychotherapy but also contributions of attachment theory, object relations, self-psychology, and the findings of neuroscience. This is being combined with an integration of spiritual/religious concepts and beliefs. This has led to a new level of interest and commitment by faculty, staff, and residents and will hopefully lead to a renewed level of scholarships, innovation, and publication.

But psychiatrists alone do not make up the mental health treatment team. We must also recognize the value of added treatment carried out by a team of dedicated mental health professionals: psychiatrists, nurses, psychologists, social workers, counselors, chaplains, activity therapists, and others.

Richard Nies, Ph.D., and Vernon Shafer, Ph.D., are Adventist psychologists who have contributed not only to a theoretical and clinical understanding of patients and the development of a therapeutic approach, but also to emphasizing the added benefit of integrating the spiritual/religious aspect into treatment. Both were among the first Adventists to receive a Ph.D. in clinical psychology from a major university, although there were earlier psychologists with degrees in educational psychology. Both had a deep interest in spiritual matters, clinical evaluation, treatment, and education. Vernon Shafer contributed much to articulating an Adventist perspective on the importance of a spiritual/religious approach and developing and nurturing a well-functioning treatment team with whom the treatment plan and psychodynamic information were shared. A treatment team has been found to be very effective and can enable staff to experience the support so necessary to sustain treatment over the time needed to bring about change in patients with highly complex problems.

Another important educational activity and an effective bridge between Adventist mental health professionals and church pastors and conference leaders was the Institute on Mental Health for Seventh-day Adventist Clergy, held annually at the Harding Hospital from 1955 to 1984. Sponsored jointly by the Seventh-day Adventist Theological Seminary (Andrews University) and Harding Hospital, this annual institute brought to the hospital campus pastors, chaplains, teachers, and conference officers to study how the mind works and how clergy—whether pastors, teachers, or chaplains—can increase their effectiveness with parishioners and others.

The idea of such an institute occurred during a General Conference Spring Meeting in Washington, D.C., in the early 1950s. Speaker Charles Wittschiebe, a pastor and professor of pastoral care at the Seventh-day Adventist Theological Seminary, caught the attention of psychiatrist Charles Anderson with this statement: "It is just as important for the pastor to assure that his sermons are emotionally sound as it is that they are theologically sound." In his devotional message, he described his experience as a clinical pastoral education (CPE) trainee at St. Elizabeth Hospital in Washington, D.C., and the understandings he developed as he interacted with patients and attempted to understand what they were seeking to communicate. Charles Anderson and Charles Wittschiebe talked far into the night. Then with the support of George Harding III, Harrison Evans, L. Harold Caviness, and Dr. Vernon Hendershot, dean of the Seventh-day Adventist Theological Seminary, the first of these institutes was advertised for the autumn of 1955. The announcements inviting conference presidents to send pastors to this mental health institute evoked concern and hesitation on the part of some. That first year, a number of conference presidents attended. T. H. Unruh, at that time president of the Pennsylvania Conference, acknowledged an initial uneasiness and a need to hear what was being taught before exposing any of the pastors in his field to the program. After attending the first institute he became a strong supporter. From that year on, more pastors applied to attend than could be accommodated.

Over the next thirty years, more than five hundred Adventist clergy attended. Psychiatrists, psychologists, social workers, nurses, and chaplains gave lectures, demonstrations, and discussions on how the mind works, the importance of relationships, and how ministry could be more effective. With the patients' permission, patients were interviewed. Charles Wittschiebe—a gifted teacher and pastoral counselor—would lead the discussion on topics of greatest interest to the participants. Pastors were enthusiastic and a number asked to return a second time. Lowell Bock, Ontario/Quebec Conference President when he first attended and later Lake Union President and Assistant to the President of the North American Division, wrote:

> My attendance at the Institute on Mental Health changed my ministry. I knew the Lord, theology and the church organization, but I was ill-equipped to deal with the personal problems my parishioners were struggling with. I had no concept of transference. Learning something about transference, and helping pastors to avoid some of the pitfalls they sometimes fell into was only one of many helpful concepts and practices presented during the two Institutes I attended. I thank the Lord for having this life-changing and ministry-changing experience. The Institute opened my eyes and enabled me to deal with many difficult situations in a far more constructive way than I had known before. (Bock, personal letter, 2008)

Adventist psychiatry has contributed to the concept of treating the whole person, a mind-body connection that includes the psychological when dealing with the physical and the physical when dealing with the mind. It has also recognized the importance of integrating religion into psychiatric practice and the synergy achieved by having a team of committed clinicians working together rather than each working in a silo. Adventist psychiatry has recognized the importance of an effective educational program for professional growth and replenishment. This is true not only of psychiatrists but of all mental health professionals. Perhaps of greatest importance is having ongoing liaison with pastors, teachers, chaplains, and colleagues in other medical specialties and mental health professions.

There remains one important question. What record have Adventists made through publications to disseminate their approach to treating the whole person, using the treatment team effectively, and maintaining an abiding interest in and compassion for patients? Harold Shryock, a long-time Loma Linda professor and Dean of the School of Medicine, although not a psychiatrist, wrote many articles and books on topics of interest to psychiatrists and other mental health professionals. One of his most important contributions was developing a syllabus on psychobiology for use in teaching first-year medical students. In 1939, Walter E. McPherson, Dean of the School of Medicine, asked Dr. Shryock to develop a course on psychological functioning and human relationships, which had recently become a requirement for medical schools. Although Loma Linda medical students had received lectures in psychiatry from the institution's beginning in 1909, this was the first course to deal with the daily mental and emotional challenges of living. Earlier, psychiatry had been taught at Patton State Hospital where patients with severe mental illness were paraded before the students. The term "psychobiology," which had been coined by Adolf Meyer of Johns Hopkins, the father of American psychiatric education, seemed an appropriate course title to Dr. Shryock (Shryock, personal communication, 2004).

Dr. Shryock's additional publications were widely read, including *Happiness for Husbands and Wives, Happiness and Health, Highways to Health, The New Modern Medical Counselor,* plus 621 articles in sixteen publications for lay readers (Schaefer, 2005). In 2007, Carlos Fayard, with William Murdoch, John Brunt and George Harding IV, published an article titled "Clinical Implications for Psychotherapy from the Seventh-day Adventist Tradition" in the *Journal of Psychology and Christianity*. A paper on spirituality assessment by Hall, Reise, and Haviland (2007) from nearby UCLA and Biola University appeared in the *International Journal for the Psychology of Religion*. Mark Haviland has published more than sixty papers in peer review journals, including *Archives of General Psychiatry, The American Journal of Psychiatry, Academic Medicine,* and other health care journals. We are encouraged by the increase in publications and especially by the publications in the area of religion and psychiatry. Nevertheless, rather than a trickle, there needs to be a stream of research and publications in this important area.

Needless to say, countless people have been treated and helped in Adventist hospitals, clinics, and individual doctor's offices around the world. The church has articulated the concept that the human body is the temple of the Lord (1 Cor. 6:19) and that it is the religious/spiritual duty of the individual to protect and care for the body in a way that will provide for maximum health, both physical and mental. It is also emphasized that the human body is one body (Rom. 12:4), not divided up as body, mind, and spirit, but that each part of the body interacts with and influences every other part (1 Cor. 12:12). The motto of Loma Linda University ("To Make Man Whole") and the mission statement ("To Continue the Healing Ministry of Jesus Christ") have been specific contributions to the entire medical and healing professions. And the fact that the Loma Linda University Department of Psychiatry Residency Program offers the only medical school and Department of Psychiatry program in the United States with a Christian orientation is a unique and valued contribution.

Seventh-day Adventists have demonstrated that mental health is an integral part of medicine, an idea reaffirmed in recent years by organized psychiatry after dallying with jettisoning our medical roots in favor of closer ties with non-medical mental health professions.

Adventists have also given a demonstration of how integration of religious/spiritual belief and psychiatric practice can be accomplished.

The value of individualized personal care is recognized and emphasized but has to be adapted to the reality of twenty-first-century medicine. Other important elements include graduate (residency) education of newly graduated physicians, and encouragement to graduates to scatter to underserved areas in the United States and abroad where they can provide clinical leadership and thus enable many dedicated but lesser trained people to also contribute to whole person healing care and increased mental health education to the public.

Another element is the treatment team concept and how effective a well-functioning treatment team can be. On the other hand, a treatment team can become dysfunctional unless there is mutual respect, common purpose, regular communication, team meetings, and the importance of keeping up with cutting-edge developments.

PRESENT

Where are we now? Driven by managed care, psychiatric treatment has increasingly utilized psychopharmacology and deemphasized the time spent in building a relationship and in psychotherapy. Many who desperately need treatment, but whose illness prevents them from recognizing it, receive no treatment or only brief psychotherapy, bricf hospitalization, hurried programs, and discharge when treatment has only been initiated and little improvement has occurred.

Nevertheless, there are increasing signs of dissatisfaction with this approach. There is an increasing interest on the part of psychiatric residents in taking time to know their patients, developing a working relationship, empathizing, and interacting in a therapeutic way. Treatment guidelines are being developed to show the kinds of illnesses best treated with pharmacology, those most effectively treated by psychotherapy, and those which respond best to combined psychotherapy and psychopharmacology. There is an interest in going beneath the superficial and understanding the underlying cause—to helping the patient make both superficial and structural changes rather than symptomatic changes only.

Today the Loma Linda University Department of Psychiatry is the only School of Medicine Psychiatric Department in the United States which acknowledges a Christian orientation and commitment to integration of the spiritual/religious and scientific psychiatry. However, like other medical centers, Loma Linda has given increasing emphasis to psychopharmacology over the past twenty-five years. Among physicians electing psychiatric residencies, only a small proportion have demonstrated a deep commitment to spirituality or religion. This is not unlike other students in the School of Medicine. Ten years ago there were almost no medical students preparing to go overseas as medical missionaries, and few Loma Linda graduates had a commitment to Adventist institutions and hospitals. Today we see the beginning of a change—a resurgence of commitment to spiritual/religious values and a larger percentage of dedicated Adventist and other Christian applicants for psychiatric residencies. Residents in psychiatry are more involved in spiritual discussions and seeking spiritual opportunities. The global mission experience is an increasingly popular elective for residents in psychiatry. Domestically, residents are expressing more interest in being part of Adventist Health Care institutions. We aim to forge a closer relationship with Adventist Health Care that will encourage these institutions to actively recruit dedicated Christian psychiatrists to lead out in the psychiatric programs in these important health care institutions.

We are hopeful that this will lead to increased scholarly exploration, research, and publication on the reciprocal interaction of spirituality/religion in psychiatry and the added value this has for the future. We see Loma Linda University's Department of Psychiatry assuming an increasing role in clinical care, education of residents, collaboration with other mental health professionals, and continuing education of pastors who frequently are the first to be consulted for mental health assistance. Christian psychiatry, with an Adventist perspective which was initiated in the Battle Creek Sanitarium, was developed and refined at the Harding Hospital which many considered to be the center of Adventist psychiatry from its opening in 1916 through the remainder of the twentieth century. Today the leadership has shifted to Loma Linda University. It is important that the clinical services keep up with developing treatments and techniques and remain solidly Adventist Christian. We look to the Department of Psychiatry to give leadership and to demonstrate that it has a vision of what can be accomplished with dedicated leadership and a committed staff, including support staff, who share the commitment to sound psychiatry and Christian values. In addition, Loma Linda University needs to enlarge its training of psychiatric physicians and other mental health professionals, providing the opportunity for Christian growth in their educational program. High priority must be given to people with spiritual interest and a commitment greater than toleration. Residents need to be encouraged to go to under-served locations in the United States and around the world and to see the multiplication of efforts that can occur when a dedicated psychiatrist joins with other mental health professionals and staff to provide a comprehensive treatment program utilizing a team approach.

And, of course, research into how this can be done most effectively and what Christian values are most useful in developing growth in patients must be increasingly explored. Findings need to be published so that the impact of wholistic, spiritual/religious thinking from a Christian Adventist perspective will inspire others to integrate this added value into their teaching and practice.

REFERENCES

Alexander, F., & Selesnick, S. T. (1966). *The history of psychiatry*. New York: Harper and Row.

Ashworth, W. (1983). Chapter 9: Edward A. Sutherland: Reformer. In G. Knight (ed.), *Early Adventist educators*, p. 179. Berrien Springs, MI: Andrews University Press.

Blazer, D. (1998). *Freud vs. God: How psychiatry lost its soul and Christianity lost its mind*. Downers Grove, IL: InterVarsity.

Bowlby, J. (1990). *A Secure Base: Parent-child attachment and healthy human development*. New York: Basic Books.

Butler, M., Thornton, F., & Stolz, G. (1994). *The Battle Creek Idea: John Harvey Kellogg and the Battle Creek Sanitarium*. Battle Creek, MI: Heritage Publications.

Daniells, A. G. (1930). Personal communication: Letter to George T. Harding III.

Engel, G. L. (1980). The clinical application of the biopsychosocial model. *American Journal of Psychiatry, 137*, 535–544.

Fayard, C., Harding, G. I., Murdoch, W., & Brunt, J. (2007). Clinical implications for psychotherapy from the Seventh-day Adventist tradition. *Journal of Psychology and Christianity, 26*, 207–217.

Foskett, J. (1996). Christianity and psychiatry. In J. Bhugra (Ed.), *Psychiatry and religion: Context, consensus, and controversies*. London: Routledge.

Frankl, V. E. (1987). *Man's search for meaning* (5th ed.). London: Hodder and Stoughton.

Freud, S. (1935). The future of an illusion. In E. Jones (Ed.), *The international psychoanalytic library, No. 15* (W. B. Robson-Scott, Trans.). London: Hogarth Press.

Friedman, L. J. (1990). *Menninger: The family and the clinic*. New York: Alfred A. Knopf.

Fromm, E. (1950). *Psychoanalysis and religion*. New Haven, CT: Yale University Press.

Harding, G. II (1919). *Prospectus of the Sanitarium Realty Co.* [Pamphlet]. Worthington, OH: Author.

Harding, G. III (1934, January). *In memoriam: A life sketch of George Tryon Harding II*. Presented at G. T. Harding II Funeral Service, Worthington, OH.

Harding, G. IV (1987). Adventists and psychiatry: A short history of the beginnings. *Spectrum, 17*, 2–6.

Harding, G. IV (2001). Aspects of religion and psychiatry. In *Encyclopedia of the Social and Behavioral Sciences*. Oxford: Elsevier.

Harding, G. IV, & Shafer, V. (1959, November). *Harding Sanitarium: 40 years in Worthington*. Paper presented at the 40th anniversary of the Harding Sanitarium in Worthington, OH.

Heritage Battle Creek (2009). *The Battle Creek Idea*. Retrieved January 18, 2011, from http://www.heritagebattlecreek.org

Jung, C. (1959). *The undiscovered self*. New York: Signet.

Knight, G. R. (1983). *Early Adventist Educators.* Berrien Springs, MI: Andrews University Press.

Larson, D. B., & Greenwold, M. M. (1997). Making the case for spiritual interventions in clinical practice. *Mind/Body Medicine, 2,* 20–30.

Larson, D. B., Lu, F., & Swyers, J. (Eds.) (1996). *Model curriculum for psychiatric residency training programs: Religion and spirituality in clinical practice.* Rockvile, MD: National Institute for Healthcare Research.

Mengh, H., & Freud, E. (Eds.) (1963). *Psychoanalysis and faith: The letters of Sigmund Freud and Oskar Pfister.* New York: Basic Books.

Menninger, K. (1973). *Whatever became of sin?* New York: Hawthorne.

Menninger, W. (1982). *The Menninger hospital's guide to the order sheet.* Topeka, KS: Menninger Press.

Robinson, D. (1943). *Story of our health message.* Washington, D.C.: Review and Herald.

Schaefer, R. (2005). *On becoming [Harold] Shryock.* Washington, D.C.: Review and Herald.

Schore, A. (2003). *Affect regulation and the repair of the self.* New York: Norton.

Shafer, V. (1959). *Harding Hospital guide to treatment* [Pamphlet]. Worthington, OH: Author.

Schwartz, R. W. (1970). *John Harvey Kellogg, M.D.* Nashville, TN: Southern Publishing Association.

Schwartz, R. W. (2000). *Light bearers to the remnant.* Nampa, ID: Pacific Press.

Schwartz, R. W. (2006). *John Harvey Kellogg, M.D.: Pioneering health reformer.* Hagerstown, MD: Review and Herald.

Stevens, J. W. (2010). *God-fearing and free: A spiritual history of America's Cold War.* Cambridge, MA: Harvard University Press.

Tillich, P. (1957). *Dynamics of faith.* New York: Harper and Row.

White, E. G. (1863). *Manuscript Releases: From the Files of the Letters and Manuscripts* (Washington, D.C.: E. G. White Estate, 1981–1993).

White, E. G. (1884). *Testimonies for the church* (Vols. 1–8). Mountain View, CA: Pacific Press.

White, E. G. (1886). *Historical sketches of the foreign missions of the Seventh-day Adventists.* Basle, Switzerland: Basle Imprimerie Polyglotte.

White, E. G. (1903). *Ministry of healing.* Mountain View, CA: Pacific Press.

Section 2

Theoretical and Philosophical Foundations

Ellen White and Mental Health

Merlin D. Burt

Seventh-day Adventists are Protestant Christians who love Jesus and seek to help people know God. Based on Bible prophecy they believe that Jesus is coming soon and are intentional about proclaiming the gospel to the entire world. In doing this they have established a number of major ministries including educational and health care systems. These ministries now circle the globe and have been instrumental in preparing workers for the church and in extending the healing ministry of Jesus to a broken world. Both psychological and emotional health issues are intrinsically connected to education and medical ministry.

Ellen White, as one of the three principal founders of the Seventh-day Adventist church, was instrumental in establishing the educational and health care systems of the Seventh-day Adventist church. Her leadership role was unique in that she exhibited a gift that Adventists recognize as prophetic. Between 1844 and 1915 she received hundreds of prophetic visions and dreams. One of her major roles was to help individuals and the church organization to understand and follow God's will. Though she had no formal mental health training, Ellen White often served as a spiritual counselor for people who had various emotional and psychological needs. She touched the lives of thousands of people and gave them new hope with a healthy spiritual, mental, and emotional focus. Her extensive writings demonstrate sympathy for mental health issues. Among other material she wrote an important chapter titled "Mind Cure" in her book *Ministry of Healing*, and in 1977 the Ellen G. White Estate published a two-volume compilation titled *Mind, Character, and Personality: Guidelines for Mental and Spiritual Health.*

The purpose of this paper is to introduce Ellen White's philosophy of mental and emotional health and healing. It will briefly examine her personal experience and her writings on the subject. Certain difficulties have existed in interpreting her positions. A historical background will be provided for clarification.

ELLEN WHITE'S PHILOSOPHY OF MENTAL HEALTH

Ellen White used the term "mental health" in her writings, which she associates with "mental clearness, calm nerves, a quiet, peaceful spirit like Jesus" (personal communication, White to D. T. Bourdeau, February 10, 1895, Letter 7, 1885; see also White to D. T. Bourdeau, Letter 39, 1887). In order to understand Ellen White's observations on mental health issues, it is necessary to understand her use of terms. She uses nineteenth-century language. For example, she uses the words "diseased imagination" to refer to delusional thinking or emotional imbalance and "despondency, which increases to despair" when speaking of depression (White, 1948a, Vol. 2, p. 305). She also uses the term "mind cure" to describe mental health issues.

For Ellen White, Jesus is the great healer of the sin-damaged human mind. She departs from a purely self-actualized or human-based mental healing. She ascribed to the Christian view that human nature is inherently sinful and needs external help from God. "It is impossible for us, of ourselves," she wrote, "to escape from the pit in which we are sunken. Our hearts are evil, and we cannot change them." She quoted Job 14:4 and Romans 8:7 to support this view. She then continued: "Education, culture, the exercise of the will, human effort, all have their proper sphere, but here they are powerless. They may produce an outward correctness of behavior, but they cannot change the heart; they cannot purify the springs of life. There must be a power working from within, a new life from above, before men [and women] can be changed from sin to holiness" (White, 1948b, p. 18).

For Ellen White there is a convergence of psychology and theology. The two must interplay and when correctly integrated provide the most help for the human mind and emotions. For her the true source of mental and emotional health is God the loving Father, Jesus the "Great Physician," and the Holy Spirit as Counselor.

She strongly advocated a proper connection between the physical, mental, and spiritual in the human experience. "The spiritual life is built up from the food given to the mind; and if we eat the food provided in the Word of God, spiritual and mental health will be the result" (White, 1906, p. 8). For Ellen White, true mental health was dependent upon establishing a proper balance between the body and the mind. "We cannot afford to dwarf or cripple a single function of the mind or body, by overwork or abuse of any part of the living machinery. As surely as we do this, we must suffer the consequences. Our first duty to God and our fellow-beings, is that of self-development" (White, 1882, p. 181). Dozens of times Ellen White uses the phrase "physical and mental health." For her, the physical and mental dimensions are closely connected and require proper balance and care. Ellen White believed that a right environment, right actions, and a proper diet facilitated mental health. She was a strong advocate of the healing benefits of nature, a right attitude, and acts of service for others (White, 1932/1963).

Ellen White's philosophy on mental health, while informed by her study of Scripture and her visions, was the answer to her own experience. As a child and young adult she had to wrestle with significant physical and mental health challenges. Much of her confusion began to resolve when she came to understand the loving paternal character of God and the compassionate Savior.

ELLEN WHITE'S PERSONAL EXPERIENCE WITH MENTAL HEALTH ISSUES

Through her long life Ellen White was no stranger to emotional pain and psychological challenges. As a child she was introverted, shy, and emotionally sensitive. To this was added the complication of a physical disability. During her younger years she experienced fearfulness and hopelessness that brought protracted periods of depression. In addition to her personal struggles, her immediate family was touched with mental disability issues.

CHILDHOOD STRUGGLE WITH DEPRESSION AND CONFUSION

Ellen White's fundamental touchstone for mental and emotional health was an understanding of the loving character of God. As a child she viewed God as a "stern tyrant compelling men to a blind obedience" (White, n.d., p. 43). When preachers would describe the fires of an eternally burning hell, she personalized the horror of that experience. She wrote: "While listening to these terrible descriptions, my imagination would be so wrought upon that the perspiration would start, and it was difficult to suppress a cry of anguish, for I seemed already to feel the pains of perdition" (White, 1915, pp. 29–30). This led her to doubt her acceptance with God and caused periods of depression. She recalled one occasion: "Despair overwhelmed me, and…no ray of light pierced the gloom that encompassed me" (White, 1915, p. 32). Her "feelings were very sensitive" and at one point she feared she would "lose" her "reason." Ellen White recollected that "sometimes for a whole night" she would not dare to close her eyes but "knelt upon the floor, praying silently with a dumb agony that cannot be described" (White & White, 1880, pp. 152–154).

Ellen White's pre-teen and early teen years were complicated by physical disability. She was severely injured through an accident at about the age of nine. A broken nose with other complicating damage caused equilibrium problems and prevented her from continuing her education. She also developed a chronic pulmonary disorder that was diagnosed at the time as "dropsical consumption," or, in modern terms, "tuberculosis with complicating congestive heart failure." Her fears were exacerbated by the thought that she could bleed out at any time from an arterial rupture in her lungs (Loughborough, 1892, p. 92). Her physical and emotional trauma, combined with her introverted personality, prevented her from seeking help.

Finally, at about the age of fifteen, she talked with someone who helped her to better understand the loving character of God. She pointed to her interview with Levi Stockman, a Millerite Methodist minister, as providing her with the most help. Stockman was sympathetic to Ellen's emotional pain and even shared her tears. She wrote that she "obtained" from Stockman "more knowledge on the subject of God's love and pitying tenderness, than from all the sermons and exhortations to which I had ever listened" (White, 1915, p. 37). She specifically identified what helped her most: "My views of the Father were changed. I now looked upon Him as a kind and tender parent.... My heart went out towards Him in a deep and fervent love" (White, n.d., p. 43). The love of God became Ellen White's favorite theme throughout her life. She also believed that "Christ's favorite theme was the paternal tenderness and abundant grace of God" (White, 1941/1900; White, 1948a, Vol. 6; White, 1893). Her five-volume masterpiece series on the cosmic conflict between Christ and Satan begins and ends with this theme (White, 1958a/1890; 1911/1939). Her most popular book, published in scores of languages with millions of copies, has as its first chapter "God's Love for Man" (White, 1948b, pp. 9–15).

Ellen White's own visions and dreams confirmed her conviction of a loving God and compassionate Savior. An early personal dream that occurred before her first prophetic vision brought her into the presence of Jesus where she realized that He knew all her "inner thoughts and feelings." Yet, even with this knowledge He "drew near with a smile," laid His hand on her head, and said "fear not" (White, 1915, pp. 33–34). During an interview with C. C. Crisler, during the last year of her life, Ellen White said, "I find tears running down my cheeks when I think of what the Lord is to His children, and when I contemplate His goodness, His mercy, [and] His tender compassion" (White, 1914).

MENTAL HEALTH CHALLENGES IN ELLEN WHITE'S FAMILY

Besides her own emotional struggles during childhood and at times during adulthood, Ellen White faced mental health challenges within her family. Her second son, James Edson, evidenced some of the characteristics of a person with attention deficit/hyperactivity disorder. Her husband suffered from a series of strokes during the 1860s and 1870s that altered his mental state and brought marital conflict. In 1879 Ellen White realized her husband did not "have sufficient physical and mental health" to give counsel and advice (Burt, n.d.). At one point she wondered if he was a "sane man" (personal communication, White to Lucinda Hall, May 16, 1876, Letter 66). Her niece, Louisa Walling, became so mentally unstable that she was admitted to a mental facility. Out of concern for Louisa's two children, Addie and May Walling, James and Ellen White brought them into their home. Ellen White ended up raising the girls and they called her "Mother" (Burt, n.d.).

Ellen White's personal experience combined with her visionary guidance to give her a unique ministry to individuals who also suffered with mental and emotional brokenness. Her writings reveal a consistent compassion for people who sometimes have serious life dysfunction. She engaged to a remarkable degree in close personal work with many people.

ELLEN WHITE AS A COUNSELOR TO PEOPLE WITH SERIOUS MENTAL HEALTH ISSUES

Throughout her life, Ellen White addressed mental health and social dysfunction issues. Her scope of interaction with various people was diverse. Four examples of her interaction with people are provided in this section to show her way of addressing serious mental health issues. They include obsessive behavior, emotional abuse, alcohol addiction, and sexual dysfunction. Ellen White's writings demonstrate that much of her time was spent in direct personal work to help people with mental, emotional, social, and spiritual dysfunction.

OBSESSIVE BEHAVIOR

Ellen White's letter to "Brother Morrell" shows her perception of his mental condition. She described this man as having "large conscientiousness" and "small self-esteem." It seems that Morrell was obsessive and pathologically perfectionistic about his conduct. He felt guilty for the smallest perceived mistake to the point of mental instability. Ellen White wrote of this man's condition thus:

> Brother Morrell's nervous system is greatly affected and he ponders over these things [his perceived sins and failings], dwelling upon

> them. His imagination is diseased. It has a morbid imagination. The mind has suffered beyond expression. Sleep was driven from him. (personal communication, White to "Brother Morrell," December 28, 1867, Letter 20)

She wrote directly:

> I saw, Brother Morrell, you must cast away your fears. Leave consequences with the Lord and let go. You try too hard to save yourself, to do some great thing yourself which will commend you to God.... Jesus loves you, and if you will consecrate yourself and all you have to Him, He will accept you and will be your Burden-bearer, your never failing Friend....Believe Jesus loves you and in your efforts to obey the truth, if you err, don't feel that you must worry and worry, give up your confidence in God, and think that God is your enemy. We are erring mortals....You cannot cleanse yourself from impurities; carry all your burden to Jesus. (personal communication, White to "Brother Morrell," December 28, 1867, Letter 20)

As a complement to her spiritual and emotional counsel, she urged this man to adopt health reform and avoid stimulants. "Then," she wrote, "can the brain think more calmly, sleep will not be so uncertain" (personal communication, White to "Brother Morrell," December 28, 1867, Letter 20).

EMOTIONAL ABUSE

Ellen White has several letters of counsel to women who were either emotionally or physically controlled by their husbands. In December 1867 she visited the Washington, New Hampshire, Seventh-day Adventist church with her husband and J. N. Andrews. She first gave oral counsel and followed up with a written "testimony" based on a vision she had received. She provided pointed counsel to Harriet Stowell. After the death of her first husband Joshua Goodwin—who was the minister who brought Adventism to Washington—Harriet married Freeman S. Stowell. He was about twelve years younger than her and apparently was not practicing the faith of his father, John Stowell (identities confirmed by 1850, 1860, and 1870 Federal Census records for Washington, NH; Committee Chosen by the Town, 1886, pp. 535, 630). John Stowell was one of the founders of the church in Washington. Ellen White's words are clear and explain the situation:

> I was shown the daughter-in-law of Brother Stowell's, the sister of Brother Mead. She is beloved of God, but held in servile bondage, fearing, trembling, desponding, doubting, very nervous. Now this sister should not feel that she must yield her will to a godless youth who has less years upon his head than herself. She should remember that her marriage does not destroy her individuality. God has claims upon her higher than any earthly claim. Christ has bought her with His own blood, she is not her own. She fails to put her entire trust in God and submits to yield her convictions, her conscience to an overbearing, tyrannical man fired up by Satan when his Satanic majesty can make it effectual to intimidate the trembling, shrinking soul who has so many times been thrown into agitation that her nervous system is torn to pieces and she nearly a wreck. Is this the work of the Lord that this sister should be in this state…? (White, 1868)

Ellen White supported individuality in marriage and rejected the idea that a woman must give up her personality and self-identity. This testimony was an encouragement and help to this woman who was driven almost to emotional collapse.

ALCOHOL ADDICTION

Ellen White recognized the effect of alcohol addiction and an induced emotional state on the cognitive process in a letter to a troubled young man while she was in England. Henri Frey worked as a translator for the European mission in Basel, Switzerland. He was probably also an alcoholic. Because of his actions, he was removed from his position as translator. He then wrote Ellen White that he was being persecuted. She supported the decision of the mission but personally appealed to this man. "I feel the tenderest feeling of pity, and of love for your soul; but false words of sympathy to sustain you in rebellion and defiance of those whom God has placed in responsible positions in His work shall never be traced by my pen." She cogently described his condition.

> You find your emotional nature untrue to your best resolutions, untrue to your solemn pledges. Nothing seems real. Your own inefficiencies lead you to doubt the sincerity of those who would do you good. The more you struggle in doubt, the more unreal everything looks to you, until it seems that there is no solid ground for you anywhere. Your promises are nothing, they are like ropes of sand, and you regard the words and works of those whom you should trust in the same unreal light.

She continued by emphasizing the power of the will in meeting emotional dysfunction. "You may believe and promise all things, but I would not give a straw for your promises or your faith until you put your will over on the believing and doing side." Her letter of counsel is interwoven with appeals for this young man to see the help Jesus can give.

> I tell you that you need not despair. You must choose to believe, although nothing seems true and real to you....Your part is to put your will over on the side of Christ in the matter of faith. Just as you yield up your will to the will of Jesus Christ, God immediately takes possession of that will, and works in you to will and to do of His good pleasure; and all of your nature is brought under the control of the spirit of Christ, even your thoughts are subject to Him.

Ellen White concluded this letter with words of hope.

> A life of usefulness is before you, if your will becomes God's will. Then you may stand in your God-given manhood an example of good works....Will you try Henri, will you now change square about? You are the object of Christ's love and intercession." (personal communication, White to Henri Frey, July 21, 1887, Letter 49)

SEXUAL DYSFUNCTION

Ellen White often dealt with sensitive issues. One of these was child abuse. In 1896, she wrote to a leading minister in South Africa. He was guilty of sexually abusing young girls and perhaps boys and had written to Ellen White of his struggles. He believed he was not guilty of adultery or breaking the law of God. She began her letter with a prayer, "May the Lord help me to write you the very words that will be for your restoration and not for your destruction." She then wrote most directly to him:

> I feel sorry, very sorry for you. Sin, my brother, *is sin*; it is the transgression of the *Law*, and should I try to lessen the sin before you, I would not be doing you any good....Your mind and heart are polluted else all such actions would be loathsome.

She described for this man the longterm effect of sexual abuse on children including the generational effect. She cited several cases and described how psychological damage was often life long. "How can I frame words to express the enormity of this awful sin?" she wrote. "How can I present it in such a manner that you will no longer look upon it, as you have done, as no great wrong?" After a lengthy direct and sometimes painfully graphic description of his conduct, she appeals to the man with these words:

> You are a free moral agent. If you will repent of your sins, and be converted, the Lord will blot out your transgressions and impute unto you His righteousness....If you will take hold of Christ by living faith, and humble your soul before Him, He will undertake your case, and angels will guard you. But you must resist the devil. You must educate yourself to a different train of thought. Put no confidence in yourself. Never seek the companionship of women or girls. Keep away from them. Your moral taste is so perverted, that you will ruin yourself and ruin many souls if you do not turn square about....Everlasting life is worth a life-long, persevering, untiring effort.

Finally she urged him to make himself accountable to "brethren who know this terrible chapter in your experience" (personal communication, White to a Prominent Minister, June 1, 1896, Letter 106a).

These four examples illustrate the level of involvement Ellen White had in the lives of many people. Those who are familiar with Ellen White's writings are not always aware of the extensive nature of her work with people who had emotional and mental health difficulties. One of the remarkable characteristics of her work is her consistent optimism that a person can recover no matter how broken he or she may be. Ellen White always points the person to God as the great healer of the mind and soul.

MENTAL HEALTH THERAPEUTIC ISSUES IN ELLEN WHITE'S WRITINGS

There are several important clarifications that need to be made in terms of Ellen White's therapeutic approach to mental healing. It is imperative that one understands the nineteenth-century historical context of her writings. This is particularly important because she writes strongly against the use of drugs and against "psychology." Some have concluded that this therefore means that the modern application of these modalities should be avoided. In order to correctly understand Ellen White on these issues, one must understand what she actually means when she rejects these modalities.

Ellen White pointed to the vital importance of mental health. "The mind controls the whole man [person]. All our actions, good or bad, have their source in the mind. It is the mind that worships God and allies us to heavenly beings." She also recognized the effect of physical health on the mind. "All the physical organs are the servants of the mind, and the nerves are the messengers that transmit its orders to every part of the body, guiding the motions of the living machinery" (White, 1897, p. 33).

USE OF DRUGS IN THERAPY

Because of the confused and problematic state of drug therapy during most of Ellen White's lifetime, she has little or nothing to say about the medicinal treatment of mental illness. Her philosophical basis for healing and mental health therapy is more wholistic with an emphasis on the spiritual, hydropathic, and natural remedy dimensions. She wrote:

> Pure air, sunlight, abstemiousness, rest, exercise, proper diet, the use of water, trust in divine power—these are the true remedies. Every person should have a knowledge of nature's remedial agencies and how to apply them. It is essential both to understand the principles involved in the treatment of the sick and to have a practical training that will enable one rightly to use this knowledge. (White, 1942, p. 127)

In her application of healing modalities, Ellen White sought to "understand the principles." The nineteenth century was a time of confused and fallacious philosophies of healing. The default treatment modality was the "traditional" heroic therapy advocated by Benjamin Rush. He advocated bloodletting, blistering, and the use of emetics to relieve "fevers" or "vascular tension" that he believed caused illness. This included the internal use of drugs such as calomel and the topical use of caustic chemicals. Calomel was a mercury compound used as a purgative. The poor person's alternative to "traditional" physicians was the Thompsonian approach. Samuel Thompson said that all disease was caused by cold. He therefore sought to increase the body's natural heat. He used lobelia, an American plant that had sedative and emetic characteristics. Other philosophies of healing included homeopathy, which said that small doses of drugs that produced the symptoms of a disease in a healthy person could cure the same disease. By the time of the Civil War, homeopathy was the preferred method of treatment for physicians who had rejected "heroic therapy." Beyond heroic therapy, the Thompsonian approach, and homeopathy, there were many other treatments that had little philosophical basis and used drugs such as opiates, arsenic, and quinine, together with various plant and root products of often-unknown origin. These were usually suspended in alcohol.

Little wonder that Ellen White wrote against the use of drugs during her lifetime. This is a classic statement by her: "There are more who die from the use of drugs, than all who could have died of disease had nature been left to do her own work" (White, 1864, p. 135). She was not opposed to the use of drugs when they had lifesaving results even when the drug was dangerous. For a time in the treatment of malaria, quinine was the only known drug. Ellen White indicated, "We are expected to do the best we can" and "If quinine will save a life, use quinine" (White, 1958b, p. 282).

The modern use of drugs in psychiatric treatment has a more physiological basis and would follow Ellen White's position that doctors understand the "principles involved in the treatment of the sick." Were she present today she would probably still argue that natural methods are best where possible but that physiologically-based drug therapy has its place.

ELLEN WHITE'S STATEMENT AGAINST PSYCHOLOGY

There were three philosophies of healing current in Ellen White's day that influenced her comments on psychological and mental health issues. They were mesmerism, phrenology, and the rest cure. Ellen White was strongly opposed to all three. In 1862 she wrote: "The sciences of phrenology, psychology, and mesmerism are the channel through which he [Satan] comes more directly to this generation and works with that power which is to characterize his efforts near the close of probation" (White, 1948a, Vol. 1, p. 290).

Mesmerism. During her early years of ministry, Ellen White was forced to repeatedly confront mesmerism and its mind-manipulating methods. In the United States during the mid-nineteenth century, Animal Magnetism was a popular philosophy of healing. Originated by

Viennese physician Franz Anton Mesmer (1734–1815), it taught that an invisible magnetic fluid permeated the universe. Mesmer theorized that disease produced an imbalance of this fluid within the human body, which could be cured through the use of magnets and electrical current. He eventually abandoned the use of magnets and proposed that the "healer's body" "permeated with animal magnetism, could redirect the patient's magnetic fluid without the use of magnets." The goal was to induce a "crisis" by altering the subject's mental state through fever, delirium, convulsions, uncontrolled weeping, and nervous twitches. Mesmer saw these manifestations as healthy symptoms of healing. Suggestibility and dominance were used to produce a trance and thus re-align the body (Kirsch, Lynn, & Rhue, 1993, p. 5; Burnham, 1977). James Braid later redefined the term "mesmerism" as hypnotism, and Mesmer became known as the father of modern hypnosis (Skinner, 1949, p. 186).

During 1845 Ellen White was forced to confront a prominent Millerite Adventist minister in Maine, named Joseph Turner, who was using mesmerism. He even tried to mesmerize or hypnotize her. On one occasion in Poland, Maine, she was at a meeting where he sought to manipulate her. She recollected: "He had his eyes looking right out of his fingers, and his eyes looked like snakes eyes, evil." Her experiences in confronting this man, together with her visionary guidance, placed her in opposition to hypnotic mind-controlling modalities that removed a person's God-given mental independence and freedom. She wrote very directly and specifically on this topic. "It is not God's purpose that any human being should yield his mind and will to the control of another, becoming a passive instrument in his hands.... He is not to look to any human being as the source of healing. His dependence must be in God" (White, 1942, p. 242).

In a series of letters during 1901 and 1902 to A. J. Sanderson and his wife, who were the medical directors at St. Helena Sanitarium, Ellen White warned of the dangers of hypnotism. "Cut away from yourselves everything that savors of hypnotism, the science by which satanic agencies work" (personal communication, White to Arthur J. and Emma Sanderson, February 16, 1902 [typed], Letter 20). She identified the feature of hypnotism that most concerned her and revealed one of her core values in mental healing: "The theory of mind controlling mind is originated by Satan to introduce himself as the chief worker to put human philosophy where divine philosophy should be.... The physician must educate the people to look from the human to the divine" (personal communication, White to A. J. Sanderson, September 12, 1901 [typed], Letter 121).

Phrenology. Phrenology was a theory popularized in America during the mid nineteenth century. Popularized by Orson S. Fowler and his brother Lorenzo N. Fowler, phrenology said that the shape of a person's head determined his or her character and personality. Though based on a fallacious premise, it was widely accepted as authentic during the nineteenth century. Ellen White became settled in her opposition to this modality. In 1893 she wrote of phrenology as "vain philosophy, glorying in things they do not understand, assuming a knowledge of human nature which is false" (personal communication, White to E. J. Waggoner, January 22, 1893, Letter 78).

Rest cure. The "Rest Cure" modality was championed by Silas Weir Mitchell as the answer to nervous disorders. Mitchell advocated complete rest and an absence of any sensory stimuli. This method demanded that the subject have no visitors, letters, reading, writing, washing, exercise, or even the presence of light or sound. Rest was to be enforced, uninterrupted, and prolonged. Ellen White contradicted this view: "The sick should be taught that it is wrong to suspend all physical labor in order to regain health" (White, 1948a, Vol. 1, p. 555).

The philosophical basis of these three nineteenth-century modalities, though popular in their day, has been shown to be fallacious. When Ellen White used the terms "psychology" and "science," she was speaking of these spurious and erroneous movements and not the modern definitions of these terms. On one occasion she even wrote positively when using the term "psychology" in a more general sense.

"The true principles of psychology are found in the Holy Scriptures. Man knows not his own value. He acts according to his unconverted temperament of character because he does not look unto Jesus, the Author and Finisher of his faith" (White, 1899). For Ellen White, correct "psychology" had a high view of the value of human beings as understood in the light of the gift of Jesus and the love of God. For her, the goal of psychological study was how to reconnect the person with God as the great healer of the mind and soul.

Receiving psychological guidance from a counselor. While it has been shown that Ellen White centered her philosophy of mental health and healing on God, she did not exclude the role of humans in cooperating with God. She is clear that God can use counselors to assist in bringing those with mental and emotional illness to healing. "Christ's servants are His representatives, the channels for His working. He desires through them to exercise His healing powers" (White, 1940, pp. 823–824). In another similar statement she wrote: "God designs that the sick, the unfortunate, those possessed of evil spirits, shall hear His voice through us. Through His human agents He desires to be a comforter, such as the world has never before seen" (White, 1952, p. 22). She even gives an imperative for counseling. "When a crisis comes in the life of any soul....It is the consistent life, the revelation of a sincere, Christlike interest for the soul in peril, that will make counsel effectual to persuade and win into safe paths." She continues that those who neglect this work "will have to give an account for their neglect of those whom they might have blessed, strengthened, upheld, and healed" (personal communication, White to "Brethren in responsible positions in the Review and Herald office," January 13, 1894, Letter 70). Ellen White's own experience, as a counselor, is an application of this statement. Though not trained in psychology, she helped many to better emotional and mental health during her lifetime. To this day, her writings provide a helpful philosophical and theological framework that supports "medical missionary" activity, as she called it, in the fields of psychiatry and psychology.

Some well-meaning Christians have been unwilling to speak to mental health professionals out of fear that God does not want them to tell another human of their sins or weaknesses. They think that seeking psychological help is a betrayal of their faith by looking to humans for help rather than to God. But Ellen White is clear that there are venues where it is correct and proper to confide in others (White, 1977, Vol. 2). She was a frequent listener and counselor to those with sorrows and perplexities. She wrote the following words of comfort to a man in Australia who confided in her.

> If the human agents from whom we might be led to expect help fail to do their part, let us be comforted in the thought that the heavenly intelligences will not fail to do their part. They will pass by those whose hearts are not tender and pitiful, kind and thoughtful, and ready to relieve the woes of others, and will use any human agent that will be touched with the infirmities, the necessities, the troubles, the perplexities, of people for whom Christ died." (personal communication, White to J. R. Buster, August 3, 1894, Letter 4)

A review of her many statements on the role of human counselors shows that Ellen White remained confident that Jesus was the ultimate helper and healer. Yet human counselors, whoever they may be—whether friend, parent, pastor, physician, or psychologist—are to help the person to Jesus as the "never-failing Friend in whom we can confide all the secrets of the soul" (White, 1948a, Vol. 1, p. 502).

Mental and emotional healing, like physical healing, is a process that takes time. A reading of Ellen White's writings reveals a remarkable degree of sensitivity to the sometimes-lengthy process psychological help requires.

CONCLUSION

This paper has provided a brief overview of Ellen White's philosophy regarding mental health. Ellen White was keenly aware that the broken human condition included the mind and emotions. She found from her own experience the redemptive and restoring power of God to heal damaged and wounded minds. She never saw any persons as beyond restoration if they would reach out to God. She believed in the vital importance of fellow humans who were able to assist those in need to mental health.

Ellen White was wholistic in her approach to healing. She realized that the mind was linked to the body and that God intended humans to have restored social relationships. The most important connection was a spiritual one with a loving and holy heavenly Father. She rejected the idea that true mental and emotional healing could occur apart from God.

Ellen White's approach to therapeutic treatment of the mentally ill focused on an application of principles. She supported counseling and natural healing methods. She never developed a physiologically based view on drug treatment except to acknowledge that certain drugs such as quinine—though having negative side effects—might be used if they had a necessary therapeutic effect. Her sweeping rejection of drugs is based on the erroneous philosophies of healing that were current in her day and the dangerous chemicals and drugs that were used. She was particularly opposed to the use of mesmerism or hypnotism. She saw it as dangerous in that it placed a person's mind under the control of another person. Her statements against "psychology" and "science" are related to her opposition to mesmerism, phrenology, and the "rest cure."

Ellen White as a counselor effectively applied her philosophy of mental health. She had extensive interactions with people throughout her lifetime and dealt with various types of psychological dysfunction. She remained sympathetic and redemptive even when the condition was particularly objectionable. She had no mental health training and lived at a time when mental health science was still rudimentary. Nevertheless she was able to be remarkably effective in helping many people. She understood that emotional and mental brokenness was not cured instantly and that a person could be walking with God but still need support and guidance. She believed in the necessity of direct intervention by others who were able to counsel and guide. Though she did not directly write about the role of mental health practitioners, she did write positively of the type of help that can be provided by these disciplines. We cannot precisely say what her reaction would be to the modern practice of these disciplines, but a study of her life, writings, and activities suggests that she would be supportive of Christian psychological practice that was in harmony with a biblical philosophy of healing.

REFERENCES

Burnham, J. C. (1977). Franz Anton Mesmer. In B. B. Wolman (Ed.), *International encyclopedia of psychiatry, psychology, psychoanalysis, and neurology* (pp. 7–213). New York: Aesculapius Publishers.

Burt, M. D. (n.d.). *Caroline True Clough Family and Ellen White.* Unpublished manuscript. Ellen G. White Estate Branch Office, Loma Linda, CA.

Committee Chosen by the Town. (1886). *History of Washington, New Hampshire, from the first settlement to the present time 1768–1886.* Claremont, NH: Claremont Manufacturing Co.

Kirsch, I., Lynn, S. J., & Rhue, J. W. (1993). Introduction to clinical hypnosis. In *Handbook of clinical hypnosis* (p. 5). Washington, D.C.: American Psychological Association.

Loughborough, J. N. (1892). *Rise and progress of the Seventh-day Adventists with tokens of God's hand in the movement and a brief sketch of the advent cause from 1831 to 1844.* Battle Creek, MI: General Conference.

Skinner, H. A. (1949). *The origin of medical terms.* Baltimore, MD: Williams & Wilkins.

White, E. G. (n.d.). *Life sketches.* Unpublished manuscript.

White, E. G. (1864). *Spiritual gifts* (Vol. 4). Battle Creek, MI: Seventh-day Adventist.

White, E. G. (1868). *Manuscript 2.* Unpublished manuscript.

White, E. G. (1882, April 20). The primal cause of intemperance. *Signs of the Times, 8,* 181.

White, E. G. (1893, June 6). The New Zealand camp meeting. *Review and Herald, 17,* 354–355.

White, E. G. (1897). *Special testimonies on education.* Battle Creek, MI: Review and Herald.

White, E. G. (1899). *Manuscript 56: Following Jesus.* Unpublished manuscript.

White, E. G. (1906, March 22). Search the Scriptures. *Review and Herald, 83*(12), 8.

White, E. G. (1914, July 21). Interview with C. C. Crisler.

White, E. G. (1915). *Life sketches.* Mountain View, CA: Pacific Press.

White, E. G. (1923). *Fundamentals of Christian education.* Nashville, TN: Southern Publishing Association.

White, E. G. (1939). *The great controversy between Christ and Satan.* Mountain View, CA: Pacific Press. (Original work published 1911)

White, E. G. (1940). *The Desire of Ages.* Mountain View, CA: Pacific Press.

White, E. G. (1941). *Christ's object lessons.* Washington, D.C.: Review and Herald. (Original work published 1900)

White, E. G. (1942). *The ministry of healing.* Mountain View, CA: Pacific Press.

White, E. G. (1948a). *Steps to Christ.* Mountain View, CA: Pacific Press.

White, E. G. (1948b). *Testimonies for the church* (Vols. 1–6). Mountain View, CA: Pacific Press.

White, E. G. (1952). *Welfare ministry.* Washington, D.C.: Review and Herald.

White, E. G. (1958a). *Selected messages: Book two.* Washington, D.C.: Review and Herald.

White, E. G. (1958b). *The story of patriarchs and prophets.* Mountain View, CA: Pacific Press. (Original work published 1890)

White, E. G. (1963). *Medical ministry.* Mountain View, CA: Pacific Press. (Original work published 1932)

White, E. G. (1977). *Mind, character, and personality* (Vols. 1–2). Nashville, TN: Southern Publishing Association.

White, J., & White, E. G. (1880). *Life sketches.* Battle Creek, MI: Seventh-day Adventist.

Faith-Science Issues: An Epistemological Perspective

E. Edward Zinke

I was standing before a large memorial boulder in a quiet section of the city of Constance, Germany. On one side was inscribed the name Huss, and on the other Jerome. I was deep in concentration for a number of minutes—what would it be like to surrender one's life rather than compromise the authority of the Bible as the Word of God?

After moments of meditation, like any good tourist, I got out my camera to take a picture. It was not until then that I realized that an elderly woman was sitting on a park bench beside the boulder. The camera startled her. She immediately stood up, circled the boulder several times with her gaze constantly fixed back and forth between the camera and the stone, and then took off down the street in bewilderment, wondering why any American would be interested in the rock. I imagined this woman growing up just a block from the boulder, yet never realizing its significance.

I then thought of our church. We grew up with the Rock, the Word of God. But did we understand its significance? We were the people of the book. Our mission was tied to its message. But did we comprehend what it meant to say that the Bible was the authority not only for our theology but also for life?

For example, we acknowledge that secularism and materialism are fundamentally opposed to the biblical message, for they are humanistic[1] at their foundation. Yet we often accept other ideas equally such as empiricism and rationalism as a foundation for life and thought. We may see them as producing criteria for our acceptance of truth in the Bible and as providing the foundation for our understanding of the world. We make a clear distinction between

---

1. For this paper, humanism is defined as any system of thought that is grounded in some aspect of humankind or the natural world rather than in biblical revelation.

the material world that God has given us to use and enjoy and the materialism that makes material goods the god of our lives. Yet we fail to make that same distinction between reason and rationalism, the five senses, and empiricisms. We critique the world within which we live for its commercialism, immorality, and materialism, yet we accept its humanistic epistemologies as providing the framework within which the world should be known and understood, and in which our lives should be lived.

We seek a rock-solid foundation upon which to build our faith—a foundation built upon the unmovable successes of reason, science, and mathematics. However, in so doing, we fail to recognize that we have just made them the foundation of our lives.

This paper does not argue against the use of reason and science. It does not deny the value of understanding the structure of our existence. But it does speak against rationalism, empiricism, existentialism, and any other form of humanism that makes some aspect of humankind the foundation and measure of all things. That role should be reserved for God and His word alone. The Bible provides the foundation and structure for our understanding of the natural world, rather than the other way around.

The fundamental issue in the discussion of the relation between faith and learning is the question of foundational authority. Such authority provides one's worldview which makes possible a cohesive understanding of the world in which we live. How do we know what we know, and what foundation provides the lens through which we understand the world?

Epistemology is the path we take. Our destination is determined by our epistemology. This in turn has implications for our self-understanding, the purpose of our existence, our knowledge of the world in which we live, our concept of what the universe is like, and finally, our understanding of who God is. When our epistemology changes, our concept of the universe, of ourselves, and of God changes as well.

We live in a world that is bombarded from all sides with humanistic ways of thinking. From the classroom, to the news media, to everyday life in the workplace, we are taught to think humanistically. This paper will call for a paradigm shift from humanism to biblical thinking. We will start with a brief history of intellectual thought followed by a critique of the resultant humanistic methods from the perspective of the Bible and E. G. White.

HISTORICAL OVERVIEW: THE IMPACT OF GREEK THINKING ON CHRISTIAN WORLDVIEWS

The early church was dominated by Neo-Platonic thinking. For Plato, the truly real was the Form or the transcendent Idea. The Form was perfect and eternal, whereas the concrete phenomena were transient and imperfect. The material world was transient, something to be left behind on the way to absolute knowledge.

For Neo-Platonism, the universe was ordered by a hierarchy, from perfect eternal forms to earthly imperfect instances of these forms. Knowledge emanated from the eternal forms through the hierarchy, and the goal of earthly instances was to return to the eternal form.

Neo-Platonic thinking had a major impact on the theology of the early church. The allegorical method of interpretation, which was borrowed from Neo-Platonism, allowed the imposition of Neo-Platonism upon the Bible. For example, rather than affirming the biblical notion of the unity of the human being, a dualism of mind and body was asserted. Since the truly real was not the material, but the eternal Form, the idea of the natural immortality of the soul was introduced into the Christian church. The material body, that is, the imperfect instance of the perfect form, was of less consequence. This led on the one hand to asceticism: the denial of bodily pleasure to assure that the body did not hinder the soul from returning to the eternal Form. On the other hand, this led to lack of restraint since the body was material and therefore of no consequence.

The Neo-Platonic worldview also put a distance between God and humans. God was approachable only through intermediaries. This found its way into the church through intermediaries such as Mary, the apostles, and other saints.

Scholasticism of the Middle Ages was dominated by Aristotelian philosophical understanding of the world. The empirical world was fully real. Reason was employed to discover the order inherent within the empirical world itself. Yet, the mind was regarded not only as activated by sensory experience, but also by something eternally active, immortal, and divine, totally apart from the sensory world.

Thus, in spite of Aristotle's empiricism, it was his rationalism that dominated the history of Aristotelian thought. Aristotle posited an ideal Form, a pure Mind, a Supreme Being toward which everything was drawn—what he called the *Unmoved Mover*. The *Prime Mover* was the cause of all other celestial movement including that of the planets, moon, and, finally, movement on earth. Earth was at the center of the universe, not because of its grand importance, but because things moved according to their intrinsic nature. Heavier elements such as water and earth moved to the center of the universe, and lighter elements such as air, fire, and anything divine moved intrinsically upward.

Partaking of divinity, the sun and the planets moved in perfect circles around the earth. Since a circle is perfect, the natural path of non-earthly (divine) things was circular rather than linear. A very complex mathematical formula was used to explain the observed elliptical orbit of the planets. Finally, the Hellenistic astronomer Ptolemy codified this earth-centered view by positing epicycles and eccentrics to explain what was observed. The theory was self-sustaining since the discovery of new discrepancies could be explained by additional epicycles. Thomas Aquinas represents the most developed theology of the Middle Ages. For him, the task of the theologian was to synthesize the truths of nature, that is, the philosophy of Aristotle, who obviously described the nature of the natural world, with the spiritual insight of the Bible. Aristotle's model was the Bible *and* nature. Thus he was within the tradition of the

Roman Catholic Church, where theology was of necessity based upon the Bible *and* nature, tradition, the pope, *and* philosophy. Aquinas's God began to take on the character of the Unmoved Mover of Aristotle instead of the active God of the Bible. The Bible, while considered the supreme authority, became encased within the philosophy of the age.

The Reformation Era responded to the scholastic synthesis of the Middle Ages with the assertion that the Bible and the Bible alone was the foundation and guide to life. The slogan "the Bible alone" did not rule out other methods of knowing. However, it asserted that the Bible *alone* was the foundation. This meant that the Bible was not to be interpreted by alien philosophies or hermeneutical methods. The Bible was to be its own interpreter. That is, it was to provide the worldview for its own interpretation.

The principle of "the Bible alone" brought about new freedoms and responsibilities, and a renewed understanding of the individual and God. The individual was no longer beholden to his or her place in the universe, subject to king, pope, church, the ideal Form, or Pure Mind. That person was now personally accountable to God, and God was personally interested in humans and directly accessible to them. The structures of existence that had encased human thought and life were challenged by the Word of God, resulting in human freedom and individual direct personal relationship with God. As mentioned above, humanity was freed from the structures of the external world which were felt to be imposed upon humankind by Neo-Platonism and Aristotelianism. Humans were now accountable directly to God as revealed in His Word. The Bible *alone,* rather than the philosophical systems of the Greeks, was seen to be the *sole* foundation for understanding God, humankind, and the world.

ARISTOTELIAN SCHOLASTICISM

At the time of the Counter Reformation, there was a resurgence of Aristotelian scholasticism within both Catholicism and Protestantism. Tradition was *the* authority, not simple church tradition, but in particular the philosophical tradition stemming from Aristotle. The cosmology of Ptolemy reigned supreme. It was obviously true because it coincided best with the Aristotelian scholastic synthesis that so perceptively described the nature of reality. Scripture and nature were to be understood by the presumptive authority of the past, the traditions of the church, and particularly the intellectual traditions of the scholastics. Things were categorized by their degrees of perfection, which defined a great chain of being which allowed one to know contemplatively the value of all things. The scale of perfections placed God at the top. There was a divide between the mutable things of the earth and the immutable things of the heavens.

The earth was at the center of the universe, not because it was at the center of God's activity, but because mutable things fall to the earth, while divine things rise to the heavens. The heavenly bodies were higher on the scale of perfection and therefore operated by different laws than earthly objects, which were imperfect.

THE SCIENTIFIC REVOLUTION, THE ENLIGHTENMENT, AND COSMOLOGY

The era of the Enlightenment took place within the context of the freedoms opened up by the Reformation on the one hand, and as a reaction to the authority and rigidity of scholastic philosophy on the other. This new freedom opened the world to the development of modern science and new philosophical understandings.

A series of observations made by Copernicus, Kepler, Galileo, and Newton brought an entirely new understanding of cosmology. The earth was not the center of the universe with all planetary bodies revolving around it. Rather, the earth was itself a planet in orbit with the other planets around the sun.

This new understanding brought into question the entire scholastic tradition. The planetary movements were discovered to be elliptical rather than the implied perfection of circular motion. Stars were discovered that had not been seen by Aristotle. The moon had mountains (and therefore was not perfectly circular, i.e., divine), and the sun had spots and thus did not partake of divine perfection. Therefore, these bodies were not the incorruptible and immutable heavenly objects of Aristotelian-Ptolemaic philosophy. Objects fell to the ground because of gravity, not because they were trying to find their natural and rightful place in the universe. Circular motion was not natural to heavenly bodies, for they also would move in a straight line if it were not for the pull of gravity upon them. Thus planets remained in orbit by the same laws that caused rocks to fall to the ground. The dichotomy between the celestial and terrestrial realms was broken. The same laws that applied on earth also applied to the heavens. The heavens were also composed of material substances, their movements impelled by natural mechanical forces according to mathematical laws.

The absolute authority of Aristotelian tradition was called into question. Scholasticism had sought a synthesis between nature and religion. When scholasticism fell, a schism developed between science and religion. The Bible had been so fully reinterpreted by Greek philosophy that it also was caught in the undertow. Science was now seen to be autonomous not only from human tradition but also from any biblical foundation and guidance. The freedoms opened by the reformation were detached from God and His Word. Humanity now had its own independent epistemological foundations.

PHILOSOPHY

Francis Bacon. Bacon rejected the stale orthodoxies inherited from Scholasticism as airy speculation in magic and alchemy. Experience and experimentation were the only legitimate methods for arriving at knowledge of the natural world. As historian of western thought Richard Tarnas writes,

> The true basis of knowledge was the natural world and the information it provided through the human senses. To fill the world with assumed final causes, as did Aristotle, or with intelligible divine essences, as did Plato, was to obscure from man a genuine

> understanding of nature on its own terms, solidly based on direct experimental contact and inductive reasoning from particulars. No longer should the pursuer of knowledge start from abstract definitions and verbal distinctions and then reason deductively, forcing the phenomena into prearranged order. Instead, he must begin with the unbiased analysis of concrete data and only then reason inductively, and cautiously, to reach general, empirically supported conclusions. (1991, p. 273)

The spiritual and the natural realms had their own laws and appropriate, distinct methods. Science must not be hampered by irrelevant assumptions from the religious imagination of scholastic theology. Science and religion will both be better served if they are kept entirely separate.

Descartes. The crumbling fortification of the scholastic synthesis produced a new skepticism about the possibility of certain knowledge. Descartes set about solving this problem of skepticism by systematically doubting everything, including the existence of the physical world and his own body. At the end of this exercise, there was one thing that could not be doubted—the certainty of his self-awareness: "I cannot doubt that I am a doubting self, therefore I exist" popularized by the slogan "I think, therefore I am." From the certainty of his self-awareness he argued for the existence of God. From the existence of God he argued for the reality of the natural world, for a perfect God who lets humans discern self-evident truths through reason would not deceive humanity.

In contrast to mind, all physical phenomena are to be comprehended as machines. The laws of mechanics are identical to those of nature. Nature can be measured, and therefore mathematics, available to the light of human reason, was the tool for understanding the universe. Analytic reason *alone* was the basis for understanding the natural world. Tarnas (1991) summarizes Descartes' philosophy as follows:

> Thus human reason establishes first its own existence, out of experiential necessity, then God's existence, out of logical necessity,

and thence the God-guaranteed reality of the objective world and its rational order. Descartes enthroned human reason as the supreme authority in matters of knowledge, capable of distinguishing certain metaphysical truth and of achieving certain scientific understanding of the material world. Infallibility, once ascribed only to Holy Scripture or the supreme pontiff, was now transferred to human reason itself. In effect, Descartes unintentionally began a theological Copernican revolution, for his mode of reasoning suggested that God's existence was established by human reason and not vice versa. Although the self-evident certainty of God's existence was guaranteed by God's benevolent veracity in creating a reliable human reason, that conclusion could be affirmed only on the basis of the clear and distinct criterion, in which authority was fundamentally rooted in a judgment by the individual human intellect. In the ultimate religious question, not divine revelation but the natural light of human reason had the final say. Until Descartes, revealed truth had maintained an objective authority outside of human judgment, but now its validity began to be subject to affirmation by human reason. The metaphysical independence that Luther had demanded within the parameters of the Christian religion, Descartes now intimated more universally. For whereas Luther's foundational certainty was his faith in God's saving grace as revealed in the Bible, Descartes' foundational certainty was his faith in the procedural clarities of mathematical reasoning applied to the indubitability of the thinking self.

Moreover, by his assertion of the essential dichotomy between thinking substance and extended substance, Descartes helped emancipate the material world from its long association with religious belief, freeing science to develop its analysis of that world in terms uncontaminated by spiritual or human qualities and unconstrained by theological dogma. Both the human mind and the natural world now stood autonomously as never before, separated from God and from each other.

Here, then, was the prototypical declaration of the modern self, established as a fully separate, self-defining entity, for whom its own rational self-awareness was absolutely primary—doubting everything except itself, setting itself in opposition not only to traditional authorities but to the world, as subject against object, as a thinking, observing, measuring, manipulating being, fully distinct from

> an objective God and an external nature. The fruit of the dualism between rational subject and material world was science, including science's capacity for rendering certain knowledge of that world and for making man "master possessor of nature." In Descartes' vision, science, progress, reason, epistemological certainty, and human identity were all inextricably connected with each other and with the conception of an objective, mechanistic universe; and upon this synthesis was founded the paradigmatic character of the modern world. (pp. 279–280)

Humankind was now free not only from the dictates of tradition, church, and king, but also from the foundational authority of the Bible. Reason *alone* was foundational for understanding.

John Locke. Locke was the reigning epistemological authority in Europe during the seventeenth century. He provided the epistemological foundations for its scientific achievements. For Locke, ideas are not innate, as with Descartes, but rather our mind is a *tabula rasa,* a blank slate to be written upon by our sense experience of the world. We know because our experience of the world is imprinted upon our own mind by the senses and reflection. We cannot know apart from our experience. The authority of *experience alone* over against intuition, reason, and the Bible is the foundation of our knowledge both of the external and internal worlds.

Deism. The new epistemology brought a new view of God and humankind. God was now the divine architect who set the universe in motion, but he was not the Man of Calvary who is active in history and who will return in a literal manner a second time. The universe was to be explained on mechanical and mathematical principles. These principles were to be sought through observation and analysis, not by scholastic ideas or divine revelation. Providence and God's love were now reinterpreted to mean God's action in the creation and design of the ordered universe, but not His action with particular individuals or specific historical events. God did not reveal Himself to a particular people at a particular time; His revelation of Himself is universal through nature.

Humanity was now autonomous—free to determine its own foundational worldview apart from the Bible. Morality, knowledge, and the existence and nature of God were all to be determined independently from God's self-revelation in scripture.

EFFECTS OF THE ERA OF ENLIGHTENMENT

1. The nature and source of knowledge of humankind and the natural world was not to be determined by special revelation. It is to be discovered by some aspect of humanity, primarily by science.
2. Doubt was crucial to the process of acquisition of knowledge. Everything was to be questioned until one arrived at an absolute starting point.
3. "Faith," if it had any meaning at all, was founded upon and harmonious with the results of the scientific process.
4. In general, there was a radical separation of theology and natural inquiry. If there was a relationship between science and theology, the foundation was scientific. Special revelation could not be used as a starting point for the study of the natural world.
5. Science was king. Historian of science Bernard Cohen put it in almost religious terms: "The greatest achievement of Newtonian science must ever be the first full explanation of the universe on mechanical principles. One set of axioms and laws of universal gravitation applied to matter everywhere on earth as it did in the heavens. Who, after studying the contribution to thought, could deny that *pure science* [emphasis added] exemplifies this creative accomplishment of the human spirit at its pinnacle? What an exalted view of science. What a transforming view Newton gave to all humans. In all different endeavors the optimistic view that humans could deduce the order of the natural world had a significant trickle down effect in other human endeavors." Science had become the way, the truth, and the life. It was the foundation of all thinking and the basis of all worldviews.

6. Freedom was absolute. Humanity was no longer under the bondage of Greek metaphysics, scholastic theology, the church, tradition, or the authority of the Bible. As Tarnas (1991) puts it,

> While the classical Greek world view had emphasized the goal of human intellectual and spiritual activity as the essential unification (or reunification) of man with the cosmos and its divine intelligence, and while the Christian goal was to reunite man and the world with God, the modern goal was to create the greatest possible freedom for man—from nature; from oppressive political, social, or economic structures; from restrictive metaphysical or religious beliefs; from the Church; from the Judeo-Christian God; from the static and finite Aristotelian-Christian cosmos; from medieval scholasticism; from the ancient Greek authorities; from all primitive conceptions of the world. Leaving behind tradition generally for the power of the autonomous human intellect, modern man set out on his own, determined to discover the working principles of his new universe, to explore and further expand its new dimensions, and to realize his secular fulfillment. (p. 290)

Humanity had come of age. There was no need for God to look over our shoulder telling us how to live or what to believe about our nature and origins. The tutelage of God our Father was not necessary to understand ourselves or the universe. That can be done on our own, for we are autonomous from God and His Word. Whoever or whatever God is, if He exists at all—we will decide that—He must conform to whatever we discover to be true in the natural world.

POSSIBLE RELATIONS BETWEEN SCIENCE AND SCRIPTURE

This very brief history of the theory of knowledge as it relates to our concept of God and humanity has pointed to several possible relations between human studies and the Bible.

1. Human studies—science, philosophy, history, psychology, etc.—are *alone* the absolute foundation for all knowledge, whether it comes from nature or from the Bible. In this view, whatever is truth in the Bible (if anything at all) must be verified by, and interpreted within, the context of humanism. Nature can be understood completely on its own terms. There is no valid truth in the Bible apart from human verification. Human study alone provides the way, the truth, and the life.
2. Truth is truth wherever it may be found. Nature *and* the Bible both bring a valid approach to knowledge. It is the task of the theologian to integrate the truths of these two sources of knowledge. Both of these disciplines may be understood completely separate from each other; but since there is truth in both, there is value in synthesizing these truths. Human *and* religious sources provide the way, the truth, and the life.
3. The realms of nature and of the Bible are radically separate. Science deals with nature alone, and the Bible deals with religion alone. The two do not intersect. Both may be understood completely on their own. Since there is no connection between them, it is useless to try to synthesize them. The Bible has nothing to do with the realm of science.
4. God has revealed Himself both in nature and in the Bible. Nature by itself is misleading. Both may be legitimately studied from the standpoint of the Bible and the Bible *alone.* Christ *alone* as He is represented in His Word is the way, the truth, and the life.

THE BIBLE AND EPISTEMOLOGY

The contrast between living by humanistic methodologies and living by the Word of God is illustrated many times in the Bible. For example, Eve, the antediluvians, and the ten spies at Kadesh-Barnea each brought the Word of God into question based upon their own humanistic empirical and philosophical methodologies (Zinke, 2004).

By contrast, Noah[2] (White, 1895), Abraham[3] (White, 1890), and Christ[4] (Zinke, 2004) made their decisions to live by the Word of God *alone*.

BIBLICAL EPISTEMOLOGY

The biblical understanding of truth is quite different from that of scholasticism and the era of the Enlightenment. Understanding of reality is not imposed by the objective external world of the ideal form or the transcendent idea. Nor does it come from analysis of the human subject or empirical methods. The gospel of John uses the language of Greek philosophy to describe a completely different

---

2. Heb. 7:11; "The wise men of this world talked of science and the fixed laws of nature, and declared that there could be no variation in these laws, and that this message of Noah could not possibly be true. The talented men of Noah's time set themselves in league against God's will and purpose, and scorned the message and the messenger that He had sent. When they could not move Noah from his firm and implicit trust in the word of God, they pointed to him as a fanatic, as a ranting old man, full of superstition and madness. Thus they condemned him because he would not be turned from his purpose by reasonings and theories of men. It was true that Noah could not controvert their philosophies, or refute the claims of science so called; but he could proclaim the word of God; for he knew it contained the infinite wisdom of the Creator, and, as he sounded it everywhere, it lost none of its force and reality because men of the world treated him with ridicule and contempt" (White, 1895, pp. 243–244).

3. "'By faith Abraham obeyed when he was called to go out into a place which he should after receive for an inheritance, obeyed; and he went out, not knowing whither he went.' Hebrews 11:3. Abraham's unquestioning obedience is one of the most striking evidences of faith to be found in all the Bible. To him, faith was 'the substance of things hoped for, the evidence of things not seen.' Verse 1. Relying upon the divine promise, without the least outward assurance of its fulfillment, he abandoned home and kindred and native land, and went forth, he knew not whither, to follow where God should lead....He could not even explain his course of action so as to be understood by his friends. Spiritual things are spiritually discerned, and his motives and actions were not comprehended by his idolatrous kindred" (White, 1890, p. 126).

4. Matt. 4:4, 7, 14.

worldview of the source and nature of truth. The Logos is not an abstract metaphysical concept. It is a person—Jesus Christ who is Himself God (John 14:1–18).

When Pilot asked, "What is truth" (John 18:38), he did not realize that he was standing in the presence of the One who is the way, the truth, and the life (John 14:6).

God wants us to know Him, the only true God (John 17:3). This knowledge is available in Jesus Christ and His Word, the Bible. Paul warns that knowledge of God does not come through human means of achieving knowledge. In its wisdom the world does not know God (1 Cor. 1:21). We will be cheated if we attempt to know God through philosophy, the traditions of human beings, or the basic principles of the world (Col. 2:8–10). It is only in Christ that all the treasures of wisdom and knowledge are hidden (Col. 2:3; cf. 1 Cor. 1:30; John 1:17; 1 John 5:20).

Truth is not merely an intellectual concept. We know the doctrine when we choose to do God's will (John 7:17), and we know the truth when we walk in it (Ps. 26:3). Since we can be blinded by the gods of this age (2 Cor. 4:4), we must cast down arguments and every high thing that exalts itself against the knowledge of God (2 Cor. 10:5). Empiricism is not the foundation for knowledge, for if we are not willing to listen to Moses and the prophets, neither will we be persuaded though one come back from the dead (Luke 16:31). The Jews seek empirical knowledge, and the Greeks philosophical knowledge, but God will destroy the wisdom of the wise and the understanding of the prudent, for knowledge of God does not come through human wisdom, but through Christ, who is the power and the wisdom of God. The cross of Christ is foolishness and a stumbling block to those who seek empirical and philosophical foundations apart from Christ (1 Cor. 1:18–25).

ELLEN WHITE AND EPISTEMOLOGY

A major theme of Ellen White's writings was the authority of the Bible. She addressed this topic in many different contexts. For her, the Bible was the foundational framework and authority for every aspect of our lives.

Ellen White specifically affirms the authority of the Bible in a number of areas. All human teaching is to be subordinate to the oracle of God. The Bible and the Bible alone is our rule of faith. The authority of the Bible encompasses the whole of knowledge and life. The Bible provides the criteria of religion, the test of inspiration, the basis of faith, the test of the manifestation of the Holy Spirit, the basis of morality, the rule of conscience, the standard of character, the foundation of the home, the basis of true happiness, and even the cornerstone of the nation's prosperity (Zinke, 2004).

The Bible is the basis of truth, of all study, of all education, and of knowledge of God. It is the foundation for our understanding of Christ, the natural world, and history. It is the key to true philosophy and the basis of true principles of psychology (Zinke, 2004).

In a summary paragraph in *The Great Controversy*, Ellen White envisions a church in which God's people will build upon the reformation principle of *the Bible alone*:

> God will have a people upon the earth to maintain the Bible, and the Bible only, as the standard of all doctrines and the basis of all reforms. The opinions of learned men, the deductions of science, the creeds or decisions of ecclesiastical councils, as numerous and discordant as are the churches which they represent, the voice of the majority—not one nor all of these should be regarded as evidence for or against any point of religious faith. Before accepting any doctrine or precept, we should demand a plain "Thus saith the Lord" in its support. (White, 1911, p. 595)

In summary, as contrasted with scholasticism and the era of the Enlightenment, Ellen White sees the Bible as providing the authoritative foundation and worldview for the totality of our lives including our understanding of God, humanity, and the natural world.

FAITH AND FREEDOM

The principle of *sola scriptura* has implications for the nature of faith and freedom. The biblical concept is distinct from the humanistic concepts of the Enlightenment and beyond.

Faith. The humanistic concept of faith may be outlined as follows: The process generally starts with doubt, by attempting to prove the validity of an assertion in order to offer it as truth as worthy of one's faith. It relies upon genius, creativity, initiative, freedom of exploration, and capabilities of humankind. It relies upon the five senses as a basis for collecting the relevant data. It looks for patterns and integrates the data and interprets it on the basis of a paradigm which interprets our common experience and understanding of the world. A hypothesis is formed which leads to testable predictions which result in a new round of observations. The result is a probability statement as to what things are like or as to how new pieces of data entering the system will relate to the old.

In summary, the data is brought together in such a way as to yield a conclusion—a faith statement as to how things probably are. The conclusion is in the hand of humankind. It is under human control. It is a human achievement, and it is created upon an autonomous human foundation such as reason or some other faculty of humankind.

The biblical concept of faith is just the reverse: Faith is not a human creation; it is the gift of God (Eph. 2:8) in order that faith might not rest on the wisdom of human beings but in the power of God (1 Cor. 2:4–5). For Christ Himself is the author and finisher of our faith (Heb. 12:2).

> No man can create faith. The Spirit operating upon and enlightening the human mind creates faith in God. In the Scriptures faith is stated to be the gift of God, powerful unto salvation, enlightening the hearts of those who search for truth as for hidden treasure. (White, 1957, p. 940)

Faith is not built upon an external foundation, but is itself the assurance, the conviction, the substance, the evidence of things not seen (Heb. 11:1). Faith itself is the foundation of knowledge. "By faith we understand that the worlds were framed by the word of God" (Heb. 11:3, NKJV). "Only in the light of revelation can it [nature] be read aright" (White, 1952, p. 134). "Faith is the key of knowledge" (White, 1898, p. 139; White, 1952, p. 24). It is the basis for discerning between truth and error (White, 1958, Book 1; White, 1962).

Faith comes by hearing the Word of God (Rom. 10:17). It relies upon the power of the Word of God rather than upon the empirical methods of the Jews or the philosophical methods of the Greeks (1 Cor. 1:18–2:14). The assurance and evidence for faith is God's Word (White, 1958, Book 2).

To attempt to use humanistically founded methods as criteria for determining whether Scripture is the Word of God is to doubt that which has already been declared by God. It is similar to Christ's temptation in the wilderness, namely, to doubt that He was the Son of God after "it had already been affirmed by the Word of God. Genuine faith has its foundation in the promises and provisions of the Scriptures" (White, 1898, p.72; cf., White, 1962, p. 260; White, 1945, p. 72).

Freedom. The humanistic concept of freedom is also radically different from the biblical concept. The humanistic concept of epistemological freedom is that of autonomy. Not only are we free from every human institution, but we are also free from the authority of the Bible, the Word of God. The possibility of truth in the Bible must be determined on a humanistic basis rather than by its divine inspiration.

The Enlightenment taught that we are absolutely free. We start from a position of complete neutrality and objectivity to decide for or against God. But Christ said, "If you are not for me you are against me" (Matt. 12:30; Luke 11:23, CEV). We are either servants of Satan and sin, or of Christ; there is no neutral ground (John 8:34; Rom 6:15–23). Humanistic methodology states that we are absolutely free to discover the truth. Christ turns this idea one hundred and eighty degrees: "Ye shall know the truth, and the truth shall set you free" (John 8:32, KJV; see also Rom. 6:22, 8:3; Gal. 5:1).

MISSION FOR THE SEVENTH-DAY ADVENTIST CHURCH

The mission of our church stands upon a unique and specific epistemology. The call to give the totality of God's message to the world at the end of time is not a call for an epistemological synthesis of what is available in the cafeteria line—a little empiricism here, a little rationalism there, combined with bits and pieces of postmodernism. It is a specific call for a people who are willing to take, as the foundation of their message, the Bible and the Bible *only,* as opposed to all other epistemological systems.

The doctrines of *sola scriptura,* and *sola gratia—sola fidea,* are parallel doctrines. They were understood in tandem with each other at the time of the Reformation. If one is lost, the other will eventually be lost as well. For example, if one must go through a humanistic foundation to determine that salvation is by grace, salvation is no longer by grace, but by the system that founded that knowledge.

SOLA GRATIA	SOLA SCRIPTURA
There is nothing I can do on my own to obtain righteousness.	There is nothing I can do on my own to obtain special revelation.
Righteousness is not to be manipulated by humans.	Revelation is not to be manipulated by humans.
Righteousness rests completely upon the Gift of God.	Revelation rests completely upon the Gift of God.
Works follow naturally from the receipt of the gift of God's salvation.	Epistemological works follow naturally from the receipt of God's foundation.
Works never form the basis of our salvation.	Humanistic epistemologies are not the true foundation of our knowledge.

The two doctrines are analogous and they are really one: God's gift of Himself to us in order that we might know Him, the only true God (John 17:3).

The precious understanding of righteousness by faith alone will stand only so long as we place beside it the twin doctrine of the foundational authority of the Bible alone. Just as in 1888 the church made a new commitment to the doctrine of righteousness by faith, today we must reaffirm our commitment to the authority of the Bible.

God has given us reason, senses, emotions, aesthetic appreciation, material goods, talents, and much more for our use and enjoyment to His glory. *Sola scriptura* does not take away from the important role that each of these plays in our lives. But it does mean that God has provided a foundation and structure within which each of these gifts may be properly used. When we use them apart from the foundation of God's Word, we act autonomously from Him.

The foundational authority of the Bible may be illustrated by my house. It has a foundation upon which it is built and a set of plans that guided its construction. It also has a front door, windows, a kitchen, bedrooms, a study, and a roof. All of these features and many others are important to my house, but they will never become the foundation. If my house were to be turned upside down so that it rested upon its roof, my house would collapse. So also, God has given us reason, our five senses, emotions, talents, friendship, and many other things. He wants us to enjoy them and use them to their fullest to His glory (1 Cor. 1:31). But if we make one or all of them the foundation of our life, our world will collapse.

It is tempting to found our understanding of the world upon a synthesis of two epistemologies, as did the scholastics. Some prefer to build their house on the rock *and* the sand rather than on the Rock *alone*. But we cannot serve two masters (Matt. 6:24). Humanism and biblical authority do not mix. It is like asking the Redskins to play the White Sox. Whose field will be used? Whose ball will be in place? Who will umpire the game? Whose rules will be used? Imagine kicking a football to a baseball batter. There is no synthesis between the two games. Either we will invite the one to join the other or vice versa.

Paul warns us not to be "conformed to this world," but to be "transformed by the renewing" of our mind (Rom. 12:2, KJV). The

Greek verb translated "transformed" comes from the same verb used in Mark 9:2, when Jesus was "transfigured." It is through the truth that we are sanctified—not the "truth" that we generate ourselves, but the truth that comes from the Word of God (John 17:17–19). While we once walked according to the course of this world, according to the prince of the power of the air, we have been made alive together with Christ (Eph 2:1–9). We tend to emphasize conversion of the heart. But conversion also involves transformation of the mind. It is a change of direction in one's thinking: a direction that is no longer energized by the humanism of the world, but is directed by God's Word. God invites us to be converted in our mind, to make a change in direction, so that we see things from the perspective of His Word rather than from the perspective of this world.

The epistemological path that we take will determine our concept of God, ourselves, nature, and history. As a church we have a mission to look at the world from God's perspective rather than at God from the perspective of the world. We have the challenge to teach our children how to think biblically rather than humanistically. We can only do that when we have been converted in heart and mind.

The acceptance of the biblical worldview as foundational to human understanding has many implications for the study of human nature and mental health. We will suggest a sampling of areas that may be fruitful for further consideration: The gift of God's self revelation in His Word; submission to the Word of God for understanding rather than reliance upon human autonomy; the unity of mind and body; creation in the image of God, the fall from and partial distortion of that image caused by sin; the conditional immortality of the individual; salvation founded solely on God's saving grace rather than human ingenuity or effort; God's sustaining grace; God's eternity, knowledge, and power combined with His personal interest in each individual; individual direct access and responsibility to God; the converting power of the Word of God, the role of the Holy Spirit in comfort, fellowship, understanding, conviction, conversion, and sanctification; the role of the Sabbath; the effects of giving to God and fellow humans of our time, talents, and resources; the nature, origin, and end of evil and its association with choice and with a being called Satan; the end of sin and sinners; and the promise of eternal life with God and fellow humans.

Some of these topics are given consideration in these symposia. Understanding ourselves from the standpoint of God's revelation of Himself, ourselves, and the universe in which we live will contribute to the restoration of the image of God in humankind and to the fullness of life that God originally intended for us.

REFERENCES

Tarnas, R. (1991). *The passion of the Western mind.* New York: Harmony.

White, E. G. (1890). *Patriarchs and prophets.* Oakland, CA: Pacific Press.

White, E. G. (1895, April 18). An example of saving faith. *Signs of the Times,* 243–244.

White, E. G. (1898). *The Desire of Ages.* Oakland, CA: Pacific Press.

White, E. G. (1911). *The great controversy.* Mountain View, CA: Pacific Press. (Original work published 1888)

White, E. G. (1945). *Early writings of Ellen G. White.* Washington, D.C.: Review and Herald.

White, E. G. (1952). *Education.* Mountain View, CA: Pacific Press. (Original work published 1903)

White, E. G. (1957). Ellen G. White Comments. In F. D. Nichol, R. F. Cottrell, D. F. Neufeld, J. Neuffer (Eds.), *Seventh-day Adventist Bible commentary: Vol. 7.* (pp. 903–990). Washington, D.C.: Review and Herald. (Original work published 1899)

White, E. G. (1958). *Selected messages, Books 1 & 2.* Washington, D.C.: Review and Herald.

White, E. G. (1962). *Testimonies to ministers and Gospel workers.* Mountain View, CA: Pacific Press. (Original work published 1923)

Zinke, E. E. (2004). Faith-science issues: An epistemological perspective. *Journal of the Adventist Theological Society, 15,* 71–90.

Christian Epistemological Foundations for the Behavioral Sciences

Miroslav M. Kiš

Epistemology as a philosophical science of knowledge investigates the origins, sources, structure, methods, possibilities, scope, and general basis of knowledge. The relation between psychology and epistemology is particularly intimate because the two sciences share an interest in the cognitive processes of perception, memory, imagination, conception, and reasoning. Yet their approaches and tasks are different. While psychology seeks to describe and explain particular acts or perceptions in the context of other conscious events, epistemology is interested in the cognitive process which conceptualizes perceptions, structures, methods, possibilities, scope, and foundations. In other words, epistemology critically analyzes and evaluates the validity of processes and warrants for claims as well as the conclusions of what is perceived as true in psychology (Runes, 1980, p. 94).

EPISTEMOLOGY IN MODERN PSYCHOLOGY

EPISTEMOLOGICAL FOUNDATIONS OF MODERN PSYCHOLOGY

As a historical survey of the philosophy of the mind reveals (Honderich, 1995; Johnson & Jones, 2000), there are several components requisite for the work of epistemological validation of the claims of knowledge. The task requires an understanding of the nature of the *subject* of inquiry, reliable *sources* of information, a proper *method*, awareness of the *worldviews* of both the subject and the researcher involved, principles of interpretation (*hermeneutics*), and a goal (*telos*) of the whole enterprise.

THE SUBJECT

The subject of study is of primary importance since, as we shall see, it has significant impact on all other elements of structure outlined above. If the human mind and its functions, structure, and behavioral effects are the proper focus of inquiry for psychology (Runes, 1980, p. 258), then it is of crucial importance to define the nature of the human mind. If, however, our focus is on the human being as a person whose mind we seek to understand, then a more comprehensive outlook is required. Yet, a consensus on the nature of the human mind is hard to find. Plato, for example, understood it as a repository of innate, *a priori* knowledge. Descartes saw it as a non-material substance standing in dualistic relation to the material body (Honderich, 1995, p. 570). So, while Plato considered human nature in terms of a body-soul dualism, the contemporary behavioral sciences owe their isolation of the mind as their subject of study to Descartes' shift to body-mind dualism. Descartes' contributions led to further developments in the twentieth century issuing in Reductive Materialism (Brown, Murphy, & Malony, 1998, pp. 87–88), which conceives of the mind simply as a material, neural center where physical states produce mental events.

SOURCES OF KNOWLEDGE

Mainstream psychology finds its data in the realm of the observable aspects of the function of the human mind. Analysis of relevant information from personal histories, plus observation of a person's immediate context and relationships, may yield specific patterns which lead to the formation of a cumulative, composite picture. This information forms the basis for describing in scientific terms the state of a person's mental health.

PROPER METHOD

The rise of the natural sciences since the Enlightenment shared in the developments of the philosophy of the mind at the beginning of the twentieth century, resulting in a new understanding of the subject and sources of knowledge. The materialistic view of the human mind coupled with the rise of an empirical method of study ruled out any data coming from faith or revelation as highly unreliable. Thus psychology as an empirical, natural science uses procedures on which all rational persons can agree and which deliver the same knowledge outcomes, regardless of the researcher's assumptions. Moreover, psychology forbids straying from a strict description of humans exclusively in terms of natural processes (Johnson, 2004) under the threat of finding their efforts relegated to the level of "folk psychology"(Honderich, 1995). Standard research uses mostly an inductive approach, empirical observation, quantitative measurements, and statistical analysis.

WORLDVIEW

But from whence come all of these changes and pressures towards a neo-positivist and secular outlook? To find the answer to this question we must go back some four centuries to a time when an increasing number of individuals from among leading intelligentsia in Italy and all over Europe spearheaded a new way of understanding reality. Without formal organization, the Renaissance and later the Enlightenment initiated slow but resolute steps aimed at emancipation of the arts and sciences from under the firm grip of the institutional church's control. On a dubious traditional basis, the church for centuries proscribed the painting or sculpting of all non-biblical subjects and prohibited all scientific theories or activities that could not be squared with the official position of the church. Subsequently, additional restrictions emerged as a consequence of a close connection between the powers of church and state. Hence the experiences of Galileo and Copernicus, as well as the difficulties of artists like Michelangelo and da Vinci, who wished to study the human body through dissection but could do so only under the threat of exile or death.

This situation, more than any other developments, yielded a secular worldview in the arts and sciences by the beginning of the twentieth century. Several aftereffects followed: (1) Since the Bible became relegated to the level of any other book, as in the writings of Albrecht Ritchel, such traditional loci of authority as revelation and dogma were rejected as roadblocks to true knowledge. (2) The existence of the supernatural was rejected in favor of pervasive secularization. (3) Pursuit of personal happiness set aside any absolute and universally valid moral norms. (4) Exaggerated optimism about the capacities of human nature to improve and transform itself became the order of the day.

HERMENEUTICS

Epistemology calls for interpretation of data. But an interpretation of any kind betrays the worldview in which it occurs, and bears the marks of the understanding of the subject, the sources, and the method used. These serve as parameters that delineate and define what is considered acceptable and respectable research. Scholars today are compelled to conduct their research as detached and objective observers, to use methods of logical naturalism, to describe human beings in terms of natural processes, to use inductive and hypothetico-deductive methods and quantitative measurements, and to interpret and evaluate their data with statistical procedures (Johnson, 2004). Yet this approach is adequate only if the human mind possesses no other capacities worth learning about but the rational faculty, as Cartesian anthropology mandates. If, however, this view of the human subject is only a part of a larger whole, then such an evaluation will be partial, and insufficient indeed.

THE GOAL (*TELOS*)

The ultimate assignment of psychology is to describe and explain the human mind, its states, and its functions in a scientific way. Data are carefully identified, counted, measured, and classified, and the mechanisms of the mind are isolated, described, and labeled, disclosing the ways in which the mind functions. The findings are then communicated to the rest of the scientific community, where specialists formulate categories needed for diagnosis, and ultimately for therapy.

This is a brief sketch of the epistemological system used by mainstream scientific and secular psychology today. Psychology's contribution to the philosophy of the mind is enormous and enduring. Yet, Christians involved in any branch of behavioral sciences can profit from the fruits yielded by over two millennia of hard and creative work if, and to the extent that, these fruits are critically assessed, and as long as they relate in a balanced and holistic way to the understanding of the human being as an indivisible, multidimensional unity, as presented in Scripture.

CHRISTIAN EPISTEMOLOGICAL MATRIX

HISTORICAL APERCU

Predating the philosophy of the mind, and alongside of it, there exists another history of epistemology. We encounter its inception in the second chapter of Genesis where the first reported activity of the first man consisted of his becoming involved in learning. "So out of the ground the Lord God formed every beast of the field and every bird of the air, and brought them to the man to see what he would call them; and whatever the man called every living creature, that was its name" (Gen. 2:9, NKJV). It is important to note several crucial points here. (1) It is God who initiates this learning experience. Contrary to Promethean claims and the policies of the medieval Christian church, God is not ill disposed toward learning; on the contrary, there is safety and richness in scholarly research under His mentorship. To have "that joy of discovery mixed together with the joy of worship is truly a powerful moment for a Christian who is also a scientist" (Alexander & White, 2006, p. 66). (2) Giving names in the biblical sense involves much more than placing a label for the purposes of identification. A name actually describes the very character of the subject under study. This implies that God wanted Adam to know the very nature and character of animals and birds before he could become qualified to rule over them (*Seventh-day Adventist Bible Commentary*, 2005, p. 226).

In chapter 3 of Genesis we encounter the issue of knowledge for the second time. Here, though, God has no input in carrying out the research, not even at an assistantship level. The Serpent knew the power of knowledge and its temptation to autonomy, and for that reason he used it as bait with which to separate humanity from itself and from God. Outside of God's protective presence, the very power which can help people grow and learn became the cause for evil, yielding confused knowledge and ignorance (2 Tim. 4:3–4). "So when the woman saw that the tree was good for food, and that it was a delight to the eyes, and that the tree was to be desired to make one wise, she took of its fruit..." (Gen. 3:6, NKJV). For the first time the human mind knew shame, a need for a coping mechanism (fig leaves, v. 7), fear and guilt (v. 10), detachment from others, a need to lay blame (vv. 12–13), and, most significantly, homelessness and separation from God (vv. 22–24). These are the very same cases of troublesome human histories and states of mind that behavioral scientists encounter today.

However, the mind alone, functioning simultaneously as the subject of study, the instrument of research, and the tool of interpretation in academic psychology, proves to be too narrow a basis for understanding the richness of the human psyche. Paul at the Areopagus in Athens urged the intelligentsia of Greece to consider the fact that human life does not exist in itself, by itself, or for itself. "[F]or 'in him [God] we live and move and have our being'; as even some of your poets have said, 'For we are indeed his offspring'" (Acts 17:28, NKJV). In Hebrews 11:3, Paul includes faith as a necessary tool in search for knowledge. On that basis a significant number of philosophers of the mind, behavioral scientists, and theologians call for a holistic approach to the study of the human being. Mental health in the context of physical and spiritual health is the strongest epistemological foundation, and it is the one rooted in Scripture.

In the middle of the twentieth century, an influential movement arose in Europe fostering a Christian holistic approach to mental health. It sprung out of the growing conviction among physicians that psychosomatic unity is an undeniable truth, and for that reason psychological states must be taken seriously when attending a physically ill patient. Such titles as "Psychophysische Korrelationen" by F. Georgi, R. Fischer, R. Weber, & P. Weis (1948); *Medecine Sans Frontieres* by Georges

Menkes (1945); *The Healing of Persons* by Paul Tournier (1965); and *La Personne du Médecin, un Agent Psychothérapeutique* by A. Maeder (1953) are but a sample of writings from that period. During that time, annual conferences were organized to exchange ideas that actively promoted healing of the total human being.

As the collective work of this movement continued, the inclusion of the spiritual dimension of the human being gained legitimacy as well. It is the spiritual that makes a person, writes A. Stocker (1949). Paul Tournier insists:

> I often ponder over the nature of true human sincerity, true transparency....It is a rare and difficult thing; and how much it depends on the person who is listening to us! There are those who pull down the barriers and make the way smooth; there are those who force the doors and enter our territory like invaders; there are those who barricade us in, shut us in upon ourselves, dig ditches and throw up walls around us; there are those who set us out of tune and listen only to our false notes; there are those to whom we will always remain strangers, speaking an unknown tongue. And when it is our turn to listen, which of these are we for the other person's sincerity? That should make us think of God, who is not only One who says: "Listen to me!" but also One who says: "I am listening to You." (1957, p. 165)

Toward the end of the twentieth century a similar change of orientation occurred on the North American scene. A very insightful history and bibliography can be found in Johnson and Jones (2000, pp. 11–53).

EPISTEMOLOGICAL FOUNDATIONS OF CHRISTIAN PSYCHOLOGY

What would a Christian epistemological foundation look like? More specifically we ask, "What is the basis for a Seventh-day Adventist (SDA) Christian theory of knowledge"? Certainly there may be similarities with other approaches, but what would be the unique SDA contribution to knowledge in psychology?

Psychology is defined generally as a science of the human psyche. Christian psychologists tend to agree that psychology is a science that studies the functioning of the human soul. It is a knowledge emerging from close observation, which includes numerous theories of personality representing different understandings of the human soul, and it encompasses many psychotherapeutic models aimed at redressing ills defined by a particular theory (David Powlison, in Johnson & Jones, p. 198, and Robert C. Roberts in Johnson & Jones, p. 152).

THE SUBJECT

The human being as defined in the Bible is the subject of study for Christian psychology. Genesis 1:26–28 and 2:7 contain several important elements which signal the uniqueness and dignity of human nature scarcely found in other philosophies of religions.

First. The planning phase preceding the creation of Adam, which concludes with the words, "Let us make man" (v. 26, KJV). The Bible views humans as worthy of careful planning, especially in the context of childbearing. God, too, is engaged in planning and preparation.

Second. The Trinity then makes another decision. This new creature will be "in our image, after our likeness" (v. 27, KJV). There is no hint here of the idea that humanness resulted from random mutation or from some amorphous accident of cells hanging loosely together. A likeness to God is what we all, female or male, share in common.

Third. "And God blessed them, 'Be fruitful and multiply'" (v. 28, KJV). He blessed humans with pro-creative powers, that is, with a responsibility to create "for" ("pro") Him. Conception, while explainable in physical/physiological terms, cannot be evaluated in those terms alone.

Fourth. Then God introduces the pair to the ample provisions He has made for them (vv. 29–30). Malnourishment, hunger, and poverty, as well as abuse, loneliness, neglect, and trafficking, which de-humanize millions today, are an affront to the God who will call humanity to account (James 5:1–6).

Fifth. Genesis 2:7 magnifies for us the creation of the first human beings, Adam and Eve. It signals a change in the method of creation. While animals appeared in response to a detached command, God's direct involvement in creating Adam and Eve is very far from detachment. God *touches* the clay in forming Adam, and touches Adam to extract a rib and subsequently construct Eve. Second, God *breathes* the breath of life. Third, God *converses* using a language that is audible and understandable to humans.

Sixth. "And man [*adam*] became a living soul" (Gen. 2:7, KJV). Body plus breath become more than the sum of the two; they become one: he, Adam. We know the *origin* of the body and we know the *origin* of the breath of life, but when the two unite we know the *beginning* of the soul. The appearance of the soul labels the body as Adam's body; it identifies the breath as Adam's breath, until death. But more than that, the soul also expresses an individualized being: it affirms and articulates the "once-for-all-ness" of every person. Every cubic millimeter of the human body, together with every breath, are his/her soul. And because they are so masterfully united, the capacities that become possible transcend the capacity of each component.

The concept of the soul as an integrated whole, as the core unity of a human being, is very important to SDAs. From it proceeds our stand on stewardship of the totality of human life. Integral to the Christian lifestyle are healthful nutrition, exercise, and family relationships, together with the traditional spiritual disciplines like communion with God, prayer, Bible study, and worship. A healthy holistic lifestyle enhances a more vigorous physical, mental, and spiritual experience.

Scripture also reveals the true human condition. It reminds us that the totality of a human being is affected by sin (Rom. 7:18), that all humans have sinned (1 Kings 8:46; Rom. 3:23), and that the chasm created by sin has separated humans from the Source of life (Isa. 59:1–2) and alienated them from themselves (Luke 15:17). Sin entices men and women to act in suicidal ways; hence, all of us are fallen and to a certain extent abnormal.

Here is where a Christian interpretation of symptoms and data will make a difference. It is not infrequent that mental conditions and even physical illnesses stem from complex causes and that some aspect of a religious or spiritual antecedent participates in the mix. A psychiatrist friend of mine shared with me the situation of a woman with a severe case of herpes who was referred to him by a physician. No medical treatment proved satisfactory. After a short period of exploring her memories and experiences in young adulthood, it became clear that she had been a victim of abuse by her recently deceased father. "He slipped away before I had enough courage to confront him!" she lamented. The psychiatrist suspected deep scars because of the way even her spiritual life was affected. He wondered if a pastoral perspective could be of help. At first separately and then together, he and her pastor explored such themes as forgiveness of past injustices, and grace for the future. She was encouraged to write a factual and straightforward letter to her father. Nothing should remain unexpressed. After she read it at their next session, she was asked to write her father's repenting and apologetic response to her. The more vivid understanding of grace and forgiveness, not just as a theory but now as the very gate to her complete health, brought healing. She became conscious of God before whom her father stood guilty, God who needed no help from police or witnesses or earthly judges, God who knows how to make human wreckage whole again, and God who holds in His hand the responsibility to right all wrongs and to make a new person from the ashes of the past. It was this cooperation between medical, psychiatric, and pastoral approaches that resulted in her complete restoration. The indivisible human nature requires unsegregated expertise.

SOURCES OF KNOWLEDGE

Ever since Descartes "improved" on Plato's body-soul dualism with body-mind dualism, the concept of the mind has slowly become a thing detachable from the rest of the human being. That view of the nature of the subject of study has produced a very valuable corpus of information to date, but in the process some important dimensions of the human mind and an indivisible human nature have eluded researchers' observation. Tournier explains in *Meaning of Persons*: "In this depersonalized state of mind man himself becomes a thing. Anatomy and physiology study his body as a thing, and psychology his mind as a thing, a mechanism. Economics studies him as a thing, an instrument of production and consumption, while sociology studies him as an element of society. He is a pawn on the chess board of politics, a cog in industry, a learning-machine, everywhere a fraction of the mass" (1957, p. 180). But humans are more complex than this, and much more intricate. Tournier again:

> The person always eludes our grasp; it is never static. It refuses to be confined within concepts, formulae and definitions. It is not a thing to be encompassed, but a point of attraction, a guiding force, a direction, and attitude, which demands from us a corresponding attitude, which moves us to action and commits us. The world of things does not commit us. It is neutral, and leaves us neutral. We are cold, objective, impersonal observers, watching the operation of blind and inexorable mechanisms. (pp. 179–180)

Empirical data, which have been painstakingly tested, acquired, and recorded, are but a part of the picture. A Christian psychologist focuses on the mind as it affects and is affected by other dimensions of the human subject. Thus a Christian understanding of the human being involves richer and more complete insight in the light of biblical and Christian sources.

The Bible. The revelation of God the Father, Son, and Holy Spirit discloses a presence of the supernatural in human life. God the Father with all His transcendent attributes is "Our Father" in heaven (Luke 11:1–4). He who is holy and majestic, who does not trifle with our self-abusive attitudes and actions (Exod. 34:7), and who cannot overlook injustices made to others (James 5:1–6) does not relate to us only in a diagnostic way by contrasting our puny wretchedness with His excellencies. He is at the same time our Savior; that is, He not only relates to our sin with uncompromising thoroughness but He relates to us as persons in therapeutic (redemptive) ways. "God was in Christ reconciling the world to Himself" (2 Cor. 5:19, NKJV).

The revelation of Jesus Christ as a true human being (John 19:5) provides the Christian psychologist and counselor with a vision of a healthy person.

- ◊ Jesus models true humanity when He allows the full expression of His emotions, such as sadness (John 11:35), anxiety (John 12:27), joy (John 17:13), and compassion (Matt. 9:36). Real people need not be ashamed and expected to repress their feelings.
- ◊ Jesus models the formation and maintenance of a good support system, so essential for mental and emotional health (Luke 10:38–41), but He also shows how clinging to our Father in heaven helps us to survive when such a system fails (Matt. 26:36–46).
- ◊ His mind actively engages the minds of doubters (John 20:24–28), scholars (John 3:1–15), and tax collectors (Luke 19:1–10), but He never ridicules ignorance.

Revelation of the Holy Spirit communicates to us the importance God places on our mind, mental states, thoughts, feelings, attitudes, and moods. It is the Holy Spirit who has access to our spirit (Rom. 8:16), who is our Counselor and Guide (John 14:16–17), who assists us in our weakness and intercedes for us (Rom. 8:26–27), who convinces us (John 14:8–11), and who brings about in us a fundamental change when no fixing or repairing would do. He brings about a new birth (John 3:5–8) and a new creature (2 Cor. 5:17). Any psychiatrist, psychologist, or counselor knows the feeling of the limits of human endeavors. Yet Christians know how to refer to and confer with the Divine Advocate from the outset of therapy.

Biblical cases of mental and emotional distress display both human ambivalence toward, and vacillation between, doubt and faith, distress and courage, foolishness and wisdom. We can easily identify with biblical men and women, learn from their mistakes, and be inspired by their virtues and victories (cf. Heb. 11).

Publications of Ellen G. White such as *Mind, Character, and Personality* (1977), *Steps to Christ* (1956), *Ministry of Healing* (1942), and *Medical Ministry* (1963) contain valuable information about ministering to human needs in a holistic way. A full understanding of her corpus would require a special project but would prove of enormous help for mining out biblical insights relevant to psychology. One quote must suffice for now:

> To know oneself is a great knowledge. The teacher who rightly estimates himself will let God mold and discipline his mind. And he will acknowledge the source of his power....Self-knowledge leads to humility and to trust in God, but it does not take the place of effort for self-improvement. He who realizes his own deficiencies will spare no pains to reach the highest possible standard of physical, mental, and moral excellence. (White, 1943, p. 419)

THE PROPER METHOD

Method is defined as a systematic procedure—a chosen path of dealing with facts, phenomena, and hypotheses (Wolman, 1973). Our task is to sketch a method suitable for Christian psychology. This is an intimidating and daunting task, but a worthy challenge to pursue.

Christian psychologists, who consider the human mind as an integrated dimension of the human being, feel uncomfortable and restricted with empiricism as the only or the dominant method of research. We must ask: is it tenable to affirm that human complexity, creativity, dynamism, and yearning for the transcendent are but a mirage? If they are legitimate dimensions, can we commit to observation alone the task of grasping and encompassing the totality? If it is true that a man cannot step into the same river twice (Heraclitus), is it not too far from truth to say that the same human cannot step into the same river even once?

Consider the words of Victor Frankl:

> I do not believe that the gas chambers of Auschwitz…have to be traced to some ministry of state in Nazi Berlin. I think that they are ultimately the outcome of what philosophers and scientists have been preaching in their lecture halls and cynically writing on their desks. Consider for instance, what one world famous Nobel prize winning Anglo Saxon author once wrote: "Man is defined as nothing but an accumulation of complicated, complex molecules of prothane, and this complex runs around some unimportant planet called Earth for about 70 years to dissolve itself afterwards." Then small wonder if you plead for euthanasia and so forth, and also for gas chambers. And something parallel holds for what I have tried to convey to you. If you do not recognize that man is self-transcendentingly reaching out for other human beings, reaching out meanings to fulfill, but see him just as a closed system dominated by the wish to maintain homeostasis and inner equilibrium, small wonder that your youngsters who have been indoctrinated that way think: "Now, I don't like tensions, I would like to restore my homeostasis, let us use dope." Small wonder, if you instill in them the notion that life is nothing but what we project into it out of our unconscious wishes, reaction formations, and defense mechanisms. And, finally, if you teach them that man is not really free, but is beyond freedom; if you teach your youngsters what I used to call "pandeterminism," there's no freedom at all, everything is totally determined, then it is small wonder if they end up in violence, because they regard themselves the victims of their childhood experiences—of their oedipal situations, of their castration, fears, and so forth. (as cited by Joy, 1983, pp. 43–44)

Given the multidimensional indivisibility of human nature, Christian psychology is called to profit from a "cluster of methods" working together as an organic whole. Information received from biblical exegesis, theology, philosophy, and psychology all will contribute to a deeper understanding of human beings and their needs, and will provide a Christian orientation for therapy. As psychologists listen and gather data to formulate clinical judgment, their Christian minds will urge them to go beyond mere description to identify causes and their effects. Biblical knowledge will remind them to explore deeper causes. They will recall that the pains and traumas of their clients are evils which are caused by sin, even if not necessarily the patients' own sin. Of course, at the onset, these theological and axiological explorations may not be apparent to the patients. They should be the inner workings of the mind of the Christian psychologists.

For the sake of clarity let us think of Mary. Initial psychotherapy points to a young lady sexually abused by her friends. Her marriage is in trouble because of her inability to be free in her relations with her husband. A mixture of guilt, resentment, and fear of being discovered separate her from her parents and her church as well. What now? The Christian therapist might remember the biblical story of a woman caught in adultery (John 8:2–11). True, any sexual intercourse outside of marriage is sin. But the woman described in John's Gospel (as well as our patient Mary) knows that very well. No one needs to rub it in. Her guilt, resentment, and fear are clearly visible on her face and in her body language. Besides, the empirical evidence of having been caught in the act removes all doubt about her guilt. But Jesus looks beyond this. Jesus does not treat symptoms, nor is He satisfied with some surface causes. He notices the accusation: "This woman has been caught *in the act* of adultery" (v. 4, ESV). How did they know where to find her? So, setting her aside for a moment, He writes on the ground a narrative of the accusers' own involvement (White, 1940, p. 461). Then, beginning with the eldest, the deeper causes of the woman's sin, her own accusers left the scene. She was left alone with Jesus.

So our patient Mary, too, can now for the first time find herself alone with Jesus. The therapist is but a facilitator. She can hear the words, "Neither do I condemn you, go and sin no more" (v. 11, KJV), as addressed to her. The past is gone forever. She has the future to make her dream come true. In Mary's case that could mean confronting her past and coming clean with her parents and church. At the deepest level, it will mean realizing her standing with her God and receiving His mercy and forgiveness, which will give her courage to face the future.

But what if Mary's abusers (or some of the Pharisees) come next week to Jesus seeking healing for themselves? Jesus, or the psychologist acting in His place, would again look deeper than those empirically discernable causes. He would lead them all to repentance, and a new life based on grace. But the way to that goal would be custom made; it would not be the same for all. In Scripture we find words of forgiveness: "You will be with me in paradise" (Luke 23:43, NIV), or "your guilt is taken away, and your sin is forgiven" (Isa. 6:7, NASB). There are also words of confrontation: "You are the man!" (2 Sam. 12:7, NIV), or "you must be born again" (John 3:3–16, NIV). Yet the results each time bring resounding positive results. The Bible-based method is not only holistic and comprehensive; it is also adaptable to individual needs, respecting the particular ways which would lead the person to victory and healing.

WORLDVIEW

The biblical view of the world in which human life exists is captured in the image of the great controversy between Christ and Satan, between good and evil. This world is not friendly to humans. The air is full of germs, pollutants, and noise; human relationships are fragile; the good and the normal are not as popular as the evil and the cruel. Cornelius J. Plantinga (1995) puts it well in the title of one of his books: *Life Is Not the Way It's Supposed to Be*. It will bring much hope to the parents of troubled children, and to the children of troubled parents, to be reminded that even the first man born on this planet, of parents who had the closest possible relationship with God and to whom God Himself made a visit for a counseling conversation—this man, Cain, did not turn out right. Why? Though we might never know the whole story behind human tragedies, Jesus gives at least a partial answer. He tells the story of a farmer who prepared his land, sowed good seed, and waited for an abundant crop. But as the plants came up, tares appeared among the wheat. When the workers queried, the master answered, "an enemy has done it" (Matt. 13:28, NKJV). The weeds grow without care, but a good and healthy mind and heart do not grow unattended.

But the Bible informs us that God is on our side, and that the victory of good over evil is assured. When Christian psychologists, psychiatrists, and counselors do their work, they are braving the onslaughts of the enemy. Yet they know that warfare on the level of the mind and psyche is not just physical/biological in nature, since human nature cannot be so neatly separated in self-contained units. God is very much concerned that the mind be set free from the dominance of evil. To the Romans Paul writes, "Do not be conformed to this world (or this age), but be transformed by the *renewal of your mind,* that you may prove what is the will of God, what is good, acceptable and perfect" (Rom. 12:2, NKJV, emphasis added). On a personal level, the great controversy is waged in our minds. "We destroy arguments and every proud obstacle to the knowledge of God, and take every thought captive to obey Christ" (2 Cor. 10:5, ESV).

Victims of addictions, abuse, broken relationships, and such must not be left to themselves after they have been freed from harmful behavior. In Matthew 12:43–45 (NKJV) Jesus warns that if an unclean spirit leaves a man, and later returns and finds the room "empty, swept and put in order," the spirit will return with seven other spirits, and the state of that man will become worse than before. Post-war recoveries are often much harder and longer than the wars themselves. There is no safety or lasting healing for our clients and patients unless they are left alone in Jesus' presence, like the woman caught in adultery. This type of referral is of paramount importance—all the more so since in this great controversy the basic issue is that of allegiance, and our clients, fragile as they may be, will have to return to the war zone. Isaiah's experience might be helpful here. As he experienced God's throne room in a vision he exclaimed, "'Woe is me! For I am lost; for I am a man of unclean lips, and I dwell in the midst of a people of unclean lips; for my eyes have seen the King, the LORD of hosts!' Then flew one of the seraphim to me, having in his hand a burning coal which he had taken with tongs from the altar. And he touched my mouth and said, 'Behold, this has touched your lips; your guilt is taken away, and your sin forgiven'" (Isa. 6:5–7, ESV). This is also where the church as a home for broken people and as a shelter and "recovery room" becomes indispensable. Every move, word, and action are aimed at healing and recovery in every church where Christ is the head.

This, then, is the Christian worldview within which we all live. Psychological illnesses are real. The focus on the states and functions of the mind is necessary. People need real help when faced with schizophrenia or depression, and psychologists have committed their lives to this work. But when we come to our clients with the understanding of deeper causes, aware that there is a spiritual environment which impacts human lives negatively, the whole approach will change. Counselors will, from the first encounter, assess clients holistically, examine what type of support system they have, and search into the strength of their belief systems and experience with God so that throughout the whole process no dimension of their beings is neglected or bypassed.

HERMENEUTICS

Hermeneutics is defined as the science of interpretation, or the science of searching for meaning, which is of crucial importance for epistemology. In this segment we examine several types of hermeneutics as they relate to Christian/SDA psychology. First, Christian psychology recognizes that human subjects are citizens of two different "cities"—the heavenly and the earthly (Augustine, trans. 1950). It also recognizes that a human being is a multidimensional indivisible unity, and that because several disciplines and methods must work together to provide more complete care, they all must learn how to hear and understand each other. Next, biblical/theological hermeneutics and behavioral sciences need to join together in an adventure not unlike that of marriage. Unless this marriage is carefully discussed and agreed upon, the two cannot become one because they will not agree on which "one" to become. Biblical/theological hermeneutics that are easily understandable by behavioral sciences will make holistic healing possible, and awareness of the issues with which behavioral sciences deal will result in a more user-friendly theology. Niebuhr says:

> The obvious fact is that man is a child of nature, subject to its vicissitudes, compelled by its necessities, driven by its impulses, and confined within the brevity of the years which nature permits its varied organic form, allowing them some, but not too much, latitude. The other less obvious fact is that man is a spirit who stands outside of nature, life, himself, his reason and the world. (Niebuhr, 1964, p. 3)

The human spirit is the realm of consciousness of the human self as the image of God (Gen. 9:6), as a son or daughter who belongs to Him (Isa. 45:4), and without this dual identification there can be no meaning worthy of human identity.

Inter-dimensional hermeneutic. The human body is physical and dependent on nature for food, water, air, warmth, and health. This point is well illustrated in the original language of the Bible: the Hebrew word for man is *adam*, and the word for earth is *adama*. Human physical and physiological health and needs must be cared for in harmony with natural laws. A broken bone cannot be mended by any counseling technique nor spiritual discipline. Psychological and spiritual dimensions are real, and they play an important role in the care for our bodies, yet it is the domain of medical, nutritional, and public health sciences to interpret physical symptoms and to care for the physical dimension of the human being.

Yet, the human body is not neutral, nor "innocent," because it is physical. It may be characterized by passivity, or "weakness" (Matt. 26:41), or may be blameworthy for "harboring" and adjusting to bad habits and evil thoughts. For example, the "boutons" which form in our brains, creating "pathways" for addictive behavior, are issues to be dealt with. The body is "passive" and "weak" because it is at the mercy of our appetites and its "loyalties." It is affected by sin, and therefore cannot, by its physical properties alone, be an active ally for human well-being.

The human mind depends on the physical dimension, but the mind has its own laws, unique activities, and specific roles in the human existence. Mental health requires its own unique way to address the needs and anomalies which hinder human development or damage relationships. As the body is not neutral on account of being physical, neither is the mind neutral and innocent because it is not physical. "For out of the heart come evil thoughts, murder, adultery, fornication, theft, false witness, slander" (Matt. 15:18, NASB). "The good man out of his good treasure brings forth good, and the vile man out of his evil treasure brings forth evil" (Matt. 12:35, ESV).

The human spirit is like a slender and high tower looking upon a large and inclusive world, in that the human spirit stands over the world, reaching out to God. But the way in which humans use their superiority becomes crucial. "The freedom of his [man's] spirit enables him to use the forces and processes of nature creatively; but his failure to observe the limits of his finite existence causes him to defy the forms and restraints of both nature and reason" (Niebuhr, 1964, p. 17). A human being is not divided against him/her self so that the essential man (soul) can be separated from the non-essential (body) and thus resolve the problem of sin, evil, and suffering, as some forms of spiritualities claim. The human being contradicts himself/herself within his/her very essence (Niebuhr, 1964, p.16). His/her essential self is the image of God whose defacement creates separation from Him, and results in sin and evil. So what would an inter-dimensional interpretation of this data look like?

Patients with physical symptoms (fever, coughing, shortness of breath) will naturally see a Christian physician. Upon examination and proper tests, a therapy will be prescribed. The Christian physician is the *primary caregiver*. If some of the symptoms persist, the physician will, as part of the therapy, ask the questions "belonging" to psychology or the life of faith. Then, if necessary, a behavioral scientist and pastor will give their support as *secondary caregivers*. Tournier in one of numerous examples recounts the case of a woman he calls Genevieve who suffered from crippling rheumatoid arthritis. Her main goal in life was success, in both the social and financial realms. As a nanny in a rich industrialist home, she tasted of a life of relative ease. When her mistress suddenly died, her master married her. Upon their return from the honeymoon they faced complete bankruptcy. She took upon herself the task of paying her husband's debts. Overstressed and desperate, she came to see Dr. Tournier. He recalls:

> She told me all about it, and then, after a moment's silence, she added that she was well aware of the fatal influence on the course of her life of her desire to succeed, to be independent, and also her fear of the future. For a long time now she...had had the feeling that the only answer to this fear would be real faith in God. (Tournier, 1965, pp. 28–29)

Tournier sent her to an institution directed by a pastor where she "learned to give herself entirely to God, to ask her family for forgiveness, to forgive her husband, and to begin to see the possibility of reconstructing her life on a basis of faith" (p. 29).

If a client has a mental or emotional problem, here the Christian behavioral scientist will gather data, and use an appropriate therapy. The behavioral scientist is here the *primary caregiver*, but will constantly "listen" for any spiritual or physical needs. Chances are that some physical or spiritual issues may be contributing to the problem. The Christian psychologist's interest in other aspects of the client's life will make great impact. If necessary, though, cooperation with a Christian physician and a pastor as *secondary caregivers* could help.

During ministerial training, students are strongly advised not to pretend to be psychiatrists or physicians, but to refer their parishioners to a Christian specialist. But when such issues as guilt, doubt regarding forgiveness of sins, or fear of consequences arise, the pastor may be the *primary caregiver* who might need help from a Christian behavioral scientist as a *secondary caregiver*.

What is important to note here is that the compartmentalization of sciences into medicine, psychology, psychiatry, counseling, and theology or ministry is not a very good thing for patients. One woman told me during the writing of this paper about her frustrations: "Why can't I go to one person who will treat my body, help my mind, and strengthen my faith in the same treatment? Or at least, why not have clinics where all the specialists work together as seamlessly as possible?"

Bridging the gap. We now turn to another type of hermeneutics: the bridging of the gap between biblical/theological hermeneutics and behavioral sciences. Theologians are trained experts in translating biblical texts and formulating doctrinal statements and systems. But they use specialized vocabulary, and the Bible itself uses expressions which are foreign today. Much work is yet to be done in this arena, but some notable efforts merit our attention.

We would do well first to revisit the writings of some scholars predating the beginning of the twentieth century. Even though they may not be behavioral scientists as we understand it today, "these are people in whom faith and psychology have an *original union* as tight as between faith and theology. In them, psychological thought and practice is simply an aspect of faith" (Roberts, 2000, p. 152). These include Evagrius, Augustine, Thomas Aquinas, Richard Baxter, Søren Kierkegaard, and Jonathan Edwards. These writers have been reviewed by several contemporary authors who highlight psychology as a Christian science. The following is an abbreviated list: Diogenes Allen, Denis Okholm, Columba Stewart, Benedict Groeschel, Eric Johnson, Walter Sundberg, and C. Stephen Evans. For an extended bibliography, see R. C. Roberts (2000, pp. 152–155).

As we explore Christian psychology, two important tasks call our attention. (1) We need to "bracket" the *substance* of twentieth-century secular psychology (Roberts, 2000) so that Christian psychology can regain its proper place. (2) We need to rewrite Christian psychology in a form that is recognizable to today's psychologists.

Thus Robert C. Roberts looks at the Sermon on the Mount with "psychological glasses." The Sermon's approach is not to describe actions, which is the data most familiar to psychology, but rather character, which belongs more to ethics. Here is how Roberts (2000) conceptualizes the Sermon in psychological terms:

Personal well-being is composed of several traits of character with their implied actions and attitudes: gentleness, righteousness, mercy, purity, peacemaking, love for enemies, forgiveness, poverty of spirit, endurance during persecution, mourning, humility, self-unawareness, treasuring of the kingdom of God. "A person who had these traits or was disposed to these actions and emotions would, according to the psychology of the Sermon be 'mature,' 'perfect' (*teleios*) or 'blessed,' 'happy' (*makarios*)" (Roberts, 2000, p. 160–161).

Personal pathology is defined as a disposition to anger, spite, adultery and divorce, hatred, greed, slavery to Mammon, hypocrisy, ostentation, judgmentalism, or blindness to personal faults.

Psychological explanation is not as empirically evident, but some patterns are visible: Inward lust and anger manifest themselves in adultery and revenge; blindness to personal faults is expressed by judgmentalism and ostentation.

Therapeutic interventions are clearer:

> Be poor in spirit, mourn, behave gently, hunger for righteousness, be merciful, be pure in heart, make peace, allow yourself to be persecuted for the sake of Jesus, let your light shine before people, keep the commandments, take responsibility for your own anger, control your lustful eye, do not seek revenge on those who offend you, do not be ostentatious in your piety, do not fret about daily needs but seek the kingdom, focus chiefly on your own shortcomings rather than on those of others, do not hold others in contempt because of their shortcomings. (Roberts, 2000, p. 160–162)

IDEAL OR GOAL (*TELOS*)

Without doubt, personal well-being and a life in abundance (John 10:10) would rank as ultimate goals of the Christian behavioral scientist. The SDA church has from the very early days of its existence recognized the medical work as a "medical ministry." There is no doubt that mental and emotional illnesses diminish the fullness of life Jesus has come to bring. Ultimate well-being is wholistic health if we remain faithful to the biblical view of the indivisible nature of the human being.

The ultimate goal of Christian psychology, Christian psychiatry, and Christian counseling should be to join ranks with pastoral and medical ministries. The classic summary passage is Ephesians 3:14—5:2, where the people of God are called to mobilize as a transformative countercultural community (Powlison, 2000, p. 217). The Christ who wants to make humans whole cannot sanction compartmentalization of ministry into disconnected units. Both church and parachurch must come squarely under His oversight.

CONCLUSION

Here we are, facing an exciting project. There is still much good that can happen as SDA theologians and behavioral scientists work together. There are still many questions that face us as we think about this close relationship. For example, what principles of interpretation of the biblical text should guide behavioral scientists as they seek inspired insights into mental and emotional issues? Where do we find cases where the Bible addresses mental illnesses or emotional disorders? How can biblical/theological studies and behavioral sciences develop a cross-disciplinary discourse so as to communicate better with each other? What does it mean when we say that the Holy Spirit, the third Person of the Trinity, is fully involved in the daily life and trials of human existence? We have touched briefly on some of these earlier, but more is needed in order to make such statements meaningful and useful (John 3:8).

Our challenges are many. First of all, we must overcome the temptation to stereotype either theologians or psychologists. Mutual trust and teachability for the sake of bringing people into intimate personal relationships with Christ is worth our effort, even our sacrifice. Second, it is of crucial importance to recognize that Scripture should occupy a position of primacy as the Christian epistemological foundation for several reasons. (1) Scripture defines the nature of the subject of study: it is the human being, with a focus on the human mind and its states and functions. (2) The nature of the subject determines all other basic elements in epistemological theory. Thus, the method, worldview, hermeneutics, and ultimate goal in Christian psychology is strongly rooted in Scripture. (3) Using the Bible as the beacon leading ahead and defining the edges of our path will bring us to greater usefulness to humanity. We all, as behavioral scientists and theologians, as disciples of Jesus our Teacher, can learn and grow endlessly.

REFERENCES

Allen, D. (1997). Ascetic theology and psychology. In R. C. Roberts & M. R. Talbot (Eds.), *Limning the psyche: Explorations in Christian psychology* (pp. 297–316). Grand Rapids, MI: Eerdmans.

Alexander, D., & White, R. S. (2006). *Science, faith, and ethics.* Peabody, MA: Hendrickson.

Augustine. (1950). *City of God.* New York: Doubleday.

Brown, W. S., Murphy, N. C., & Malony, H. N. (1998). *Whatever happened to the soul?* Minneapolis, MN: Fortress Press.

Frankl, V. (1973). Youth in search of meaning. Presented at the 1973 National Catholic Education Convention, New Orleans, LA. Waco, TX: World Cassette Library 1973 [#0205].

Georgi, F., Fischer, R., Weber, R., & Weis, P. (1948). Psychophysische korrelationen; schizophrenie und leberstoffwechsel. *Schweizerische medizinische Wochenschrift, 78,* 1194–1200.

Groeschel, B. (1983). *Spiritual passages: The psychology of spiritual development.* New York: Crossroads.

Honderich, T. (Ed.). (1995). *The Oxford companion to philosophy.* Oxford: Oxford University Press.

Johnson, E. L. (1998). Whatever happened to the human soul? *Journal of Psychology and Theology, 26,* 16–18.

Johnson, E. L. (2004). Towards a philosophy of science for Christian psychology. *Education: Journal of the Society for Christian Psychology, 7,* 5–20.

Johnson, E. L. & Jones, S. L. (Eds.). (2000). *Psychology and Christianity.* Downers Grove, IL: InterVarsity Press.

Joy, D. M. (Ed.) (1983). *Moral development foundations.* Nashville, TN: Abingdon.

Maeder, A. (1953). *La personne du médecin, an agent psychothérepeutique.* Neuchatel, Switzerland: Delachaux et Nestlé.

Menkes, G. (1945). *Medecine sans frontieres.* Geneva, Switzerland: Mont Blanc.

Niebuhr, R. (1964). *The nature and destiny of man* (Vol. 1). New York: Charles Scribner's Sons.

Plantinga, C. J. (1995). *Not the way it's supposed to be: A breviery of sin.* Grand Rapids, MI: Eerdmans.

Powlison, D. (2000). A biblical counseling view. In E. L. Johnson & S. L. Jones (Eds.), *Psychology and Christianity.* Downers Grove, IL: InterVarsity Press.

Roberts, R. C. (2000). Christian psychology view. In E. L. Johnson & S. L. Jones (Eds.), *Psychology and Christianity.* Downers Grove, IL: InterVarsity Press.

Roberts, R. C., & Talbot, M. R. (Eds.) (1997). *Limning the psyche: Explorations in Christian psychology.* Grand Rapids, MI: Eerdmans.

Runes, D. D. (Ed.). (1980). *Dictionary of philosophy.* Totova, NJ: Littlefield & Adams.

Seventh-day Adventist Bible Commentary (Vol. 1). (2005). Hagerstown, MD: Review & Herald.

Stocker, A. (1949). Structures affectives ou hierarchie de la personne. In *Archivio di Psicologia, Neurologia e Psichiatria.* Milan: Anno X Fasc. III September.

Tournier, P. (1957). *The meaning of persons.* New York: Harper and Row.

Tournier, P. (1965). *The healing of persons.* New York: Harper and Row.

White, E. G. (1940). *The Desire of Ages.* Boise, ID: Pacific Press.

White, E. G. (1942). *Ministry of healing.* Boise, ID: Pacific Press.

White, E. G. (1943). *Counsels to parents, teachers, and students.* Mountain View, CA: Pacific Press.

White, E. G. (1956). *Steps to Christ.* Boise, ID: Pacific Press.

White, E. G. (1963). *Medical ministry.* Mountain View, CA: Pacific Press.

White, E. G. (1977). *Mind, character, and personality.* Nashville, TN: Southern Publishing Association.

Wolman, B. R. (Ed.). (1973). *Dictionary of behavioral sciences.* New York: van Nostrand Reinhold.

Mental Health and Human Wholeness: Implications from Biblical Anthropology

Richard Rice

Steven Callahan is the only man in history who survived more than one month alone at sea in an inflatable raft. In early 1982 his sailboat capsized near the Canary Islands, and for the next 76 days—from February 5 to April 21—he drifted 1,800 miles across the Atlantic in a five and a half foot raft he named *Rubber Duckey.* He survived by collecting water in two solar stills and spearing fish, which he ate raw. During the two and a half months, he drove off a number of sharks, and nine ships passed without noticing him. He was finally picked up by three fishermen from a little island in the West Indies. On day 58 of his incredible voyage, Callahan made this entry in his log:

> I have often thought that my instincts were the tools that allowed me to survive so that my "higher functions" could continue. Now I am finding that it is more the other way around. It is my ability to reason that keeps command and allows me to survive, and the things I am surviving for are those that I want by instinct: life, companionship, comfort, play. (Callahan, 1986, pp. 258–259)

Callahan's observation overturns the conventional view that mental qualities are far more important than physical ones and suggests that there is an intimate connection between the two. On both counts, his comments coincide remarkably with the biblical portrayal of human nature. According to the Bible, as we shall see, everything about us is connected to the physical, but nothing about us is merely physical. And to properly understand any facet of human life, we must see it in relation to the whole.

Among the many descriptions of the human in biblical literature, there are four essential constructs that bear on everything the Bible says about humanity. And while the biblical record as a whole presupposes all four, three are introduced in the opening chapters of the Bible, and the fourth is particularly evident in the ministry of Jesus. We will describe these four constructs below and then ask what they can contribute to a Christian perspective on mental health.

I. THE HUMAN AS CREATURE

We can summarize the Bible's most basic descriptions of human beings with the expressions "creature" and "image of God." "Then God said, 'Let us make humankind in our image, according to our likeness'" (Gen. 1:26, NRSV). These descriptions point, respectively, to the basics and the distinctiveness of human existence—to what we have in common with other forms of life and to what distinguishes us within the natural world.

When the Bible describes human origins, it places us squarely within a larger created order. On the one hand, this means that we are finite. We belong to the natural world, and we share the conditions and limitations that characterize all creaturely life. While our existence depends ultimately on God, we depend moment by moment on the world around us to provide for our physical needs. The biblical writers remind us of this when they emphasize the contingency or frailty of human existence. The Psalms, especially, remark on the transitory nature of human existence. "As for mortals, their days are like grass; they flourish like a flower of the field; for the wind passes over it, and it is gone, and its place knows it no more" (Ps. 103:15–16, ESV). "The days of our life are seventy years, or perhaps eighty, if we are strong; even then their span is only toil and trouble; they are soon gone, and we fly away" (Ps. 90:10).

Though God's creatures are contingent and finite, human beings included, they nevertheless have great value. According to Genesis 1 God repeatedly saw that what He made was "good," and when the process was complete He saw that it was "very good" (Gen. 1:31, NIV). The Bible thus opposes all forms of metaphysical dualism. It does not denigrate material existence. Although the physical world is not divine, it is not evil because it is not divine. It represents a realm of being that is good.

This emphasis on the body also appears in biblical descriptions of human destiny. For New Testament writers, life after death begins with bodily resurrection. "So it is with the resurrection of the dead. What is sown is perishable, what is raised is imperishable....It is sown a physical body, it is raised a spiritual body" (1 Cor. 15:42, 44, ESV). For the apostle Paul, the transition from this life to the future life involves a dramatic transformation, but it does not leave the body behind. In the life to come human beings will continue to exist in concrete, physical forms.

Bodily existence, therefore, is essential to our humanity. When God made human beings, He created physical organisms and placed them in a physical, material environment. Accordingly, the Bible knows nothing of human life in disembodied form. Humanity and corporeality go together. We not only have bodies, we *are* bodies.

Although the Bible affirms the importance of the body, it does not exaggerate it. It never reduces people to their physical appearance or their physical condition. For the biblical writers, a person is never merely a body—never merely a physical organism. On the other hand, the body has great importance, not just because it is vital to our existence, but because it is the bearer of personal meaning. A person's body is both the vehicle by which a person receives the world and the means through which a person projects him or herself into the world. For this reason, the human body serves as "the symbol of the person," recalling Paul Tillich's (1951) famous comments that, unlike a sign, a symbol *participates* in that to which it points. We naturally think of people, for example, by remembering what they look and sound like.

Something else that emerges from the biblical account of creation is the social nature of human existence. When God made humanity, He created two persons, not just one, as described in Gen. 1:27 "So God created humankind in his image, in the image of God he created them; male and female he created them"(NRSV). Community is an essential characteristic of humanity. We exist as groups, not merely as individuals.[5] The Bible affirms our basic sociality when it describes our destiny as well as our origins. The biblical accounts of resurrection emphasize the corporate nature of the life to come. The dead rise together to receive immortality. It isn't bestowed on them one by one. And when Christ returns, the living and the dead will be united. According to the apostle Paul, "the dead in Christ will rise first. Then we who are alive, who are left, will be caught up in the clouds together with them to meet the Lord in the air; and so we will be with the Lord forever" (1 Thess. 4:16–17, NRSV).

From the biblical perspective, we are thus fully human only as we associate with other human beings. The social dimension of our humanity is easy to overlook in a society that values nothing more highly than individual accomplishments, but several things underscore this dimension of our lives. We are biologically dependent on others, of course—each of us is the product of two other people—but we are also dependent on others for our intellectual and cultural development. Indeed, we owe our identity to other people. We learn to speak, for example, because we are spoken to and listened to, and our basic sense of self emerges from the way others interact with us.

Indeed, the fact that we are "persons," and not merely organisms, is due to the social nature of our existence. A person exists only in relation to other persons. An essential characteristic of personal existence is reciprocity, the capacity to interact with other persons, to affect them as they affect us. We could even define a "person" as a self-conscious unity capable of relationships with other persons.

II. THE HUMAN AS THE IMAGE OF GOD

Although human beings share many characteristics with other forms of life, they are remarkably different as well. In the Christian view

5. According to Paul Tillich (1951), "individualization and participation" are "ontological elements." They form one of the essential polarities of finite existence (p. 174).

of humanity, these distinctive qualities are embodied in the enigmatic and provocative designation "image of God." To bring to a conclusion His creative work in Genesis 1, God said, "Let us make humankind in our image, after our likeness" (Gen. 1:26, NRSV).

There have been innumerable attempts to specify just what it is that makes humans unique. Some people see it in the distinctive position that humans occupy the world, in their relation to the rest of creation. Right after God said, "Let us make humankind in our image," He said, "And let them have dominion…" (Gen. 1:26–27, NIV). On this view, the image of God essentially refers to the sovereignty that humans enjoy over the rest of creation. To use Wolfhart Pannenberg's expression, it consists in humanity's "creative mastery of existence" (1970, p. 15).

A more familiar approach is to associate the "imago" with a distinctive human quality or capacity, such as "reason." We often speak of humans, in contrast to animals, as "rational" beings capable of general concepts and abstract thought. For some thinkers, however, the most remarkable thing about us is not reason, but imagination. Compared to other life forms, they observe, human beings have very few instincts, and we respond to stimuli in a myriad of different ways.[6] With imagination, we can always envision new possibilities. So, while animals occupy an environment—the physical surroundings that provide them with life's essentials—the range of human experience extends far beyond our immediate situation. The world we inhabit is as large as the universe.

Many would say that the central, most essential, human quality is freedom. On the simplest account, freedom consists of making choices. If you are really free, *you* decide what you are going to do. Your action is not determined by factors over which you have no control. Freedom is the quality that makes us persons, because it

---

6. Wolfhart Pannenberg is one who sees imagination as the key to our distinctive humanity.

means that we are self-determined or self-creating to some extent. To a significant degree, we decide our own destiny. Over time, our choices form a pattern. They eventually flow into the ongoing stream that we designate with words like "personality" and "character." Thus, our choices both contribute to and reflect the sort of persons we are.

There are different sorts of freedom that appear in the biblical account(s) of creation. The more familiar is moral freedom—freedom to obey or disobey God: "And the LORD God commanded the man, 'You may freely eat of every tree of the garden; but of the tree of the knowledge of good and evil you shall not eat, for in the day that you eat of it you shall die'" (Gen. 2:16–17, NRSV). But God also gave humans what might be called "aesthetic freedom," that is, freedom to select among various equally good possibilities: "So out of the ground the LORD God formed every animal of the field and every bird of the air, and brought them to the man to see what he would call them; and whatever the man called every living creature, that was its name" (Gen. 2:19, AMP). Presumably, God would have been equally pleased with any number of choices on Adam's part. He was free to express his creativity.

Another term for the distinctive quality of human life is "spirituality."[7] Spirituality is not easy to define, but its most basic form is the capacity we have to appreciate and experience ultimate reality. It is our awareness of and openness to the mystery and meaning of the universe as a whole and the sense that we have a significant place within it. Although we are physical organisms in a physical environment, we cannot reduce our existence to a succession of physical experiences that comes to an end, at best, after seven or eight decades. To the contrary, we have an abiding conviction that

7. For Paul Tillich (1963), "spirit" as a distinctive dimension of life "comes to its full actualization only in man, in whom as the bearer of the spirit the conditions for it are present" (p. 25).

our lives contribute to a larger purpose, that in some measure they are the bearers of profound meaning.[8]

We could extend our description of the human in light of the opening chapters of Genesis. The fact that God placed Adam in a garden and gave him the task of caring for it—"to till and keep it" (Gen. 2:15, NRSV)—suggests that human beings have domestic and "industrial" qualities. In order to flourish, they need homes to live in and work to occupy them. In addition to providing them food, the trees God planted in Eden were "pleasant to the sight" (Gen. 2:9, AMP), suggesting that human beings have aesthetic needs. To enjoy life to the fullest we need beauty around us. We cannot thrive in the midst of chaos and ugliness.

Reason, along with its attendant qualities, generally receives more attention than any other facet of human existence. Yet we are most likely to equate the quality of our lives with the affective domain, with the area of emotion or feelings. No matter how talented, intelligent, beautiful, rich, and famous you are, if you still feel lousy about yourself, life will seem empty. Conversely, positive feelings seem to compensate for any other deficiency. People can learn to be happy in a great variety of circumstances. Feelings are important because they are comprehensive and complex. Our feelings relate us to the totality of our existence, and they display enormous subtlety. In both respects, feelings differ from concepts or ideas. Conceptual activity sometimes seems immune to concrete circumstances, and thought never matches

---

8. While this inherent spirituality lies behind the world's many religions, it need not take the form of adherence to a particular religious tradition. Many people are spiritual in a non-religious way: they are not adherents of any specific religious tradition. The fact that human spirituality takes many different forms does not mean, however, that the world's various religions all boil down to the same thing. In recent years, scholars have become particularly resistant to the idea that the world's religions are simply different ways to express an experience that is essentially the same for every person. This notion obscures the unique insights and manifestations that make each religion what it is.

the subtlety of feeling. We can never put our feelings precisely into concepts[9] (Pannenberg, 1985).

THE INTRICACY AND INTEGRITY OF HUMAN EXISTENCE

To do justice to human complexity, we must also note the important ways in which the different dimensions of human existence affect each other. We are physical beings, obviously, but nothing about us is merely physical. There are layers of meaning involved in every aspect of our physical nature. As we have seen, the human body is not just a thing, an object in the physical world. It is a symbol of the person whose body it is. Moreover, we manifest ourselves in bodily ways. Our actions have meaning because they give expression to thoughts and attitudes. Like all organisms we need food to live, for example, but when we eat we do more than just ingest enough nutrients to survive. A meal is often an occasion for personal fellowship, a typical way of celebrating an important event, such as a wedding, and in certain settings an act of worship. In fact, there is nothing about human behavior that is merely or purely physical. The "more" that characterizes human existence imparts a spiritual or symbolic dimension to every aspect of our physical existence.

The insights of modern science, particularly neuroscience, support the "wholistic" view of humanity found in the Bible. Studies have demonstrated that various mental functions are directly connected to specific regions of the brain—the phenomenon of "localization." And if these regions are damaged, our ability to do things like remember faces, or use proper nouns, may be impaired. Indeed, mind and body are so closely connected that it is impossible to imagine what disembodied human existence would mean.

This obviously conflicts with the long-standing philosophical conviction that the two are separate entities. As Antonio Damasio explains, "Descartes' Error" was the philosopher's influential belief

9. "When a pianist finished performing a Beethoven Sonata, someone asked him to explain what it meant. He paused for a moment and then, without a word, turned to the piano and played the piece again" (Pannenberg, 1985, pp. 248, 252).

that mind and body belong to separate realms of being—the physical and the spiritual—and the two are essentially disconnected. To the contrary, science now assures us, whatever mind may ultimately be, it has no existence apart from the body.

Other areas of inquiry also show that mind and body are intimately connected. "Cognitive linguistics" reveals that the basic structure of human thought arises from our corporeal experience in the world. In *The Body in the Mind,* Mark Johnson notes that we instinctively, spontaneously, employ metaphorical terms to communicate, and he demonstrates that many of the "basic metaphors" we use—such as "good is up, bad is down"—reflect the fact that we exist as physical forms within a physical world. So, the body not only influences the mind, but it provides the mind with its fundamental conceptual structure.

The intimate contact between mind and body—the interaction of mental and physical—underscores the fact that nothing about us is isolated from the rest of us. Touch any part of a person, or any aspect of human life, and you touch the person as a whole. The dimensions of human life are not separate, independent items glued together in some sort of collage. Instead, they are extensively connected, like strands in a vast and intricate web of being.

In summary, the Christian view of humanity attributes great complexity to human beings. As creatures, we share many characteristics with other forms of life on this planet. We, too, are finite and corporeal, physical, social, sexual, and emotional. But we are "more than nature" in certain ways as well. Our intelligence is superior to that of other creatures. More important, we have the quality of freedom, which gives us the capacity for self-determination, elevates us to the realm of the personal, helps us to master our environment, and enables us to touch the divine. We are creatures, then, and never lose our creatureliness, but we are unique creatures. We are created in the image of God. We bear the imprint of the divine.

In order for human beings to be fully human, that is, to be fully healthy, or whole, all the dimensions of human existence need to be present in their full measure and in their proper relation to each other. To tell the whole truth about humans, however, we must acknowledge that none of us is, in fact, whole. In each of us, all the dimensions of essential humanity are diminished to one degree or another, and they are never perfectly in balance. There is thus a tragic discrepancy between essential humanity and actual human existence—between what we are meant to be and what we actually are. This brings us to what many believe is the most profound, and certainly most complex, biblical anthropological construct, namely, the concept of sin.

III. SIN: THE FUNDAMENTAL HUMAN PROBLEM

According to the Bible, we are not only creatures in the image of God. We are also sinners. In other words, there is something profoundly wrong with us. As the classic expressions "total depravity" and "original sin" indicate, sin touches us all, and it touches all there is of us—physically, socially, spiritually, and of course mentally. And its influence is irresistible. As Ellen White states:

> Not only intellectual but spiritual power, a perception of right, a desire for goodness, exists in every heart. But against these principles there is struggling an antagonistic power. The result of the eating of the tree of knowledge of good and evil is manifest in every man's experience. There is in his nature a bent to evil, a force which, unaided, he cannot resist. (1903, p. 29)

Although sin diminishes us, however, it does not destroy us. Even in sin, everything essential to our humanity is still present—we are still creatures in God's image. But even though sinful human beings are fully *human*, they are not *fully* human. Everything about them is damaged. Like broken-down automobiles, we may have all our parts, but they no longer work as they were designed. As sinners, we are no longer together; we are no longer "whole." Because our humanity comprises a number of different dimensions, and all of them are intimately connected, a problem anywhere in our lives creates a problem everywhere.

Sin not only diminishes our various capacities; it fragments and fractures us. Creatures in sin are creatures in conflict,[10] and this conflict involves all the essential dimensions of our nature, beginning with our relationship to God. Adam and Eve "heard the sound of the LORD God walking in the garden at the time of the evening breeze, and the man and his wife hid themselves from the presence of the LORD God among the trees of the garden" (Gen. 3:8, CSV). Although human beings are essentially related to God, they find themselves out of harmony with His will. They resent the interest He takes in them and resist the plans He makes for them.

The most obvious conflicts that beset us involve our relations with each other. We are essentially social beings. We need companionship. But if life alone is not worth living, life together is extremely difficult. The clearest example of our social disease is the perpetual unrest that engulfs peoples and nations. In the twentieth century human beings arguably made more technological progress than in all previous history, yet we killed one another at a rate that defies comprehension—by the tens of millions, in two global wars and dozens of other ones. In fact, mass destruction is the most conspicuous legacy of our time.[11]

The conflicts and rivalries that take such tragic and vivid form in war are universally at work in human relationships. Sin prevents us from seeing the true worth of human beings, our own or anyone else's. We typically exaggerate our own importance at the expense of others, and, as feminist thinkers emphasize, we sometimes exaggerate the

---

10. It is natural to think of sin as conflict, but the symbolism of evil includes a host of metaphors, among them symbols of isolation and defilement. Sin interrupts all the essential relationships that constitute human existence, and it leaves us feeling guilty and stained. An influential portrayal of sin as defilement is Paul Ricoeur, *The Symbolism of Evil,* trans. Emerson Buchanan (Boston: Beacon Press, 1967).

11. An interviewer once asked Leonard Bernstein, famous director of the New York Philharmonic, why he held the music of Austrian composer Gustav Mahler in such high regard. Bernstein answered, "Because he realized before any else did that this would be the century of death."

importance of others to our own detriment. Either way, sin isolates and alienates us. And because sin distorts our perspective, we view other people as threats, and we instinctively act to protect our own interests. What is true of individuals is even more true of communities. Groups, like individuals, typically pursue their own interests at all costs, and the selfishness of groups is less obvious and more difficult to counteract.[12]

The most pathetic manifestation of our brokenness, and the one perhaps most directly related to mental health, is the fact that we are in conflict with ourselves. In *Man Against Himself,* Karl Menninger asserts that there is a self-destructive tendency in all of us, and it takes many different forms. "Each man has his own way of destroying himself," says Menninger; "some are more expedient than others, some more consciously deliberate than others" (Menninger, 1938, pp. 311, 343). This tendency can lead to voluntary death, but it can also lead to things like self-mutilation, purposive accidents, and organic illnesses.

Sin thus affects us physically and mentally, and it can work in either direction. Physical illnesses often have spiritual and emotional causes, and they almost always have spiritual and emotional effects. The man whose four friends brought him to Jesus suffered in a variety of ways, and Jesus recognized that he needed both physical and spiritual restoration (Mark 2:1–12). But whether physical illness has mental, emotional, spiritual, or social causes or mental, emotional, spiritual, or social symptoms, the fundamental truth is the same. A problem anywhere is a problem everywhere. Nothing about us is merely physical, or merely anything else.

---

12. As Reinhold Niebuhr argues, large institutions can make extravagant claims seem plausible in ways that mere individuals never could. In addition, human institutions lack the moral resources that individuals have. Human collectives—whether families, races, classes, nations, or even churches—are notoriously incapable of self-criticism. When a group feels threatened, it inevitably acts to protect itself, and the individuals who belong to it typically subordinate their personal values to those of the larger community (*Moral Man and Immoral Society* [New York: Scribner's, 1932]).

This wholistic view of sin gives illness a spiritual identity. Sin is the ultimate cause of all our problems, and an adequate solution to any of them must include a spiritual dimension. The relation between sin and suffering is not one to one, of course. Few people suffer in direct proportion to their misdeeds; reality is more complicated than that.[13] But every illness, accident, and injury is a manifestation of human brokenness, and each one can leave a person feeling anxious, vulnerable, and diminished. And because illness affects the whole person, effective healing must do the same.

IV. HUMANITY, SALVATION, AND HEALING

As we have seen, a wholistic view of essential humanity affirms all the dimensions that make us human—physical, mental, emotional, social, and spiritual—and a wholistic view of our actual existence acknowledges that every aspect of our humanity is unfulfilled and damaged by sin. Similarly, a wholistic view of salvation will envision the eventual restoration of our humanity—in all of its essential aspects. Salvation involves physical, emotional, social, spiritual, social, and mental renewal.

The theme of restoration appears throughout the Bible. Apocalyptic literature, for example, promises restoration on a cosmic scale—new heavens and a new earth—reversing the disruption that sin brings to the universe. Jesus' preaching of the kingdom announced restoration on a political or corporate level. The doctrine of the resurrection promises restoration on a physical level. The theme of restoration runs through Jesus' ministry, particularly His miracles of healing. On one hand, these miracles anticipate the final restoration of all things at the end of history. On the other, they indicate that restoration is available here and now.

Jesus' ministry indicates that however damaged by sin we may be, our fundamental value to God remains unchanged. Jesus embraced people whom the society of His day excluded, whether for spiritual reasons,

---

13. When His disciples asked Jesus whose sin caused a man's blindness, his own or his parents, Jesus said that neither one did (John 9).

like the "sinners" mentioned in Luke 15, or for physical reasons, like the lepers He healed and the woman with the issue of blood (Mark 5), or for psychological reasons, like the demoniac who was chained and shackled (Mark 5:1–5). He saw their problems in full relief, but He also saw the person beneath them, and He never reduced people to their physical, spiritual, or mental maladies. Others surrendered to hopelessness, but He saw the possibility of restoration. Indeed, Jesus compared Himself to a physician to show that restoration was the purpose of His ministry. "Those who are well have no need of a physician," He said, "but those who are sick; I have come to call not the righteous but sinners" (Mark 2:16–17, ESV). Jesus performed a variety of miracles, indicating that the restoration He came to achieve involved all aspects of human existence, including mental as well as physical healing.

Most of the thirty-five miracles specifically described in the Gospels deal with physical illness, and since the body and the mind are connected, we may assume that the victims suffered mental or emotional distress as well. But the half dozen cases where Jesus cast out demons are directly related to our concern here. Whether demonic activity was a pre-scientific way of describing mental illness or the result of supernatural evil influences is an issue we will not address here. What is clear in either case is that Jesus reversed its damaging effects on its victims' mental functions. The mentally incapacitated became whole. After Jesus healed the demoniac in Gadara, an area on the eastern shore of the Sea of Galilee, the people in the region "came to Jesus and saw the demoniac sitting there, clothed and *in his right mind*" (Mark 5:15; YLT Bible, emphasis added). The expression is significant. It indicates that one purpose of Jesus' ministry was to restore mental health.

Some of Jesus' miracles exhibit another quality that has an important bearing on mental health. Those whom Jesus healed were made whole instantly most of the time, but not always; sometimes the healing was progressive. According to the Gospel of John, Jesus restored the sight of a man born blind and sometime later healed his spiritual blindness as well.[14] Since we are temporal beings, our significant experiences typically involve a process. We acquire physical maturity gradually, for example, and intellectual growth takes even more time. Healing can take time, too. And in the case of mental illness, a person may need to pass through several stages on the way to recovery.

The manner in which Jesus healed the man born blind—first enabling him to see and then awakening his faith—also suggests that people do not always acquire physical, mental, and spiritual wholeness at the same time. The ideal is perfect symmetry, or perfect proportion, but the ideal is seldom realized. Though all the dimensions of our lives are connected, the needs in one area may be more acute than in others.

APPLICATIONS

Our analysis of the human presents us with four things to consider in an attempt to achieve a biblical perspective on any aspect of our lives. Human beings are first of all *creatures*, second bearers of *God's image*, third *sinners*, and fourth potential recipients of *divine redemption*. To illustrate how this complex perspective illuminates our understanding of all things human, let us apply them to some important aspects of life. What do we learn about the following facets of our existence if we view them through the following interpretive lenses: creatureliness, image of God, sin, and salvation?

FOOD

The most basic needs we have are the ones we share with all other organisms. Of these, our most obvious need is food. Without enough to eat, we can't survive. Without enough of the right things to eat—vitamins, minerals, and so on—we will never enjoy optimum physical health. Many diseases, mental as well as physical, are attributable to deficiencies in diet. Others are attributable to eating too much of one thing or another, or, in the case of obesity, of just eating too much. According to the Bible,

14. John 9:1–7, 35–38.

providing food is one of the most important things God does for His creatures. Both creation accounts (Gen. 1:29–30 and 2:9) mention it, and the same idea also appears in the Psalms (e.g., Ps. 104:14, 21). Eating well was evidently a part of God's plan for all His creatures. On two occasions, Jesus miraculously provided vast multitudes with something to eat.

Food is not only one of life's basic necessities; it also has profound significance for the creatures that bear God's image. To eat bread is a physical act, as someone said, but to share bread is a spiritual act. Indeed, sharing bread with another may be the most elemental means of establishing community—the Latin for *bread* is the root of the English word *companion.* To eat with someone is to affirm the person's humanity and accept her as an equal. The Gospels contain numerous accounts of Jesus' table fellowship, as scholars refer to it. He ate with the rich—He invited Himself to Zacchaeus' house for dinner. And He ate with the poor—on more than one occasion He miraculously provided food for those who had none. Jesus' several "banquet parables" illustrate a point we are all familiar with. Special meals underscore the importance and add to the enjoyment of significant events like weddings. When He ate a final meal with His disciples, Jesus instituted "the Lord's Supper" to give them a lasting way to remember Him and to provide the Christian community with a lasting symbol of His continuing presence within it.

Sin has a profound effect on food. When Adam and Eve ate from the forbidden tree in the garden of Eden, the effects were catastrophic, and one of them was the difficulty they would face in getting food thereafter. The earth produced thorns and thistles, and, Adam was told, "by the sweat of your face shall you eat bread" (Gen. 3:19, ESV). Overeating, or gluttony, is one of the seven deadly sins of Christian tradition. There are many ways of misusing food. Some people overindulge for emotional reasons. They turn to food to compensate for a lack of satisfaction elsewhere in their lives. Some people deny themselves food for emotional reasons. Food becomes an enemy to those pursuing an unrealistic image of themselves. Anorexia is a serious medical condition, and it can be life-threatening. Then there are those who use food, or the lack of it, as a weapon. Ruthless leaders sometimes deny their people food in order to perpetuate their own power. They know that starving people have neither the strength nor the will to mount a serious opposition. It is estimated that over half the famine in the world is the result of political causes.

In spite of, or in the face of, its misuse, food remains one of God's great gifts to us, and in the light of redemption its spiritual significance can be restored. For one thing, food is a symbol of God's abiding care. As the Lord's Prayer indicates, our daily bread is a gift from God, a reminder that He can supply all our needs. For another, common meals are an important means of promoting Christian community. Jesus ate with "tax collectors and sinners" to show that He accepted them and cared for them (Luke 15:1–2, NIV 2010). The early Christian church provided meals for those in their number who needed them (Acts 6:1). Paul had a lot to say to the Christians in Corinth about the meals they ate together. He recognized that it could split the church if those who were well-off enjoyed themselves without any regard for others. The purpose of religious meals, he wrote, is not to satisfy hunger, but to focus our spiritual attention. They should eat and drink "to the glory of God" (1 Cor. 10:31, KJV).

WORK

According to Genesis 2, work was also integral to human life from the beginning. After God created man, he "put him in the garden of Eden to till it and keep it" and then told him he could "freely eat of every tree of the garden" except one (2:15–16, NASB). The mention of work and food in succession suggests that the two are closely related. As do all creatures, humans require nutrition, and they must exert themselves in order to meet this basic need. Along with many other animals, humans also work in order to acquire shelter and provide for their young.

Because human beings bear God's image, however, work means a great deal more to them. Through their work humans express themselves, give meaning to their existence, and illustrate their creativity. Along with caring for the garden, the first man was entrusted with naming the animals, an act of great significance. In the biblical world, names were more than verbal handles; they were the bearers of identity. Nothing fully existed until it had a name. By naming the animals, therefore, the man participated in God's own creative work. He brought to completion what God had begun.

The entrance of sin had a drastic effect on human work. As a result of the fall, God told Adam, "in toil you shall eat of it [the ground] all the days of your life....By the sweat of your face you shall eat bread" (Gen. 2:17–18, ESV). What was intended to be fulfilling and creative, even exhilarating, became drudgery. Instead of giving life meaning, it deprived life of meaning. Instead of enhancing life, it diminished it.

Sin not only makes work a good deal harder, but it changes our perspective on work in a number of ways. One is the tendency to identify people with the work they do. When a person's name appears in the newspaper, for example, it is almost always followed by some occupational designation, such as building contractor, school teacher, dentist, minister, truck driver, whatever. Even if the individual is unemployed or retired, the occupational designation still appears. Similarly, we often ask children what they want to be when they grow up, as if it were not enough for them to be happy five- or six-year-olds; they have to be future something-or-others as well.

Another is the tendency to equate people with their occupations, and to exaggerate or diminish their significance accordingly. We typically adulate those with outstanding athletic, intellectual, or artistic gifts, and look down on those who lack distinctive abilities or engage in mundane pursuits.

Perhaps the most striking manifestation of sin's effects on work is slavery, the complete reduction of people to their productive capacities. Slaves are less than persons in the fullest sense—they are denied the freedom of self-determination—and their value is equated with the effort that others extract from them. Work even takes the form of deliberate degradation. Ruthless totalitarian regimes often use forced labor as a calculated means of demoralizing their enemies and critics.

How does the presence of grace affect this aspect of human life, affected as it is by sin? There are several biblical passages that mitigate against the tendency to reduce human beings to their productivity. One is the fourth commandment, which enjoins a day of rest, a cessation of work, for all humans, even for slaves. While work is important it is not all-important. It is not the most important thing people do, and it is not as important as the persons who do it. Human beings have significance because of what they are, not because of what they do.

Another passage deals directly with people in a work situation, namely, the apostolic advice to slaves and their masters in the letter to the Ephesians.

> Slaves, obey your earthly masters with fear and trembling, in singleness of heart, as you obey Christ; not only while being watched, and in order to please them, but as slaves of Christ, doing the will of God from the heart. Render service with enthusiasm, as to the Lord and not to men and women, knowing that whatever good we do, we will receive the same again from the Lord, whether we are slaves or free. And, masters, do the same to them. Stop threatening them, for you know that both of you have the same Master in heaven, and with him there is no partiality. (Eph. 6:5–9, HCSB)

This passage indicates that no matter what our station in life, we can view our work as a way of doing God's will and expressing our obedience to Christ. A person's work can therefore acquire a significance that transcends his or her immediate situation. From one perspective, a slave may seem to be nothing more than a sophisticated tool, a living machine of sorts. From another, however, a slave is nothing less than an agent of divine purpose. The passage also indicates that slaves deserve to be respected and valued. Their ultimate Master dwells in heaven.

To summarize, work plays an important role in human life. It is the means of fulfilling our basic needs *and* of expressing our aspirations and creativity. Though often degraded by sin to toil and labor, work can nevertheless have great spiritual significance. Work has an important contribution to make to mental health. We all have a basic need to engage in activity that both interests us and benefits other people. As the expression "occupational therapy" indicates, finding useful things to do can play an important role in increasing mental fitness.

SEXUALITY

The same four lenses—creature, image of God, sin, and salvation—bring into biblical focus other aspects of human life, including sexuality, one of the most important. The first biblical reference to human sexuality appears in Genesis 1. God created human beings "male and female," and instructed them to be fruitful and multiply. On the biological level, human beings share with many other creatures the capacity for sexual reproduction. Presumably, God could have populated the entire planet at the beginning, but instead He gave His creatures the capacity to procreate. Sexual differentiation, and sexual activity, was an integral part of God's plan for the world.

While human sexuality has a fundamental physical function, it serves other purposes as well. The divine image imparts to sexuality a depth that surpasses its biological purpose. The second biblical passage that refers to human sexuality places it in an entirely different context. After God placed Adam in Eden and provided for his physical needs, He said, "It is not good that man should be alone." The narrative that follows includes the creation of the animals—potential but not perfect companions for the man—and concludes with the creation of Eve, Adam's perfect counterpart. "This at last is bone of my bone and flesh of my flesh." The passage ends with a clear reference to sexual activity: "They were naked and they were not ashamed" (ESV).

In Genesis 2, nothing is said about procreation. As described here, the purpose of human sexuality is to meet a profound need for companionship, or intimacy. Accordingly, sex employs a physical union to unite human beings psychologically and spiritually as well. It is the means by which two become "one flesh." Sexual contact establishes a relationship that surpasses all others in permanence and significance—

even the relationship between parents and children: "for this cause a man shall leave his father and mother, and be joined to his wife" (NASB).

Just as no aspect of human life illustrates the connection between the physical and the "more than physical" more vividly than sexuality, no aspect more vividly illustrates the corrupting, distorting effects of sin. It is significant that Paul describes sexual perversion as a clear manifestation of human life apart from God (Rom. 1:26–27). Sexual perversion runs in different directions. One form is pure sensuality; it denies the spiritual significance of sexuality, reducing it to the mere gratification of physical urges. Another exploits the spiritual significance of sexuality to inflict personal anguish. Sexual brutality violates the dignity of its victims. And the pursuit of sexual gratification for its own sake does violence to both parties.

The Bible is clear in affirming the importance and value of sexual activity and equally clear in acknowledging the distorting effects of sin. At the same time, it also indicates the ways in which this aspect of human life can be redeemed. From the ministry of Jesus we learn that sin may affect the whole person, but it need not define the whole person. As His reaction to the adulterous woman indicates (John 7:53—8:11), Jesus did not reduce people to their sexual sins. He refused to condemn this unfortunate person, caught as she was in a web of human intrigue, and offered her the promise of a new and better life.

We can see the effects of redemption, the fourth lens in our perspective on the human, in the area of human sexuality by examining the New Testament contexts in which the expression "one flesh" appears. The first is Matthew 19, where the issue engaging Jesus and His questioners was divorce. On this occasion, Jesus invoked the expression "one flesh" to support the claim that marriage was intended to be permanent. Jesus' statement implies that the ideal framework for sexual activity is a relationship between two people, a man and a woman, characterized by enduring commitment. The second context is 1 Corinthians 6, where Paul urges his readers to "flee fornication" (KJV). His reason? Sex is never just a casual physical experience. According to the apostle, the expression "one flesh" indicates that sexual contact connects people on a profound personal level, whether they intend it to or not. "Do you not know that your bodies are members of Christ?...Do you not know that whoever is united to a prostitute becomes one body with her?" (1 Cor. 6:15–16, NIV).

The third context is Paul's advice to married couples in Ephesians. In this letter, Paul urges husbands to love their wives as they love their own bodies—after all, husband and wife form "one flesh." Indeed, he takes Christ's self-sacrificing love for the church as the model for husbandly care. No biblical passage elevates human sexuality more highly. It serves as a symbol of the central claim of Christian faith—that Jesus Christ was the outpouring of God's redemptive love for humankind.

What is the relation between mental health and human sexuality? In affirming that sex has a natural place in human experience, the Bible suggests that sexual activity can contribute to mental and emotional well-being. At the same time, the Bible acknowledges a persistent tendency among men and women to either underestimate or overestimate its significance, to ignore the profound personal significance that sex conveys or to equate people with their sexual situation. As the various uses of the expression "one flesh" indicate, the appropriate framework for sexual activity—arguably the only setting where sex will contribute to rather than detract from mental health—is a relationship between two people that is characterized by permanence, mutual commitment, and tender care.

COMMUNITY

We noted earlier that human beings are fundamentally social. We owe our existence to others—physically, psychologically, and culturally. We are human, beyond the mere biological sense only insofar as we interact with others, and we need human contact in order to achieve a full and well-balanced life. We also noted that the effects of sin on human existence are nowhere more apparent than in the breakdown of our relationships. Life alone may be impossible, but life together is enormously difficult. And there is no area of human society that sin does not touch. Wherever we look—whether at families, neighborhoods, communities, or nations—we see evidence of conflict.

The distortions of human community come in many forms. Some make true personal life impossible by exaggerating the importance of community. Collectives are notorious for reducing human beings to their social utility. To the collective mentality, the only thing that matters is one's contribution to the group; personal fulfillment is inconsequential. Accordingly, collectives typically suppress a sense of individuality, and in some cases, as in the fictional societies of George Orwell and Ayn Rand, they seek to eliminate individuality altogether.

There are also social units that survive by exaggerating the importance of who is inside or outside the group. The most notorious examples are gangs, groups which demand unyielding subservience from those inside, view all those outside as real or potential enemies, and often resort to violence to maintain themselves. But a strong "inside-outside mentality" is pervasive in human experience. We all have a tendency to view those who are different from us racially, ethnically, linguistically, sexually, economically, or educationally as somewhat inferior. People with this outlook sometimes bolster their own sense of importance by alienating and discriminating against the "other." Extreme forms of these distortions include Nazi anti-Semitism and American racism.

Along with views of community that make true personal life impossible, there are also views of the individual that make genuine communal life impossible. By emphasizing the individual as the be-all and end-all of human existence, individualism denies the value of community altogether. This is particularly noticeable in the United States, where the rugged individual plays a prominent role in our national consciousness. The most famous figure in American folklore is the cowboy, who in a story with countless variations rides into town alone, dispatches the bad guys with his trusty six-shooter, and rides off into the sunset. We don't know where he came from or where he's going. In some cases we never even learn his name. But we love the image of the solitary person going against the odds, and often flouting social convention, as he fulfills his individual destiny.

The fictional cowboy may be an exaggerated instance of individualism. But ever since Augustine, Western thought has been preoccupied with the discovery and the fulfillment of the human individual—discovery by introspection, by turning within ourselves, and fulfillment either through rational self-mastery, or through a celebration of personal uniqueness. Throughout its variations, however, the idea persists that the real person, the true self, is something that lies within us, and the essential unit of human reality is the individual by him- or herself. In other words, the modern self is the solitary self, detached and disconnected from others.

On this atomistic concept of humanity, society is nothing more than "a collection of autonomous, independent selves, each of whom pursues his own ends" (Grenz, 2001, p. 99). People may still form relationships, but they do so primarily to meet their individual needs. If a social connection doesn't meet their private goals, they feel free to leave. The object of their commitment is the self, not the community. Prevalent attitudes toward marriage exemplify this obsessive individualism. Many in contemporary Western societies, for example, go in and out of marriages as casually as shoppers go in and out of stores. Their goal is individual satisfaction, not true community.

Though we are fundamentally social beings, sin drastically limits our capacity for true community. Yet here, as with the other aspects of human life, divine power counteracts the effects of sin. As the Bible describes it, one of the major purposes of salvation is the restoration of community. Corporate categories play a prominent role in biblical history. The people of God occupy center stage in the Old Testament and the Christian church in the New. The central objective of the plan of salvation is arguably to restore our relationships with one another as well as with God. Jesus prayed that His disciples would be one, just as He and His heavenly Father were one (John 17:22–23). And while people often think of justification by faith as the central theme in Paul's theology, the apostle himself viewed justification as a means to the end of Christian unity. All have sinned, he argued, whether with or without an explicit knowledge of God's law; therefore all have the same need for salvation. And since salvation is provided to all on exactly the same basis, namely, through faith in God's gracious gift of Jesus Christ, there is no distinction among them, and full participation in the body of Christ is open to all. To quote Paul's letter to the Galatians, "In Christ Jesus you are all children of God through faith....There is no longer Jew or Greek, there is no longer slave or free, there is no longer male and female; for all of you are one in Christ Jesus" (3:26, 28, ESV). In another letter he makes the point even more vividly: "Now you are the body of Christ, and individually members of it." "For just as the body is one and has many members, and all the members of the body, though many, are one body, so it is with Christ" (1 Cor. 12:27, 12, ESV). By appreciating our common destiny in Christ, and realizing that what holds us together is more fundamental than what distinguishes us from each other, we can come to know true and lasting community.

THE IMPLICATIONS OF WHOLENESS FOR MENTAL HEALTH

The complex perspective on the human that emerges from these considerations has important implications for mental health. For one thing, they remind us that mental health involves the whole person.

The picture of the human that Christianity offers indicates that the list of things that makes for complete health is very long. Human beings have a number of different needs and each of them has an important connection to mental health. We will explore the implications of the Christian perspective on humanity for mental health by briefly commenting on a number of important topics.

MENTAL AND PHYSICAL HEALTH

We are physical beings in a physical world, and everything about us is connected in some way to the physical. Unless our basic physical needs are met, we cannot survive. To be healthy mentally, a person must also be healthy physically. Serious physical illness can cause mental distress, and mental illness is often accompanied by physical symptoms.

Because mind and body are integrally related, nothing about us is either merely physical or merely mental. Every aspect of physical existence is connected to the mysterious "more" that distinguishes human beings from other organisms. The human body is more than a sophisticated machine of complex parts and intricate organization. The body is the symbol of the person. Optimum mental health therefore requires a positive view of one's own body. This can be difficult to achieve in a society that places great emphasis on personal appearance and projects as "models" of ideal shape and size the images of people who are endowed with exceptional faces and forms. A positive view of one's own body has less to do with appearance than a sense of gratitude for whatever physical abilities one has and for the ability to enjoy fundamental physical pleasures, such as eating, drinking, and exercising.

THE INTELLECT AND MENTAL HEALTH

The mysterious "more" that characterizes human life is often identified with the most obvious difference between humans and other organisms, namely, superior intelligence—the capacity for abstract thought and the ability to reason. Intellectual activity is an important component of mental health. A person's ability to solve problems, meet challenges, and make decisions is essential to her sense of well-being. American schools are sometimes criticized for cultivating self-esteem rather than emphasizing academic accomplishments, but the two go together. Children love to learn and people who continue to learn through life are likely to enjoy greater mental health than those who don't.

RELATIONSHIPS AND MENTAL HEALTH

Human beings are social creatures, and nothing is more important to mental health than close and rewarding relationships. Statistics indicate that married people typically live longer and enjoy life more than singles, for example. Many people find that their greatest joys in life come from the families they belong to. By the same token, dysfunctional families are a major source of mental illness. Mental health professionals often find that it is important to consider a person's family background for any attempt at therapy to be successful. Even relationships with animals can be beneficial, as the visits of service dogs to hospitals and rest homes demonstrate.

AESTHETICS AND MENTAL HEALTH

The presence or absence of beauty in a person's life is an important and often overlooked factor in mental well-being. According to the biblical account of creation, the trees that God planted in Eden were not only "good for food," but "pleasant to the sight" (Gen. 2:9, ESV). Some people wonder if the pictures we look at as children are just as important to our growth as the stories we listen to. In recent years certain hospital administrators have been studying the effect that pleasant surroundings have on patients. Art and music have proven therapeutic benefits. It may be significant that Greek dramas were performed near temples to Aesklepios, the Greek God of healing.

OCCUPATION AND MENTAL HEALTH

Feeling productive is an important component in mental health. Humans have a deep need to feel that they are contributing to something larger than themselves. As we have seen, work is often more than a means to put food on the table, clothes on our back, and a roof over our heads. We need to express ourselves. Work activates the mind and the body. It establishes relationships. It directs us out of our immediate physical needs to participate in the larger world and increase the scope of our interests.

MENTAL HEALTH AND SPIRITUALITY

Human beings have an inherent capacity for transcendence. Unlike other organisms, we inhabit a world, not just an environment—a universe of meaning, not merely a way to satisfy our physical needs. We need to feel that we are connected to some power or purpose larger than our own existence. Spirituality and religion are often distinguished—we often hear people say that they are spiritual but not religious. But from a Christian perspective this spiritual capacity is a manifestation of the divine image. This indicates that mental health requires a spiritual component—a sense of one's place in the overall scheme of reality. It also indicates that any therapist must take into account a client's spiritual perceptions and spiritual attitudes.

MENTAL HEALTH AND THE BALANCED LIFE

We have been reviewing the factors that contribute to mental health, noting that all must be present in someone's life for one to have optimum mental well-being. To be fully healthy in any respect, one must be healthy in all respects. But it is also important that they be present in the proper proportion. Aristotle supposedly said that a gentleman should be able to play a flute, but not too well. His point was that a well-balanced life is preferable to one that emphasizes one or two faculties at the expense of others. Mental health will diminish if any of the essential components in human existence is missing, of course, but it will also diminish if one receives attention at the expense of others. We need physical and mental nourishment. We need physical and mental activity. We need work and we need recreation. We need company and we need solitude. A perfectly healthy person is one whose life is in perfect balance. True education, according to one religious leader, involves the harmonious development of all our powers.

MENTAL HEALTH AND MENTAL HEALING

One of the important implications of the biblical portrait of humanity is that no one enjoys perfect mental health. To one degree or another, sin affects all of us, and it affects all there is of us. Just as we are all physically deficient in one way or another, we also experience less than perfect mental health. We all need healing in one way or another. This means that mental health professionals should feel a sense of kinship with their clients. Our common need for healing and wholeness may not dissolve the border between therapists and clients, but it can prevent it from becoming a wall of separation.

The most important implication of Christian anthropology for mental health is the assurance that healing is possible. In its descriptions of ultimate origins and ultimate destiny, the Bible paints pictures of the ideal human situation. It is one where humans live in perfect harmony with one another, with all other creatures, and with God. As the ministry of Jesus indicates, God's ideal has practical implications for our present lives. His miracles of healing restored people physically, mentally, socially, and spiritually. Accordingly, they remind us of our essential identity as children of God. They remind us of our deficiencies and our brokenness. And they reassure us that restoration is possible.

MENTAL HEALTH AND CHRISTIAN SERVICE

The Bible also provides a strong mandate for Christians to devote themselves to healing people mentally as well as physically. As the New Testament describes it, Jesus' comprehensive ministry continued in the community He established. The apostles healed many people, including those who suffered from emotional and mental distress. And early Christians were known for their extensive care for the sick. The Christian church can promote mental health in a number of ways. By presenting the Gospel with clarity and enthusiasm, it reassures people of their essential value as God's beloved children. By cultivating community, it connects people with each other and meets their social needs. By providing opportunities to serve, it helps to meet our basic need to be industrious and productive. By promoting the Sabbath experience, it meets our needs for rest and recreation. And finally, in its worship, the church presents reassuring narratives of acceptance, forgiveness, and restoration, providing rituals of personal and social renewal.

REFERENCES

Bellah, R. N., Madsen, R., Sullivan, W. M., Swidler, A., & Tipton, S. M. (1985). *Habits of the heart: Individualism and commitment in American life.*

Berkley, CA: University of California Press.

Brown, W., Murphy, N., & Malony, H. N. (1998). *Whatever happened to the soul? Scientific and theological portraits of human nature.* Minneapolis, MN: Augsburg Fortress Publishers.

Callahan, S. (1986). *Adrift: Seventy-six days lost at sea.* New York: Ballantine Books.

Damasio, A. (1994). *Descartes' error: Emotion, reason, and the human brain.* New York: Putnam.

Gardner, H. (1983). *Frames of mind: The theory of multiple intelligences.* New York: Basic Books.

Grenz, S. J. (2001). *The social God and the relational self: A Trinitarian theology of the Imago Dei.* Louisville, KY: Westminster John Knox.

Johnson, M. (1987). *The body in the mind: The bodily basis of meaning, imagination, and reason.* Chicago: University of Chicago Press.

Menninger, K. (1938). *Man against himself.* New York: Harcourt, Brace, Javonivich.

Nussbaum, M. (2001). *Upheavals of thought: The intelligence of emotion.* Cambridge: Cambridge University Press.

Pannenberg, W. (1970). *What is man? Contemporary anthropology in theological perspective*, trans. D. A. Priebe. Philadelphia: Fortress.

Pannenberg, W. (1985). *Anthropology in theological perspective,* trans. M. J. O'Connell. Philadelphia: Westminster.

Sacks, O. (1995). *An anthropologist on Mars: Seven paradoxical tales.* New York: Alfred A. Knopf.

Schacter, D. L. (1996). *Searching for memory: The brain, the mind, and the past.* New York: Basic Books.

Taylor, C. (1989). *Sources of the self: The making of the modern identity.* Cambridge, MA: Harvard University Press.

Tillich, P. (1951). *Systematic theology* (Vol. 1). Chicago: University of Chicago Press.

Tillich, P. (1957). *Systematic theology* (Vol. 2). Existence and the Christ. Chicago: University of Chicago Press.

Tillich, P. (1963). *Systematic theology* (Vol. 3). Life and the Spirit: History and the Kingdom of God. Chicago: University of Chicago Press.

White, E. G. (1903). *Education.* Mountain View, CA: Pacific Press.

Response to "Mental Health and Human Wholeness: Implications from Biblical Anthropology"

Bruce Anderson

Anthropology is defined as the science that deals with the origins, the physical and cultural development, and the social customs and beliefs of humankind. More simply, anthropology is the study of humanity. In his paper "Mental Health and Human Wholeness: Implications from Biblical Anthropology," Richard Rice invites us to consider mental health, wholeness, and the nature of humanity from the perspective of Scripture, especially from Genesis 1 and 2, and from the healing ministry of Jesus. In doing so, Dr. Rice makes assertions about the nature of humans based on the authority of biblical revelation, including the revelation of God in Christ commonly referred to as The Incarnation.

The audacity of these assertions challenges contemporary thinking by advocating the Christian view that humanity can be understood only from the perspective of divine revelation. It suggests that as humans we have our origins in the divine and find ultimate meaning in the transcendent. Such assertions challenge current orthodox beliefs that humans are the result of the processes of natural selection, and that human personality structures reflect not heavenly origins, but are concretions growing from human aggressive and sexual impulses. They challenge the belief that culture and society are economic at their core, and are entirely the result of controlling capital and the means of production. Our modern ideas of what constitutes humanity are founded on these ideas of Darwin, Freud, and Marx.

The Christian worldview advocated by Dr. Rice is also a gauntlet thrown in the face of ideas subsumed under the term post-modernism. At their most extreme, such ideas claim that words have no intrinsic or real meaning—that meaning can be understood only from the context which assigns significance to them. Although most would find a certain common sense in the recognition that speech and language are influenced by culture, following these ideas to their extreme destroys the possibility of language bearing any fixed meaning. These ideas also imply that words expressing ideas about God or the transcendent are meaningless.

The poetic beauty and truthfulness of John 1 stands in opposition to such deconstruction of language, and responds with language which actually represents the good and true and beautiful. The inspired and resonant words "In the beginning was the Word, and the Word was with God, and the Word was God" (1:1, NIV) answer the nihilism of extreme postmodernism and assert the power of words, and the Word which first was. By this Word all creation was called to be. By this Word God enters the creation which exists because of His words. The rest of this poem asserts that by this Word a human receives an illuminating moral compass available to everyone. It further asserts that by this Word humanity may reclaim themselves as children of God, and finally, although rejected by humanity, this Word blazes the glory of the Son into eternity.

Let us consider the four perspectives of Professor Rice's paper, recognizing the breathtaking breadth of his topic. First is a consideration of the nature of human existence from a biblical perspective. This is followed by the nature of the divine imprint on humanity, which is then followed by the problem of sin separating humanity from divinity. The final perspective is that of Christ's ministry of healing and salvation, the hope of restoration, and, by implication, the hope of glory.

The first construct, the human as creature, depends on Scripture and especially on Genesis. The creatureliness of humankind puts humans in the created and divinely appointed order. God blessed the physical creation of people and animals, but human frailty and mortality resulted from the fall. The body not only symbolizes the person, but is the person until death. Humanity and individuality necessitate social reciprocity, and even resurrection assumes a social communal quality as "the dead in Christ" rise together and are reunited.

From the Christian viewpoint, the nature of humanity must include consideration of what "the image of God" implies. In this second construct, Dr. Rice considers the dominion of humankind over nature—human ability to reason and to imagine, to make decisions, and to love, to feel, to work, and to appreciate beauty. This construct points especially to the spiritual nature of humanity as evidence of the divine imprint. The complexity of the interactions of mind and body are illustrated in activities of celebration and acts of worship. Worship may involve all of the senses as well as physical acts such as standing and kneeling, or, in the case of Muslims, prostrating themselves five times daily in the direction of Mecca. This unity and connectedness of mind and body leave little room for Cartesian division between psyche and soma, or Platonic distinction between heavenly ideal and earthly reality. The fact that Adam and Eve were placed in a garden with the task of caring for it gives significance to the deep satisfaction some find in planting and tending, interacting with vegetation and the soil.

Sin as the fundamental human problem is addressed in the third construct. Christianity asserts there is something drastically wrong with us called sin, but what is it? We are broken. Who or what will mend us? Out of harmony with the divine will, we sinners fight, we compete, and we often destroy both ourselves and each other.

The awareness that we are not what we should be haunts us from our earliest years. In her Sabbath School my three-year-old granddaughter sings this song with some understanding:

> *Satan makes my heart all dark with sin,*
> *Jesus makes it white when He comes in.*

From hard-won experience we sense that the words are true. But is sin a specific breaking of the Decalogue or the consequence of our being lawless, rebellious individuals who also transgress the moral law? Or is it a broken relationship causing isolation from our peers and estrangement from God? Is sin simply humanity's state of being?

We sense it is all of these and know that we need forgiveness and healing. A lifetime of living makes us aware of the pervasive, invasive, and destructive effects of sin and leads us to yearn for forgiveness and reconciliation. Sin affects us all; none of us are undamaged or untarnished by this evil. Even the great Saint Paul said, "When I want to do good, evil is right there with me" (Rom. 7:21, NIV).

The concept of sin is neglected by modern psychology and psychiatry. Perusal of the index of any standard psychiatric text is unlikely to discover a reference to sin. I treasure an autographed copy of the book *Whatever Became of Sin?* by Dr. Karl Menninger (1973). In discussing his reasons for writing this volume, Dr. Menninger notes:

> ...I have pursued the possible usefulness of reviving the use of the word "sin"—not for the word's sake, but for the reintroduction of the concepts of guilt and moral responsibility. Calling something a "sin" and dealing with it as such may be a useful salvage or coping device. It does little good to repent a symptom, but it may do great harm not to repent a sin. Conversely, it does little good to merely psychoanalyze a sin and sometimes great harm to ignore a symptom. (p. 48)

The distinction drawn by Dr. Menninger between sin and symptom resonates with the experience of Christian psychiatrists and psychotherapists who encounter guilt in the troubled persons who consult them. Is the guilt experienced by a patient based on destructive behavior which violates the universal moral code recognized in every culture? Is this behavior actually a sin requiring repentance, confession, and perhaps restitution? Guilt may be symptomatic of major psychiatric illness or may be a sign of moral awareness and health in a patient who knows he or she should feel guilt in this circumstance. Conversely, a failure to experience guilt may represent a failure of moral judgment or of superego development.

Pathological guilt is guilt rooted in disturbed thinking and in mental illness. An extreme example of symptomatic guilt is that experienced by profoundly depressed Christians who believe that they have committed the "unpardonable sin." A troubled patient may focus on what seems a minor failure or a long-forgotten and forgiven lapse many years in the past, which becomes re-emergent with the advent of psychiatric illness. Such thinking is usually refractory to logic or good theology. The suggestion that if the individual had really committed the unpardonable sin, then he or she would be unconcerned instead of preoccupied with guilty self-recriminations, may be theologically sound. However, this sort of interpretation is certain to fall on deaf ears if the ears belong to a delusional depressed person.

Making the distinction between guilt which is irrational and guilt which represents a violation of the patient's own moral code requires the judgment of experienced therapists who are mature in their own spiritual and moral growth. Such recognition of sin as a human reality will never justify an attitude of criticism or condemnation. Rather it recalls the therapeutic intervention of our Master who in a similar situation stated, "Then neither do I condemn you." Then He furnished the injunction, "Go now and leave your life of sin" (John 8:11, NIV).

Finally Professor Rice reaches the fourth and hopeful construct—that of humanity, salvation, and healing. Salvation, restoration, and renewal are all part of the healing offered by Jesus. The miracles of Jesus, usually instant miraculous physical healing, were an affront to the religious authorities of His day as they believed that illness and poverty indicated divine disapproval. Christ indiscriminately healed sick people in need. Their only qualification appeared to be their illness and their desire for healing. Just as miraculous and just as freely offered was the healing of divine forgiveness. Jesus was especially fond of sinners and the sick and forgave and healed all who would accept His gifts. Ellen White points out that Christ longed to heal all the misery He encountered at Bethesda, but abstained from doing so because such an act performed on the Sabbath would arouse hostility and prejudice that would prematurely end His work (White, 1940, p. 201).

The concluding segment is entitled "The Implications of Wholeness for Mental Health." Here we are reminded of our human need for healing of every sort. We are reminded by the multifaceted nature of humanity that no psychiatric or psychological disease is merely mental, that every emotional disorder is also a physical illness or at least causes physical symptoms. No bodily disease is without its mental and spiritual dimensions.

Belief in the unity of mind and soul and body has characterized the philosophy advocated by Loma Linda University. This unity was a theme of the career of Dr. Jack Provonsha, physician-ethicist and founder of the LLU Center for Christian Bioethics. Psychiatrists, especially Christian ones, have long appreciated the fact that humans are not divisible into mental and physical, soul and soma. Diagnostic classifications are necessary, but can obscure the reality which is daily appreciated by psychiatric physicians. An example is the DSM (*Diagnostic and Statistical Manual of Mental Disorders)* classification "Major depressive disorder, with psychotic features." Such terminology has the virtue of being definable and descriptive, but does not begin to encompass the devastating condition which these words seek to describe. This illness pervades the entire being of a suffering patient bearing this diagnosis.

This is a disease often associated with a host of physical "vegetative" symptoms. Such patients may stop eating and suffer severe weight loss and inanition. They may become severely dehydrated; they may develop renal failure or electrolyte disturbances. Some would starve without medical and psychiatric intervention. Most are incapable of thinking clearly about what is wrong with them. The brain, the organ of awareness and self-observation, fails in these functions. Such patients may not be capable of rendering informed consent for treatment and may require the intervention of the court to confirm their inability to understand their condition or provide consent for the lifesaving treatment they may require. Some are certain that their digestion has failed and eating is pointless; delusions of poverty or guilty delusions of imagined crimes may invade their thoughts.

Such symptoms are only the most dramatic demonstrations of the reality of the mind-body unity. Every psychiatric and psychological condition may be accompanied by troubling and often disabling physical symptoms such as sleeplessness, restless agitation, and anxiety. Such conditions may be accompanied by signs such as tachycardia, tremor, and tachypnea. Just as severe and at times immobilizing are the emotions and attitudes which are so often evident in these patients, such as hopelessness and helplessness. To these demoralized souls the opportunity to end their own lives may seem the only possible escape from present misery. Suicide is a great risk and a real temptation to individuals who can imagine no other exit from their troubles.

The Christian worldview gives the believer a sense of purpose and a place in the divine will and divine creation. These priceless advantages benefit all believers, including mental health practitioners. How can such advantages be used to assist patients who do not believe? It is the task of professionals who hold such values to represent them non-coercively to their clients, while respecting the autonomy and individuality of each person. Doing so is a challenge to the conscientious Christian psychotherapist or psychiatrist. The use of spiritual methods in psychotherapy, including prayer and forgiveness, must be done in a manner which is respectful of the qualities of autonomy, decision-making, and responsibility which are so often compromised of both sin and illness.

All of us, no matter how fully we pursue a life of health and renewal, are incomplete, unfulfilled, and unwell this side of a better land, the new earth. The Christian call for wholeness and healing described so eloquently by Dr. Rice is a call for recognition of our origins in the divine purpose. It is a call to understand our creatureliness as well as the divine imprint deep within us. Human wholeness is yearned for by mortals who recognize the divine initiative and who have discovered the nature and character of the One who calls them to mental and physical health and to a glorious reunion with that Caller in a better place.

REFERENCES

Menninger, K. (1973). *Whatever became of sin?* New York: Hawthorn Books, Inc.

White, E. G. (1940). *The Desire of Ages.* Mountain View, CA: Pacific Press.

The Science of Psychology and the Ethics of Freedom: An Adventist's Perspective

Gerald R. Winslow[15]

"It is love alone which in the sight of Heaven makes any act of value."
(Ellen White, 1911, p. 487)

The science of psychology presents Adventist ethics with a distinctive set of questions. Ethics is the study of morally responsible human life. A responsible life requires freedom. Human psychology, to the extent that it adheres to the conventional norms of science, seeks explanations of phenomena based on their necessary and sufficient causes. Early in the history of Seventh-day Adventist education and health care, the church made an unusual commitment for a small, biblically grounded sectarian community of faith: we chose to link our theology to the highest possible pursuit of the sciences, especially the health sciences. For well over a century Adventists have pursued the education of students, and the care of patients, based on the conviction that Scripture and nature are both sources of truth, and that truth is ultimately unified.

With this conviction, foundational questions arise about ethics: Are advances in scientific psychology, with the gold standard of predictability, compatible with the ethics of freedom? Should the clinical application of psychology seek to be both artful *and* scientific? These questions have continued to be discussed for decades. Progress in the genetics of human behavior along with recent studies in brain imaging relative to human decisions have, if anything, deepened our puzzlement. What are the prospects for concord between belief in human freedom and completely scientific explanations of our mentation? If the science of psychology triumphs, will ethics be the casualty?

15. I acknowledge, with gratitude, long and generous conversations with two of my colleagues as I prepared this paper—Professor Henry Lamberton, theologian and psychologist, and Professor David Larson, theologian and ethicist. I would love to blame them for the mistakes here, but, alas, *mea culpa*.

This paper addresses these questions from the perspective of Seventh-day Adventist understandings of what it means to be human in the image of the Creator. In seeking answers, I will look briefly at the Adventist commitment to sound science. Then I will examine why freedom is essential to ethics, and why alliance with scientific psychology may seem tense, but should not be. In the end, I will argue that Adventists will continue to do well and do good by holding to our biblically-based theological convictions, including our strong belief in human freedom, while also pursuing the most advanced levels of science currently available to us. Even though we cannot now resolve all of the tensions between faith and science in fully coherent ways, we live best in the hope that truth is finally unitary, and the Creator will guide us continually toward better answers. The potential for squabbles between the current science of the mind and the ethics of free will are illustrative of the need for this hope. The ethical imperative to serve those who come to us for help in the best possible ways is also energized by such hope.

First, however, let me locate this paper within the context of my professional identity. I am, by calling and by choice, an ethicist. This means that I have devoted my academic life to studying the way people reason about their moral convictions. Because I am Christian, my perspectives on ethics are informed by faith in Jesus as the Messiah. My goals are essentially practical—understanding, living, and encouraging a good life, characterized by willingness to follow the way of Jesus. I side with the Christian ethics of *agapé*, or neighbor-love, made possible by the Maker's expensive gift of freedom.

I am not a scientist. Because I study neither the science of psychology nor its clinical applications, my reflections on these disciplines are suspect, and subject to correction. However, all who study ethics must incorporate some understanding of what has long been called moral psychology, because any thorough analysis of moral virtues and actions includes attention to concepts such as motivation and intention. A perspective on the dynamics of human decisions is essential to ethics.

Ethicists are also typically interested in how people come to be moral. The opening line in Plato's dialogue, *The Meno*, is illustrative. Meno queries: "Can you tell me, Socrates, whether virtue is acquired by teaching or by practice; or if neither by teaching nor practice, then whether it comes to man by nature, or in what other way?" The rest of the dialogue, exploring the central characteristics of a virtuous human life and how a person comes to an understanding of virtue, is an intriguing exercise in moral psychology. As such, it illustrates why ethicists, even those unschooled in psychology, cannot avoid the subject. This is all the more true if the conclusions of scientific psychology are interpreted to mean that the essential requirements for a morally responsible life are illusory. Thus an ethicist, who is also Adventist, has important reasons for attending to the science of psychology.

SCIENCE

Though not a scientist, I am an enthusiastic cheerleader for increasing our scientific knowledge of human psychology. I also have some interesting windows through which to observe progress in the health sciences. For years, I have served as an ethicist on federally mandated "data safety monitoring boards" (or DSMBs) whose task it is to monitor scientific experimentation with human participants. Many of these studies have involved the testing of new medications. As the lone philosopher on these DSMBs, working with some of the world's leading medical scientists and biostatisticians, I have had the privilege, and sometimes the agony, of deciding whether or not to allow a study to continue. Unlike both the medical scientists and their patients who choose to participate in so-called "blinded" studies, and unlike even the companies or government agencies who pay for the studies, members of a DSMB are permitted to look behind the "blind" and see the data as they are generated—step by often tedious step. From this experience, I know how difficult it is to be reasonably sure if an intended therapeutic intervention really works as desired. I know the joy of watching successes unfold, as I did with the drug mycophenolate mofetil that has helped greatly to enhance the success of organ transplantation.[16] I also know the keen disappointment of deciding to halt an international study involving hundreds of patients and costing over a hundred million dollars when the DSMB could see that use of an experimental drug intended to help stroke patients was, in fact, killing many of them. This effort to find a better medicine for a major cause of death and disability was, I believe, noble. But it failed.

Being a close observer of medical research in this way has fueled a passion for evidence-based care. Such experience is not conducive to patience with excuses for slapdash work in the medical sciences. Rather, it leads to more fervor for finding out what really works. In one current example, I am helping to monitor a ten-year longitudinal study in which over 2,000 patients with cryptic, unruptured aneurysms in their brains will be randomly assigned either to a group that receives the commonly accepted treatment or a group that receives no intervention other than careful observation. The letter of one patient explaining why she chose to be in this study is, to me, both touching and convincing:

> I had a decision to make. It was my life that was in risk and unfortunately, the present situation of medical knowledge couldn't help providing an answer for me. It was then, that I was proposed to participate in the research project….I meditated about it, weighted the pros and cons, and nothing was inclining me to favor one option rather than the other. Do we intervene or do we leave it alone? So, I cut it short. Chance on a randomized trial will choose for me. With this choice, at least I had ONE certitude. I will be participating in the search of a future answer. (TEAM participating patient, 2008)

Such willingness to help advance our knowledge of medical science is a remarkable affirmation of human intelligence and nobility. I could only hope that more people in our society, including more health care professionals, shared the same commitment.

---

16. Marketed by Roche as CellCept.

This hope is enlivened by another window I have on progress in the health sciences. I am one of the founding members of the California Technology Assessment Forum (or CTAF) whose membership is mostly comprised of leading medical scientists.[17] The stated goal of this publicly accountable organization is "providing credible, evidence-based information about new and emerging medical technologies." Four times a year, the group reads documents that look like a telephone book. Then they meet in open session to debate the merits of newly proposed medical therapies. They listen to the testimony of leading experts and all interested parties. At the end, they vote, in public view, to recommend adoption of these new modalities, or not. CTAF pays large sums to conduct the most thorough analyses of the published medical literature and prepare the reports. These are then made available to the health care system and the public at no charge. Time and again, medical manufacturers, patients' advocacy groups, or entrepreneurial health care professionals will argue for new treatments or diagnostic tests that have insufficient scientific evidence in their favor.

My work with CTAF for over a decade has convinced me of the profound need for greater commitment to evidence-based health care. I am, of course, keenly aware of the vast differences between, say, double-blind, randomized clinical trials with pharmaceuticals and what would be possible in the study of the clinical applications of psychology. However, to the extent that psychological interventions can be based on empirical evidence, there are both epistemological and ethical reasons to seek the evidence and be guided by it.

The conviction that we should pursue the most advanced possible science for health care is one of the best gifts of Adventist faith. Thanks significantly to Ellen White's influence, Adventists have committed to understanding both Scripture and nature, which we often call God's

17. The work of this organization is described at http://www.ctaf.org/

"second book" (Delafield, 1975, p. 127).[18] White never dismissed human reason or the pursuit of science: "The Lord does not sanction in any one of us a blind, stupid credulity. He does not dishonor the human understanding, but, far from this, He calls for the human will to be brought into connection with the divine will" (1961, p. 310). She wrote with favor about the "kingly power of reason" in human lives (White, 1905).[19] Repeatedly, she affirmed the harmony of all truth, whether from special revelation or from the study of the natural world: "All truths, whether in nature or revelation, agree" (White, 1884, p. 161). "True science and inspiration are in perfect harmony" (White, 1930, p. 189). Ellen White knew that science could be true or false, done well or poorly. She knew the same about theology. She consistently urged people to grow in their understanding of truth, whether from Scripture or from nature.

When Loma Linda University, one of the Adventist church's pioneering health sciences centers, was first established, Ellen White insisted: "The medical school at Loma Linda is to be of the highest order" (White, 1910, p. 18). At a time when other medical schools in this country were being closed because of their slipshod education, White admonished the leaders at Loma Linda to meet all the requirements so that our graduating physicians could be fully qualified and licensed. She chided leaders for their failure to support the necessary education of young Adventist scholars, thus losing important time in the development of our institutions (White, 1948, vol. 5). The fact that Loma Linda's medical school, then called the College of Medical Evangelists (CME), became fully accredited by the American Medical Association only a dozen years after its founding was nothing short of

18. Delafield (1975), p. 127: "Mrs. White loved the beauty of the natural world. To her, nature was God's second book." The metaphor of nature as God's "second book" has a long history in Western thought. Galileo used this metaphor to explain why the science that led to an understanding of a heliocentric solar system could not contradict Scripture because both nature and the Bible were God's "books."

19. White (1905), p. 130: "The kingly power of reason, sanctified by divine grace, is to bear sway in our lives."

amazing, even to the accreditors. White's influence can be felt in an early constituency meeting of the school, when its president, Dr. Wells Ruble, said: "It is the determination of the faculty to strengthen and improve the various courses in the school, constantly working toward the highest possible attainment in the sciences" (Ruble, 1912). When, a few years later, an emissary from the Association of American Medical Colleges spoke at CME, he confessed his surprise. "In my travels I have come across many a medical school operated by a Christian denomination; but never have I come across such a one as you are operating here along the highest scientific and professional lines, and yet motivated and characterized by the religious ideals you hold as a people" (Zapffe, 1925, p. 4). The reality that led to this wonderment was no accident. It was the result of much hard work and the firm determination to be a faith community making the fullest possible use of the sciences for the sake of human wholeness.

What does all this have to do with ethics and psychology? Adventists who study psychology and make use of that study in clinical practice have both theological and ethical reasons for being guided by highest quality scientific evidence. What is more, at least some Adventist psychologists and psychiatrists have obligations to advance our scientific understanding of this field. The goal of this affirmation is not to lay a load of guilt on colleagues who spend much of their time delivering people from the burdens of guilt. Rather, it is simply further encouragement for what many Adventist psychologists, working at research universities, are already doing.

However, a quick survey of the professional literature in psychology indicates that there is currently much discussion about the gap between scientific evidence and actual practice. How could it be otherwise when, by a conservative estimate, there are over 500 different types of psychotherapy currently offered (Eisner, 2000)? How would one needing psychological treatment choose from such a dizzying selection? Some, like Thought Field Therapy, appear to be rapidly gaining popularity despite the lack of any supporting empirical evidence (Lilienfeld,

2007). We might dismiss such developments as aberrations. Besides, it has often been said, even if such interventions are not helpful, they probably cannot harm patients. However, as Scott Lilienfeld observed: "There is increasing evidence from a variety of sources that certain forms of psychotherapy are directly harmful to patients, their family members, or both" (p. 216).

The author goes on to list eight popular therapies for which there is mounting evidence of harmfulness. The first on the list, "critical incident stress debriefing," caught my attention in a special way. Years ago, when I became more engaged in hospital administration, I was asked to approve a rather costly seminar titled "Critical Incident Stress Management." I looked into the matter, and found that this particular program is copyrighted and franchised out of headquarters in Texas.[20] The basic elements of the program include teaching on-site representatives how to conduct debriefing and defusing sessions, crisis management, and grief recovery following a traumatic incident in the workplace. Intuitively, the whole program made sense, so I signed the approval.

Then, mostly out of curiosity, I began to see if there was empirical evidence in the published literature that would support critical incident stress debriefings. One might imagine my own distress when I found more than one study suggesting that such debriefings led to significantly worse outcomes for the people who experienced them. Additional studies have more recently reached the same conclusion (Carlier, Lamberts, van Uchelen, & Gersons, 1998; Litz, Gray, Bryant, & Adler, 2002; McNally, Bryant, & Ehlers, 1997).

Such results are, of course, disappointing. Science is often this way. Without question, the people who promote critical incident stress debriefings mean well. Good intentions, however, do not compensate for bad facts. Unless some countervailing evidence emerges, showing benefits for most participants, it would be irresponsible to promote the practice.

---

20. The organization's web address is http://www.criticalincidentstress.com/home.

As the evidence against such debriefings has accumulated, it has been interesting to observe the responses of what might be called true believers. There is typically some expression of certainty that the studies must have been poorly done, or that the people engaged in the studies really did not know how to conduct the debriefings properly, or that future evidence will overturn the matter. Perhaps this should not surprise us. One leading physician and hospital CEO for the Mayo Clinic recently reported that it takes an average of seventeen years between finding conclusive scientific evidence in favor of changes in medical practice and the general adoption of those changes (Rupp, 2008).

There will always be some gaps between what is learned empirically and the clinical application of that knowledge. This is partly because of normal human resistance to change. More positively, it is also the inevitable result of the fact that science, when applied to fellow humans, must always be used artfully. No two humans share exactly the same biography or have precisely the same needs. Science can give us important information about what happens on average, and what the probability of error in our measurements is. But science can never tell us with complete certainty that a particular intervention will work the same way for all persons. This is reason enough for humility in making the linkage between science and its clinical application.

There are also more fundamental reasons for humility about science. Newton could show us, for example, how the laws of gravity would predict elliptical orbits for the planets of our solar system. But he could not tell us what gravity is or why it works the way it does. We still do not know. Often we must settle for sufficient evidence to achieve practical ends. Always, our attempts to explain the world empirically will face limit questions.

One of my favorite examples, from the work with CTAF, involved deliberations about "Sea-Bands." These elastic wristbands each have a little plastic bump imbedded in them.[21] The bump is designed to put

21. One can read all about Sea-Bands at http://www.sea-band.com/seaband.htm.

pressure at a specific spot on the inside of the wrist, called the Nei Kuan pressure point by traditional Chinese medicine. It was identified centuries ago and used in a practice we now call acupressure. Pressure on this point of a person's wrist, it was claimed, would eliminate or greatly reduce nausea.

Imagine the skepticism about this on the part of medical scientists in our culture. However, high-quality scientific studies showed that properly placed Sea-Bands were significantly more beneficial than sham bands that had no pressure point, or deliberately misplaced Sea-Bands, with the pressure button on the outside (or top) of the wrist (cf. Ferrara-Love, Sekeres, & Bircher, 1996). What is more, women with the nausea associated with pregnancy fared significantly better with properly placed Sea-Bands than their randomly selected counterparts who received standard medications or placebos. The CTAF panel was convinced. The evidence was elegant and powerful. But how do the little things really work? What is the mechanism? What are the pathways? No one knows. The fact that they do work, and that they have no observed, harmful side effects was good enough.

This story illustrates the deeper reason for scientific humility. Empirical evidence matters, and we have ethical obligations, when we care for others, to pay attention to that evidence. But scientific explanations always have limits.[22] This is not a bow to irrationality nor an excuse for spooky explanations. It is simply appropriate humility, and a call to push the limits.

In the case of psychology, it is my unschooled impression that the field will continue to benefit from a more thoroughly established scientific basis. An article by Alan Kazdin, a psychologist who teaches at Yale University, strengthened this impression (Kazdin, 2008). The author acknowledges the major methodological hurdles that must be

---

22. For a classic explanation of "limit questions," see Toulmin, S. (1950). *An examination of the place of reason in ethics.* Cambridge, England: University of Cambridge Press, especially the chapter on science and ethics.

overcome in order to secure adequate empirical evidence to support psychological treatments and overcome the "research-practice gap." He suggests that the use of more qualitative research methods will help, and so will a more systematic repository for the careful observations of clinical psychologists. Kazdin contends that, if we really want to improve the quality of patient care, more should be done to bridge the gulf between clinical research and practice. He concludes that "The best practice will continue to be based on the best science" (p. 157).

This makes good sense to me. But it leads to questions about what the applied science of psychology will mean for our understanding of human freedom. Will an ethical imperative to base psychological treatments on science paradoxically destroy the foundation of ethics?

FREEDOM

Though usually unspoken, one nagging reason for people of faith to have concerns about the application of scientific explanations to human behavior is that belief in human freedom may appear increasingly implausible. The more human actions can be explained in terms of sufficient causes, the less it may seem sensible to hold people responsible for their actions. This seems especially true for people whose ethical foundations are built on the conviction that our existence was made possible by a loving Creator who grants us freedom and holds us accountable for our behavior.

We, whose imaginations are shaped by the biblical narratives, are told little about the deliberation that led to God's decision to create human beings: "Let Us make man in Our image, according to Our likeness; let them have dominion…" (Gen. 1:26, KJV). It could have been otherwise. Nothing compelled the Creator to make humans in His image. It was an act of love, and, as such, freely chosen. Because "God is love" (1 John 4:7, NIV), He chose to create persons who can respond freely and creatively. In granting us dominion over the rest of creation, the Maker of heaven and earth took the risk that we might not use our freedom to trust Him or to seek the wholeness of all realms of creation. As it turned out, this was a very costly choice. As we get the story, "The Lord was grieved that he had made man on the earth, and his heart was filled with pain" (Gen. 6:6, NIV). But, as John Polkinghorne has so memorably remarked, "a world with a possibility of sinful people is better than one with perfectly programmed machines...[and] a world allowed to make itself is better than a puppet theatre with a Cosmic Tyrant" (2003, p. 14).

There are probably few, if any, passages in the works of Ellen White more frequently quoted than this: "Every human being, created in the image of God, is endowed with a power akin to that of the Creator—individuality, power to think and to do" (White, 1952, p. 15). Whatever else it means to be created in God's "image," it means that we can take responsibility for our own actions. One of the chief functions of true education is to liberate human beings from the belief that they are merely the victims of circumstances. Just a few sentences after that most familiar passage, Ellen White adds: "Instead of educated weaklings, institutions of learning may send forth men strong to think and to act, men who are masters and not slaves of circumstances, men who possess breadth of mind, clearness of thought, and the courage of their convictions" (p. 18).

Some imagine a world in which people are entirely "slaves of circumstances." Determinism pictures just such a universe. On this view, all events, including all of what appear to be human choices, are the results of prior, necessary, and sufficient causes. Such a world can be imagined, and many claim to be devout believers in determinism. But it would be very difficult to live as if this were true. Even the most avowed determinists often seem to betray hope that other people will act responsibly, and even be willing to change their beliefs to favor determinism because of arguments or evidence.

This irony first dawned on me when I read B. F. Skinner's *Beyond Freedom and Dignity*. Skinner laments the fact that "Physics and biology have come a long way, but there has been no comparable development of anything like a science of human behavior" (1971, p. 3). If we are to solve the pressing problems of our world, so many of which are caused by human misbehavior, Skinner tells us that we need a scientifically based "technology of behavior." One might think that Skinner's book would be a tedious jeremiad, decrying our foolish misbehavior and lamenting the sad fact that scientific psychology bids us relinquish our outdated notions of human freedom and dignity.

Instead, the book is mostly a cheerful discourse that celebrates the possible triumphs of science over human conduct. It is filled with the hope that scientifically based manipulation of our behavior will lead to the creation of a more humane world—a world with more rewards and fewer threats of punishment. Just as we should not blame or praise people for the genetic heritage that makes them tall or brown-eyed, we should not hold people responsible for behaviors that were surely caused by the contingencies of prior stimuli. In Skinner's words: "A scientific analysis shifts both the responsibility and the achievement to the environment" (1971, p. 23). Skinner not only describes the world as he sees it, but he also envisions and prescribes a better world. Here is the incongruity.

I was only a couple of chapters into the book when I tried to imagine vividly what it would be like to live in Skinner's (or anyone else's) deterministic world. One of the first effects, I thought, would be to lose interest in Skinner's book. If his thesis were true, then he had no choice in adopting it. His belief or disbelief in behaviorism could hardly be the only exception to his lockstep world of cause and effect. His own expressed convictions would merely be the necessary results of the accidents of his own genetic inheritance, mixed with the contingencies the various stimuli to which he had been subjected. So every idea in the book had to be the way it is. My responses to the book's thesis would be completely predetermined by the fluky influences in my life. Just so, all of his readers' reactions to Skinner's prescriptions would already be determined by their biographies. In a deterministic world, our visions of a good, better, or best life would be prefabricated for us by the forces that had already shaped us. Whether people built and used hospitals, amusement parks, or concentration camps would simply be a matter of fateful destiny.

At this point, I put the book down. I still own it, and I take it out from time to time, as I did for writing this paper, just to remind myself that I am free to read it, or not. I am at liberty to believe it, or, in my case, to find it incredible.

While a deterministic world, like Skinner's, is possible to imagine, it is obviously contrary to convictions on which ethics depends. It would be incoherent to hold ourselves responsible for our actions about which we had absolutely no choice. There would be no reason to praise heroic human actions, and none to hold scoundrels accountable. One of the truisms of ethics is that "ought implies can."[23] If, for example, a person is demented to such a degree that he or she is unaware of his or her own actions, we may find those actions regrettable but we do not find the person blameworthy. This is because we make a distinction between people who are sufficiently in control of themselves and those who, through no choice of their own, do not have self-control. It also explains why cultures typically establish a threshold in human development when a person enters the age of accountability. In our culture, we sometimes even hire psychologists or psychiatrists to tell us which persons are suitably in possession of their senses so that they may stand trial for a crime. It must be a frightful responsibility to recommend whether or not someone should be tried for a capital crime, and thus possibly be executed, based on a professional assessment of his or her capacity to be responsible for past actions. Sigve Tonstad is right to say: "The entire edifice of civilization and our most basic notions of civilized behavior rest on the conviction that human beings do have a choice and that it is right to call us to account for what we do. It will be a tall order to overturn this conviction and the institutions that sustain it" (Tonstad, 2008, pp. 37–38).

23. This expression is generally attributed to Immanuel Kant, though it is actually a pithy summary of his belief that human morality requires the autonomous action of the will. See his *Groundwork of the Metaphysics of Morals*, especially part II, many editions.

It would be a tall order indeed. This is not just because our civilization consists of so many institutions that assume human freedom and responsibility. It is also because this is how God has chosen to govern the universe.[24] Whatever their differences, the major theological treatises on *agapé* agree on this: the biblical teaching of neighbor-love presupposes human capacity to act on principle, not merely impulse, in our care for others.[25] Out of love, the Creator gave us freedom and bids us share that love. "We love," according to Scripture, "because He first loved us" (1 John 4:19, NIV). Jesus teaches that all of God's revealed will can be summarized as loving God completely and loving our neighbor as we love ourselves. Paul echoes this teaching by writing: "He who loves his fellowman has fulfilled the law….Loves does no harm to its neighbor. Therefore love is the fulfillment of the law" (Rom. 13:8, 10, NIV).

Such love cannot be bullied. It depends on freedom. Coerced love would be both conceptually incoherent and experientially impossible. When the people of God were implored to "choose for yourselves this day whom you will serve" (Josh. 24:15, NIV), it was not a charade. Like us, they could choose to serve the God of love, or not. Personal choices are real, and they matter.

This does not mean that freely chosen human actions have no causes. It means that they are *self*-caused.[26] It also means that at least some personal actions are inexplicable in terms of preceding causes other than the cause we call the *will*. Such freedom will forever be outside the realm of comprehensive explanation, except in terms of self-causation. This is true, for example, of Lucifer's decision to rebel. Of this, Ellen White claims: "It is impossible to explain the origin of sin so as to give

24. White (1905), p. 16: "Love, the basis of creation and redemption, is the basis of true education."

25. See, for example, Nygren, A. (1953). *Eros and agapé.* Westminster: John Knox Press; Outka, G. (1977). *Agapé: An ethical analysis.* New Haven, CT: Yale University Press.

26. I do not use the word "self" in order to introduce a subtle dualism, as if the self were an immaterial "soul" that pushes the body around. By self, I mean the whole person with all the dimensions of her being acting harmoniously and intentionally.

a reason for its existence" (White, 1911, p. 492). Later she adds, "In the final execution of the judgment it will be seen that no cause for sin exists. When the Judge of all the earth shall demand of Satan, 'Why hast thou rebelled against Me, and robbed Me of the subjects of My kingdom?' the originator of evil can render no excuse" (White, 1911, p. 503). The fact that Satan has no excuse and that we cannot explain sin's origin means that there was nothing in Satan's created nature or in his nurture that could explain his choice. The explanation is simply that he chose, of his own accord. Only Satan can say, "The Devil made me do it."[27]

Based both on revelation and on examination of our own experience, it is reasonable to pursue inquiry in ethics with the assumption of human freedom. All human inquiry must begin with some fundamental assumptions. We encounter every perception with some concepts already in mind. It is coherent, then, to begin with those assumptions that seem most certain to us, while acknowledging, in all humility, that they can be opened to revision. When it comes to the choice between determinism and freedom, what I find undeniable is the convergence between what Scripture says about how we are made for creativity and choice and my own inner experiences of creativity and choice. Sometimes, as I walk across the campus where I work, I deliberately take a different route even if it means taking more time. I do this, in part, just to remind myself that I am free. I am not only more like a bus than a tram, I am more like the driver of the bus.

While there is no way, outside of direct experience, to prove empirically that I am free, there is also no way to prove that I am not. All of the empirical data from brain scans that show the brain's activity just before the supposed "decision" to move a limb, for example, only beg this question: "What happened just before that?" It is possible, of course, that prior causal events led to that brain activity, and that these events were also caused through an airtight chain of events that

27. An expression used, one supposes, by multitudes but made famous by Flip Wilson (1933–1998), who also said, "What you see is what you get."

reaches all the way back to the moment of creation. I find this view incredible partly because of my direct experiences of choice and also because today's sciences, especially quantum physics with its emphasis on evidence and indeterminacy, raise doubts about the reality of such a lockstep universe.

I do not have the capacity to understand sufficiently, let alone represent accurately, the best current thinking about the relationship between quantum mechanics and the human experience of consciousness. But I do understand enough to know that some of the most accomplished scientists are now proposing hypotheses that reopen the possibility of freedom at the boundary between phenomena described by the classical physics of predictable causes and effects and the fog of decoherence and unpredictability of quantum effects. The most intriguing of the recent proposals (of which I am aware) comes from theoretical biologist and philosopher Stuart Kauffman in his latest book (Kauffman, 2008).[28] Kauffman believes that the application of quantum physics to the biology of the brain could lead us to understand that morally responsible free will is a reality. Time will tell whether hypotheses of this sort achieve support through empirical studies. But, at the very least, such hypotheses remind us of how much we still do not know, and how the future of science is not closed to the mystery of human consciousness and the reality of human freedom.

When my colleague, the neurologist Daniel Giang, contends that our understanding of human mentation must be "physics all the way down," I am inclined to respond that even physics is not physics all the way down if we are referring to the classical physics of predictable

---

28. It should be noted that Kauffman seeks a science that requires no Creator. Other scholars, working from a theistic perspective, have found quantum effects in the brain to open new potential for understanding the reality of human freedom. Among these, theoretical physicist and theologian Sir John Polkinghorne has probably been the most influential. See, for example, his *Faith, Science, and Understanding* (New Haven: Yale University Press, 2000).

effects from sufficient causes. Giang knows this, of course. He entertains briefly the possibility that we might turn to quantum physics for the explanation of our apparent experience of free will. Then he rightly concludes that "a brain that decides based on randomness is no more 'free' than a brain that decides based on other forms of physics" (Giang, 2008, p. 79). While true, this may overlook proposals, like Kauffman's, that find the possibility of intentionality and freedom at the boundary between the phenomena of classical physics and the strange world of quantum physics. In any event, I agree with Giang that what is needed for the reality of human freedom is not the randomness of indeterminacy but an opening for the emergence of self-control.

Even as we wait for scientific results from proposals like Kauffman's, we are free to describe our own inner experience of selecting one alternative future from the vast range often open to us, and then acting to realize it. As is true of the inner experience of pain, no one has more expertise on the phenomenon of free will than the person who exercises it. When I reflect at length on my facility for decisions, what I find most astonishing is the seemingly endless capacity of the human imagination. I have no exceptional gift, like that of the most creative science fiction writers, for picturing different futures. Still, I can imagine working as a stevedore or climbing Mount Denali. I can even envisage my own demise and a world without me in the future, just as it was bereft of my presence for millennia before I arrived. I can find myself in the picture drawn by the poet:

> Two roads diverged in a yellow wood
> And sorry I could not travel both
> And be one traveler, long I stood
> And looked down one as far as I could
> To where it bent in the undergrowth[29]

Imagination is the crucial engine of choice. All of us look as far as we can around the bends of many divergent paths. If this is not true,

29. Robert Frost, "The Road Not Taken."

then we are all being systematically deceived regarding our continual need to make decisions about the selection of a school, or a career, or a spouse, or reading this paper. I believe we are not so deceived. For me it is a matter of faith in God's character of love and a matter of attending carefully to the dynamics of my capacity for freedom. I know myself to be responsible. So, I contend, do the neuroscientists who design and carry out those experiments intend to describe what happens in the firing of neurons when choices are made. So do the psychologists who seek a better understanding of human thought and action. They also know that they could have done otherwise.

CONCLUSION

The key elements of my thesis can now be summarized. Evidence-based psychology is not a threat to Christian ethics, founded on God's love and made possible by His gift of free will. Failure to seek credible, empirical evidence for psychology and the practices of psychotherapy is both clinically dubious and ethically irresponsible. Because freedom is the Creator's gift to us, no amount of scientific evidence will provide a full account of why people behave the way they do. Thus, scientific psychology will always face limits. While the details differ widely, the reality of limit questions in the science of psychology is not different, in principle, from the similar limits in all empirical pursuits.

There are many ethical implications in the line of reasoning I have presented. Here are a few examples: It is ethically praiseworthy to pursue the best scientific methods for understanding human mental functioning. Psychological interventions should have carefully gathered evidence in their support. Therapies that enhance human freedom and responsibility are ethically desirable. Therapies that diminish human freedom and responsibility are ethically questionable. Psychological experiments involving human beings as research subjects require a high level of scrutiny to ensure that personal autonomy of all participants is safeguarded. Heavy use of psychotropic medications, without appropriate care for the deeply personal dimensions of mental health, is less than fully congruent with the ethical commitment to restore and preserve human wholeness with a spiritually meaningful center.

Each of these normative statements could merit its own essay of explanation and justification. That, however, is work for other times, and for other scholars who have greater knowledge about the complexities. Waiting, too, are what may be some of the thorniest ethical issues arising from the practice of coercing mentally ill and resistant patients to receive therapy. Given the perspective of this paper, forcing people to be treated for their lack of mental health must bear a heavy burden of proof. Once again, this is surely a topic deserving more space and expertise than I have here and now.

Finally, I conclude with the memorable and practical words from the Master: "If you stick with this, living out what I tell you, you are my disciples for sure. Then you will experience for yourselves the truth, and the truth will free you" (John 8:31–32, MSG Bible). The "if" points to freedom. We could choose not to follow the way of discipleship. But if we do follow, we will find that truth liberates us. With help from the Spirit, we need not fear going wherever all the truth leads. Nothing but the Creator's love is necessary to assure us of this. With this assurance, we are free to pursue the best science, including the best of scientific psychology, and we are free to live ethically responsible lives.

REFERENCES

Carlier, I. V. E., Lamberts, R. D., van Uchelen, A. J., & Gersons, B. P. R. (1998). Disaster-related post-traumatic stress in police officers: A field study. *Stress Medicine, 14*, 143–148.

Delafield, D. A. (1975). *Ellen G. White in Europe: 1885–1887*. Washington, D.C.: Review and Herald.

Eisner, D. A. (2000). *The death of pyschotherapy: From Freud to alien abductions*. Westport, CT: Praeger Publishing.

Ferrara-Love, R., Sekeres, L., & Bircher, N. G. (1996). Nonpharmacologic treatment of postoperative nausea. *American Society of PeriAnesthesia Nurses, 11*, 378–383.

Giang, D. (2008). Physics all the way down. *Spectrum, 36*(4), 41–45, 78–80.
Kauffman, S. A. (2008). *Reinventing the sacred: A new view of science, reason, and religion.* New York: Basic Books.
Kazdin, A. E. (2008). Evidence-based treatment and practice. *American Psychologist, 63,* 157.
Lilienfeld, S. O. (2007). The assault on scientific mental health. In P. Kurtz (Ed.), *Science and Ethics,* pp. 208–223. Amherst, NY: Prometheus Books.
Litz, B. T., Gray, M. J., Bryant, R. A., & Adler, A. B. (2002). Early intervention for trauma: Current status and future directions. *Clinical Psychology: Science and Practice, 9,* 112–134.
McNally, R. J., Bryant, R. A., & Ehlers, A. (1997). Does early psychological intervention promote recovery from posttraumatic stress? *Psychological Science in the Public Interest, 4,* 45–49.
Polkinghorne, J. (2003). *Belief in God in an age of science.* New Haven, CT: Yale Nota Bene.
Ruble, W. A. (1912, March). Speech to the constituency of the College of Medical Evangelists. Loma Linda, CA.
Rupp, W. (2008, July). Presentation to Loma Linda University Medical Center's clinical leadership retreat.
Skinner, B. F. (1971). *Beyond freedom and dignity.* New York: Bantam Books.
TEAM participating patient (2008, June). *A team participant testimony.* TEAMSTUDY Newsletter. Retrieved April 1, 2009, from http://www.teamstudy.org/newsletter/TEAMSTUDY_newsletter_June2008.html
Tonstad, S. (2008). Modern neuroscience and the notion of freedom. *Spectrum, 36*(4), 35–40.
White, E. G. (1884). Science and Revelation. *Signs of the Times, 10*(11), p. 161.
White, E. G. (1905). *The ministry of healing.* Mountain View, CA: Pacific Press.
White, E. G. (1910, May 19). Statement regarding the training of physicians. *Pacific Union Recorder, 9*(27), p. 3.
White, E. G. (1911). *The great controversy.* Mountain View, CA: Pacific Press. (Original work published 1858)
White, E. G. (1930). *Messages to young people.* Hagerstown, MD: Review and Herald.
White, E. G. (1948). *Testimonies for the church* (Vols. 1–9). Mountain View, CA: Pacific Press.
White, E. G. (1952). *Education.* Mountain View, CA: Pacific Press.
White, E. G. (1961). *Our high calling.* Washington, D.C.: Review and Herald.
Zapffe, F. (1925, December 24). The Most Remarkable Medical College in America. *The Medical Evangelist, 12*(26), p. 4.

Section 3

Research: Faith and Well-being

Scientific Research on the Study of Religion/ Spirituality and Mental Health: Lessons, Positive Affirmations, and Disquieting Questions

David R. Williams

This chapter provides an overview of the scientific research that examines the relationship between aspects of religious or spiritual engagement and mental health status. It begins by outlining some of the serious mental health challenges in contemporary society. Next, it reviews a growing body of scientific research which indicates that although religious involvement has positive effects on multiple indicators of mental health, under some conditions it is adversely related to mental health. The pathways linking religious involvement and mental health are identified and the chapter concludes with lessons and challenges raised by the existing research for the Christian mental health professional.[30]

AMERICA'S MENTAL HEALTH CRISIS

Mental health problems are commonplace in contemporary society. Recent national data document that 46% of adults in the United States have had a psychiatric illness at some point (Kessler, Berglund, Demler, Jin, & Walters, 2005). The lifetime prevalence of two or more disorders is 28%. One in every four (26%) adults in the United States meet criteria for a current psychiatric disorder (past year) with 60% of these disorders rated as severe or moderately severe (Kessler, Chiu, Demler, & Walters, 2005). The 2005 National Health Interview Survey found that 11% of adults reported serious psychological distress in the past year (Pleis & Lethbridge-Cejku, 2005). That distress was associated with substance dependence or abuse. Among adults with serious psychological distress, 21% were dependent on or had abused illicit drugs or alcohol, compared to 8% of adults without serious psychological distress.

30. I wish to thank Gabriel Sirota and Veronic Aghayan for assistance with preparing the manuscript and Manuela Costa for assistance with the research.

There are also large drug problems in the United States. In 2005, the national survey on drug use and health documented the magnitude of the problem (Office of Applied Studies, 2006). Some 8.1% of the population ages twelve years old or older, or almost twenty million Americans, had used illicit drugs in the past month. Illicit drugs include marijuana/hashish, cocaine including crack, heroin, hallucinogens, inhalants, or medically prescribed drugs that are used non-medically. Also, there were 10.5 million persons ages twelve or older who reported driving under the influence of an illicit drug during the past year and 29% of Americans ages twelve or older (71.5 million people) had used a tobacco product in the previous month. This survey also documented the problem of alcohol use. In 2005, 52% of Americans ages twelve or older reported being current drinkers of alcohol. One in five persons or 23% of persons ages twelve or older had participated in binge drinking in the past thirty days. Binge drinking is defined as five or more drinks on the same occasion on at least one day in the past thirty days. In 2005, 13% of persons ages twelve or older drove under the influence of alcohol at least once in the past year.

Keyes (2007) outlines some of the serious societal implications of these high levels of mental health problems. He indicates that mental illness is one of the three most costly health conditions in the United States and one of the top five causes of disability days in the world. Other evidence indicates that although the United States leads the world in the prevalence of mental health problems, evidence from the largest coordinated mental health study ever conducted reveals that mental disorders have profound social and economic effects throughout the world (Kessler & Utsun, 2008). Research has also been giving increasing attention to the protective and risk factors that can increase or decrease an individual's chances for enjoying good mental health. Many of these factors are linked to the social contexts in which people live, learn, work, and play. One factor that we now turn our attention to is the role of religion.

RELIGION/SPIRITUALITY AND MENTAL HEALTH

Some early social scientists acknowledged that religion could play a role in mental health. Emile Durkheim (1951) argued that the social regulation, integration, and meaning provided by religious groups could be health enhancing. Durkheim studied religion primarily in terms of its impact on the levels of suicide. William James (1902), an early psychologist, indicated that "healthy-minded religion could prevent certain forms of disease as well as science does, or even better." Sigmund Freud (1961) had decidedly negative views of religion. He viewed religion as an illusion and mass neurosis, but nonetheless indicated that religious ideas could reduce anxiety and serve as a source of consolation without which many could not endure life. Freud argued that a lack of religious belief would lead to chaos and additional mental anguish. Karl Marx (1844) is known for describing religion as the opiate of the people. However, in the very paragraph in which Karl Marx made the famous declaration, he indicated that religion was nonetheless "the heart of a heartless world and the spirit of the spiritless situation" (p. 42). It appears that even Marx conceded some potential health-enhancing effects of religion.

There is growing interest in the role that spirituality or religion can play in the mental health of the population; however, this is a generally neglected topic in studies in psychiatry. A systematic review of 2,348 studies published in the four leading psychiatric journals from 1978 to 1982 found that 2.5% of the studies included a quantified religious or spiritual variable (Larson, Pattison, Blazer, Omran, & Kaplan, 1986). Less than 1% assessed religion or spirituality with minimal standards of acceptability. Only one study had applied a state of the art approach to measuring religion or spirituality. The majority of studies measured religion with the use of religious denomination, which is not regarded as an optimal or comprehensive measure of religiousness. More recent studies continue to document the neglect of religion (Weaver et al., 1998).

Research on religion and spirituality is not without debate and controversy. It has been harshly criticized in recent years on both methodological and ethical grounds (Sloan et al., 2001). Methodologically, many studies have been cross-sectional in design and have utilized inadequate controls for confounding variables and covariates so that the observed associations between religious involvement and health could be overestimated. In addition, failure to control for multiple comparisons could have contributed to some inconsistencies in the empirical findings. Moreover, some researchers argue that the study of religion and health raises a large ethical issue because an individual's religious beliefs and practices are private and personal and should therefore be outside of the purview of medical recommendations. According to this view, applying any findings from research on religiousness and spirituality to clinical practice could be problematic (Sloan et al., 1999). Major researchers in the area indicate that some of the recent criticisms have not been even-handed. Specifically, they point to omitted evidence; erroneous, incorrect, or misleading statements; and arguments about ethics being based on personal opinion and straw men rather than on scientific evidence (Miller & Thoresen, 2003). For example, Koenig et al. (1999) show that Sloan et al. (1999) discuss only twenty-four of the 300+ studies of religion and physical health, none of the 900 studies of religion and mental health, only seventeen of the nearly 100 studies of attendance and mortality, and none of the nine recent high-quality studies that had been identified.

One contributor to the conflict over the study of religion and health is a clash of worldviews. Researchers as a group are markedly less religious than the general population and many feel uncomfortable with the topic. Some researchers have suggested that merely studying religion and health would be an "anti-tenure factor" for a beginning scholar (Sherrill & Larson, 1994). Similarly, Rue (1985) indicated that the study of religion is academia's "most outrageous blind spot."

Research has documented that religious variables can play an important role in physical health. The strongest association exists for measures of religious attendance. A rigorous review of the empirical evidence relating religion to health concluded that the scientific evidence is strongest for the association between religious attendance and mortality (Powell, Shahabi, & Thoresen, 2003). They indicated that there is a strong, consistent, prospective, and often graded reduction in the risk of mortality that is associated with increasing levels of religious attendance. Even after adjusting for confounders, this association exists, although the reduction approximates 25%. They also indicated that protection of religion or spirituality against cardiovascular disease is where the association is strongest, and is largely mediated through the healthy lifestyle it encourages. An example of the study of religion and health is the study by Hummer and colleagues (Hummer, Rogers, Nam, & Ellison, 1999). This national study of over 21,000 adults followed over eight years found that attendance was associated with mortality. People who never attended religious services had a 1.9 times greater risk of death than people attending more than once a week. This pattern existed for most causes of death. This study found that at age twenty, persons who attended religious services weekly or more lived on average 7 and a half years longer than those who never attended. For blacks, the difference was 13.7 years.

RELIGION AND MENTAL HEALTH

Research has also looked at the association between religion and mental health. A critical review of seventeen studies that assess the association of religion to general indices of anxiety concluded that church attendance and other religious variables are related to decreased anxiety in several populations (Shreve-Neiger & Edelstein, 2004). Some studies find that those who lived their religion (intrinsic religiousness) have less anxiety than those who use their religion (extrinsic religiousness). However, under some conditions, religion may be associated with elevated anxiety. Catholic women, for example, tended to have higher levels of anxiety than others. Sudden religious converts have been shown to have higher anxiety in some studies, and extrinsic religious persons also show anxiety in some studies.

A meta analysis of 147 studies has also examined the association between religiousness and depressive symptoms (Smith, McCullough,

& Poll, 2003). It concluded that high levels of religious involvement were associated with fewer symptoms of depression. This association was robust, but modest in size. The association was stronger for studies of persons under stress. This review also found that an extrinsic religious orientation and negative religious coping were associated with elevated symptoms of depression.

Reviews have also been conducted on the association between religion and substance use. A review of fifty-four studies of religion and drug use found that 87% showed that religious involvement predicted a lower risk of drug abuse (Johnson, 2002). Similarly, 94% of ninety-seven studies that looked at religion and alcohol use found that religious participation was associated with a reduced tendency to initiate alcohol use or have problems with alcohol, if used. These findings exist in both retrospective and prospective studies of children, adolescents, and adults.

Research also shows that religion is associated with reduced risk of delinquency (Johnson, 2002). These studies have found a lower risk of multiple delinquent behaviors, including criminal behavior associated with religious involvement. Similarly, religious involvement has been associated with preventing delinquent behavior in high-risk urban youth. It has also been related to increased pro-social behavior in adolescents that emphasize concern for the welfare of others. In some of these studies, the effect of religious involvement is evident only at the level of the group and not at the level of the individual (Stark, 1985). That is, it is not individual religious behavior that appears to be most important, but whether the individual is in a context of other religious people.

RELIGION/SPIRITUALITY AND MENTAL HEALTH: PATHWAYS

Several mechanisms have been identified by which religion might be associated with health (Williams & Sternthal, 2007). First, religious participation can discourage negative health behaviors such as tobacco, alcohol, drugs, and risky sexual practices. Second, by encouraging moderation in all things and reducing risk-taking behavior, religious involvement can reduce exposure to stress. Third, religious institutions can provide support, intimacy, a sense of connectedness, and belonging. Fourth, religious organizations and clergy engage in a range of activities that can promote physical and mental health. Other mechanisms by which religion can affect health include the effects of religious beliefs and values in providing systems of meaning that can enable individuals to interpret and re-interpret stress. Religious beliefs can also provide feelings of strength to cope with adversity. And finally, religious institutions can also adversely affect health by generating stress, time demands, role conflicts, social conflicts, and criticism.

HEALTH PRACTICES

There is striking evidence of the role of religion in enhancing healthy behaviors. A national study of high school seniors, persons in both public and private schools, found that religious high school seniors were less likely than their non-religious peers to carry a weapon such as a gun or knife to school, to get into fights or hurt someone, to drive after drinking, to ride with a driver who had been drinking, to smoke cigarettes, and to engage in binge drinking or use marijuana (Wallace & Forman, 1998). Similarly, religious seniors were more likely to wear seatbelts; eat breakfast, green vegetables, and fruit; get regular exercise; and sleep at least seven hours per night. Similarly, in the Alameda County Study an association was documented over time with levels of religious behavior (Strawbridge, Shema, Cohen, & Kaplan, 2001). This study examined the association of frequency of attendance in 1965 with improvements or changes with healthy behaviors by 1994. Adjusted for age, sex, education, and self-rated health, there were improved healthy behaviors among persons who attended religious services weekly. They were more likely over this time period to quit smoking, to start physical activity, to stop being depressed, to get and stay married, to increase social relationships, and to stop heavy drinking. There was no association between religion and starting medical checkups. Religious individuals were also more likely to continue to not smoke, not be depressed, not get divorced or separate, keep up personal relationships, and maintain medical checkups. There was no significant association between frequency of attendance and continuing physical activity or continuing to not drink heavily.

RELIGIOUS SERVICE ATTENDANCE AS THERAPY?

Research by Ezra Griffith and colleagues (Griffith, English, & Mayfield, 1980; Griffith & Mathewson, 1981; Griffith, Young, & Smith, 1984) has also documented the potential therapeutic benefits of at least some religious services. In a study of church services in New Haven, Connecticut, these researchers documented that there were several therapeutic aspects of groups that are present within the liturgy or ritual of these services. These include providing the installation of hope, group cohesiveness, altruism, social learning, and universality. These researchers argued that several major rituals could be therapeutic. For example, testimony can provide an opportunity to talk about offenders, what to do when offended, identify with the oppressed, and provide validation for the experiences described. Other rituals within the church services also provide security, renewal, installation of hope, positive sensations (feeling good, happy, and light), and reduction of tension and catharsis. Other researchers have noted that several aspects of religious services are distinctive in the provision of opportunities to articulate and manage personal and collective suffering (Gilkes, 1980). The expression of emotion and active congregational participation can promote "collective catharsis" in ways that can facilitate the reduction of tension and the release of emotional distress.

De Sousa (2005) has summarized research on the role that songs and music can play in enabling individuals to allay anxiety. Music has been shown to relax patients in critical care units and other contexts. Music has been used to alleviate grief and sadness and to combat bouts of sadness. Music therapy has also been shown to modify the behavior of children with autism and other developmental disorders and reduce agitation in patients with dementia. De Sousa (2005) argues that music can instill joy and hope and help people maintain or regain inner peace.

RELIGIOUS INSTITUTIONS: HEALTHY OR UNHEALTHY ENVIRONMENTS?

Limited research evidence also indicates that religious congregations have psychosocial environments that can vary in their health enhancing potential. Ken Pargament and colleagues (1993) studied 352 church members in thirteen congregations and found that congregational attributes were related to psychosocial well-being. There were multiple aspects of congregations examined. They included the clergy, weekly services, education programs, facilities, policies, and social programs. Leaders and members were ranked on dimensions of congregational climate (Pargament, Silverman, Johnson, Echemendia, & Snyder, 1983). Pargament and his colleagues used a congregational climate scale that rates congregations on ten different dimensions. They were openness to change, stability, social concern, autonomy, level of activity, order/clarity, sense of community, intrinsic religious orientation, extrinsic religious orientation, and expressiveness.

These researchers found that the environments of churches varied. Small black Protestant congregations had greater expressiveness, social concern, and extrinsic climate scores. Small white Protestant congregations had higher levels of a sense of community and expressiveness, but, unlike black ones, lower levels of stability and social concern. Large white Catholic parishes had lower expressiveness and sense of community scores, but a higher activity score. Importantly, the well-being of members was related to the psychosocial environment of their congregation. For example, members who perceive more autonomy in their congregations reported higher levels of self-esteem and life satisfaction. Climate may be reciprocally determined and could reflect the role of member preferences. For example, expressiveness was negatively related to well-being in some congregations, but positively related in others. This illustrates the importance of paying attention to organizational aspects of religious spiritual environments and assessing their consequences for health.

THE CLERGY: A BRIDGE OR BARRIER TO TREATMENT?

The National Comorbidity Study (NCS) documented that clergy play a major role in the treatment of mental illness in the United States (Wang, Berglund, & Kessler, 2003). This study of 8,098 individuals from a nationally representative population study in the United States found that among individuals who sought treatment for mental disorders 25% contacted the clergy, 16% contacted psychiatrists, and 16.7% contacted general medical doctors. Nearly one quarter of those seeking help from clergy had the most seriously impairing mental disorders. The majority of persons who sought help from the clergy sought help from the clergy only. Another national study found that the clergy play an important role in helping individuals cope with serious personal crises (Neighbors, Musick, & Williams, 1998). This study found that women were more likely than men to seek help from ministers and that people with economic problems were less likely than those with death and bereavement problems to seek help from clergy. Across problem types, persons who sought help from the clergy first were less likely to seek help from other professionals. Among persons seeking help from only one source, those who use the clergy were more satisfied with the support received.

There has been considerable interest in exactly what the clergy do for persons seeking help. A study of ministers in the greater New Haven area in Connecticut provides some information (Young, Griffith, & Williams, 2003). This study found that clergy on average spend 6.2 hours per week in counseling. One third indicated that they spent less time than they wanted to and more than half indicated that they had a regular schedule for counseling sessions, with a weekly schedule being the most common. In this study most of the counseling reported by clergy was short term. Two thirds reported that the duration of their typical counseling session was three months or less. Forty percent of the clergy reported that they had seen people with severe mental illness, and two thirds reported that they had dealt with substance abuse in their congregation. Two thirds of the clergy also counseled suicidal persons, and over 60% had counseled persons they considered dangerous.

RELIGION, SOCIAL SUPPORT, AND COPING WITH STRESS

The life stress paradigm is an important perspective in assessing a potential way in which religion can affect health. Research shows that exposure to psychosocial stressors is a strong predictor of the onset and the course of some mental health problems. Social resources can improve health and reduce stress in at least three ways. Social ties can directly improve health by meeting basic needs for affection, social contact, and security. Supportive social ties can also reduce social conflict and tensions, thereby reducing stress. Social ties can also buffer the negative effect of stress on health. That is, in the face of stress, social ties can reduce at least some of the negative consequences of stress on health.

Research has found that religious institutions can serve as important sources of social support (Taylor & Chatters, 1988). Taylor and Chatters (1988) report that congregation-based friendship networks can serve as a type of extended family. Another study found that church-related friends are strongly related to life satisfaction for elderly blacks and account for the advantage and subjective well-being for older blacks (Ortega, Crutchfield, & Rushing, 1983). Religious support has also been shown to provide important benefits to both blacks and whites (Ferraro & Koch, 1994). An example of a buffering effect is a study conducted in New Haven, Connecticut, of 720 adults (Williams, Larson, Buckler, Heckmann, & Pyle, 1991). This study found that attendance at religious services did not directly reduce psychological distress. However, when followed for two years, religious attendance reduced the negative effects of the stressors (28 undesirable life events and 16 health problems) on mental health.

RELIGIOUS COPING AND MENTAL HEALTH: BELIEFS MATTER

There has also been considerable interest in the ways in which religious coping can be a resource that has health consequences. Tix and Frazier (1998) studied religious coping among patients dealing with kidney transplant surgery. They found that religious coping (for example, seeking God's help in dealing with the situation, trusting God to handle the situation, and trying to find a lesson from God in the situation) was associated with higher life satisfaction and less psychological distress both cross-sectionally and when the patients were followed prospectively. Particular religious belief systems may also create expectations and anxieties that can have consequences for mental health. The role of specific religious beliefs has been understudied in the research on religion and mental health. A study of 1,139 adults in the Detroit metropolitan area found that the belief in eternal life was positively associated with psychological well-being (Ellison, Boardman, Williams, & Jackson, 2001). This study also found a buffering effect for belief in eternal life. Belief in eternal life reduced the negative effect of some stressors (such as chronic health problems and financial problems) on psychological well-being and reduced the negative effects of work-related stress on psychological distress.

The work of Ken Pargament has also highlighted the role of positive and negative religious coping. For example, a study of 296 members of two churches coping with the Oklahoma City bombing assessed both positive religious coping and negative religious coping (Pargament, Smith, Koenig, & Perez, 1998). Negative religious coping included items like wondering whether God had abandoned them, feeling that God was punishing the victims of the bombing for their sins and lack of spirituality, and questioning whether God really exists. Pargament found that positive religious coping was associated with growth and recovery over time while negative coping was strongly predictive of symptoms of post-traumatic stress disorder (PTSD) and higher levels of callousness and insensitivity to the distress of others.

LESSONS FOR CHRISTIAN MENTAL HEALTH PROFESSIONALS

The research reviewed affirms that supportive communities, health behaviors, and positive belief systems have the potential to enhance mental health. These findings are consistent with core values of the Christian faith and provide affirmation of many tenets of Scripture. At the same time, the extant research also raises some sobering questions.

WHY STAND YE IDLE?

The high levels of psychiatric disorders in the population have important implications for the work of religious congregations. Recent research consistently finds that psychiatric disorders are more disabling than physical disorders. Depression, for example, one of the more common mental disorders, is a very disabling condition. Recent analyses of data from the World Health Surveys which examined 245,000 participants from over sixty countries found that depression is one of the leading causes of disease burden worldwide (Moussavi et al., 2007). This study found that depression produces the greatest detriment in health impairment compared with the chronic diseases like angina, arthritis, asthma, and diabetes. Thus, the high levels of stress, mental disorder, and disability raise a question of the role of the clergy and religious organizations being trained to appropriately detect, screen, and refer individuals to receive help for their mental health challenges. Failure to do this will leave considerable pain and human suffering unaddressed and will leave the church with a very impaired workforce. Attention also needs to be given to the mental health needs of clergy and their families. Although the work of the clergy can be rewarding, it is also demanding and stressful and many clergy face challenges in obtaining desired levels of social support (Weaver et al., 2002).

Some research suggests that certain religious beliefs can discourage individuals from seeking help for mental help problems. In particular, persons who regard their spirituality and faith as the most effective cure for mental illness are less likely to seek treatment (Trice & Bjorck,

2006). The challenge for Christian leaders is to identify how to find the right balance in depending on God as the source of all true healing while at the same time using all of the instruments that He has provided to accomplish this.

RELIGIOUS INSTITUTIONS: MENTAL HEALTH PROMOTION CENTERS?

Churches have also been used as centers for health promotion activities. A broad range of health screenings and health inventions have been conducted at churches. These include increased fruit and vegetable consumption; reduced outdoor advertising for alcohol and tobacco; increased weight loss; lower blood pressure; reduced energy intake, dietary intake, and sodium intake; and increased screening for breast, cervical, colon, and prostate cancer. All of these things have been done by church-based interventions. At the same time, few church-based interventions have focused heavily on mental health. For example, there have been few interventions that address stress and stress management or that explicitly deal with mental health support and recovery.

Levels of stress are high and increasing in the population. The American Psychological Association (APA, 2007) conducted a survey that documented the high levels of stress within the American population. This survey found that 79% of adults in the United States reported that they live under higher than healthy levels of stress. Thirty-two percent indicated that they are living under extreme stress and 48% believe that their stress level had increased in the last five years. Almost one half (49%) also said that stress had a negative impact on both their personal and professional lives. The leading causes of stress reported by adults in the United States were work (74%), money (73%), workload (66%), children (64%), family responsibilities (60%), and health concerns (55%). These high levels of stress suggest that there is a great need within the population for strategies to effectively cope and address stressful life situations.

HOW DO WE CREATE TRUE HEALING COMMUNITIES?

Religious communities can be a source of social networks that improve health, but they can also be a source of conflict, criticism, and stress. How can our organizational structures and processes promote psychological well-being and minimize interpersonal tensions? There is some evidence in the literature that mental health varies by religious denomination, at least for some small conservative denominations. A large population-based study in North Carolina found that even after adjustment for psychosocial variables, socio-demographic factors, life events, and social support, the levels of major depression were three times higher among Pentecostals than among persons with other religious affiliations (Meador et al., 1992). How do Seventh-day Adventists fare on mental health? Some limited evidence indicates that small Christian sects that tend to follow a strict lifestyle and live apart from the world tend to have an elevated risk of psychoses but a lower risk of neuroses (Dalgalarrondo, 1993).

HOW DO WE PREPARE OUR CONGREGANTS TO COPE WITH ADVERSITY?

Religion is a widely used coping strategy by the American population in dealing with life's stressors. Some ways of using religious beliefs can lead to adaptation and adjustment over time, while other ways can lead to worsening mental health. The Alameda County Study also provides examples of how religion can have both positive and negative buffering effects (Strawbridge, Shema, Cohen, Roberts, & Kaplan, 1998). This study found that both organizational and non-organizational religiosity reduced the negative effects of non-family stressors (such as financial problems, neighborhood stress, and chronic illness) on depression. However, non-organizational religiosity exacerbated the effects of child problems on depression. And organizational religiosity exacerbated the effects of family stressors (such as marital stress, abuse, and care-giving problems) on depression. Strawbridge suggests life's problems that raise conflicts with values emphasized by religious organizations (unruly children, difficult marriages, problems caring for older parents) may be perceived as unlikely to occur, such that when they happen they can lead to feelings of stigmatization and low levels of active conflict resolution.

WHAT IS SPIRITUALITY?

A major issue in the study of religion in health has been the problem of defining and distinguishing religion from spirituality. Harold Koenig (2008) has argued that the definition of spirituality has changed in recent decades. He indicates that although historically the language of spirituality was grounded in the practice of religious beliefs and behavior, spirituality has been redefined by some more recently in terms of subjective self-fulfillment. Importantly, he argues that some of the current definitions of spirituality, which include positive mental health and human values as part of its definition, are tautological. If one defines spirituality as positive human traits, including those that reflect good mental health, one eliminates the possibility of examining the association of spirituality with mental health. Accordingly, he argues that the growing inclusion of positive psychological factors in definitions of spirituality is a troublesome development. This problem is true of the FACIT-Sp (Functional Assessment of Chronic Illness Therapy—Spiritual Well-Being) which is one of the most commonly used measures of spirituality in studies involving cancer patients. The FACIT-Sp consists of twelve statements asking respondents to indicate their agreement. These statements include, among others, these: "I feel peaceful." "I have a reason for living." "I feel a sense of purpose in my life." "I am able to reach deep down within myself for comfort." "I feel a sense of harmony within myself." "I know that whatever happens with my illness, things will be okay." Not surprisingly, studies have found that spirituality measured in this way is related with good mental health.

A national study in the United States suggests that the relationship between religion and spirituality is quite complex (Shahabi et al., 2002). The 1998 General Social Survey found that 52% of American adults rate themselves as religious and spiritual. Ten percent rated themselves as spiritual only, 9% as religious only, and 29% as neither religious nor spiritual. Self perceptions of spirituality were associated with being younger, female, and highly educated. Self perceptions of religiosity were associated with being older, an ethnic minority, less educated, and a resident of a southern state. Importantly, individuals' self perceptions of religiousness and spirituality were related to a broad range of characteristics. Spiritual and religious adults attended religious services, prayed, meditated, read the Bible, and had more daily spiritual experiences than persons in any of the other three groups. They were less distressed and less mistrusting than the religious-only group, but they (and the religious-only group) had high levels of intolerance. The spiritual-only group was politically liberal, tolerant of diverse points of view, and unwilling to claim a denominational affiliation.

CAN CERTAIN RELIGIOUS BELIEFS AND THE CERTAINTY OF BELIEF BREED INTOLERANCE?

Some types of religious beliefs and orientations can lead to rigidity in thinking, prejudice, and intolerance. There has been a long history of interest in the relationship between religion and racial prejudice. Some of the early research found that religious people were more likely to be prejudiced than non-religious people. The more religious people were on traditional indicators of theological orthodoxy the more prejudiced they were. Subsequent research indicated that the association between religion and prejudice varied by the type of underlying religious orientation (Donahue, 1985). Among persons who were intrinsically religious, there was no association between religion and prejudice, while there was a strong relationship between religion and prejudice among the extrinsically religious. How do we train our leaders and members to rise above the normal human tendencies of in-group favoritism and out-group discrimination? How can we through our individual and institutional practices create a culture that reinforces viewing every child of humanity through heaven's eyes?

Research on the relationship between religious beliefs and domestic violence provides another window on the potential negative consequences of some religious beliefs. Some evidence suggests that conservative Christians, especially women, report elevated rates of perpetrating interpersonal violence (Drumm et al., 2006). A study in the North Pacific region of the United States found high levels of intimate partner violence among Adventists. For example, 65% of respondents reported that they had experienced controlling and demeaning behavior at least once in their lifetime (Drumm et al., 2006). These researchers suggested that theological beliefs about the headship of men and the submission of women can provide the justification for some men to perpetrate violence and the rationalization for some women to accept it. Some observers have also raised the question of whether certain eschatological beliefs can have negative consequences. Newport (2006), for example, argued that Adventism's distinctive eschatology provided the seeds that led to the development of David Koresh's theology and the tragedy of the Branch Davidians in Waco, Texas. This highlights the importance of paying greater attention to the content of religious beliefs and their potential positive and negative consequences.

HOW TO IMPROVE THE ASSESSMENT OF RELIGION IN FUTURE RESEARCH

Religious rituals and symbols have been neglected in the study of religion and health (Williams, 1994). For example, the role that Sabbath observance—a weekly mini-vacation of rest and religious activity—can have in reducing stress has not been systematically examined. The promise of thinking broadly about the pervasive ways religion can affect health is illustrated in research done by Idler and Kasl (1992). In a large study of elderly persons, research found that fewer deaths occurred immediately before or during religious holidays than in the month after religious holidays. This effect existed for both Christians and Jews and was stronger among the more observant members of religious congregations. The effects for Christians were seen only for Christian holidays and effects for Jews were evident only for Jewish holidays. The ways in which religious architecture can express ideology and facilitate social support and social control has also not been explored (Williams, 1994).

IS MENTAL HEALTH MORE THAN THE ABSENCE OF MENTAL PROBLEMS?

An important direction for future research and consideration is an expansion of the concept of mental health. Keyes (2007) indicates that mental health is more than merely the absence of psychiatric disorders. He divides the United States population in terms of mental health into individuals who are languishing, moderately mentally healthy, and flourishing. In order to be flourishing, individuals have to be characterized with both the absence of mental disorders *and* the presence of positive mental health dimensions. These dimensions include positive emotions (such as being regularly cheerful, interested in life, in good spirits, happy, calm, and peaceful), positive psychological functioning (the presence of self acceptance, personal growth, purpose in life, autonomy, and positive relations with others), and positive social functioning (social acceptance, social actualization, social contributions, and social integration). Research conducted by Keyes using national data indicates that persons who are flourishing (mentally healthy) are more productive citizens and enjoy better health on multiple dimensions. Mentally healthy adults function better than adults with moderate mental health who in turn function better than adults who are languishing. Compared to their less healthy peers, the mentally healthy have fewer disability days, lower levels of health limitations, fewer chronic physical diseases and conditions, and lower levels of health care utilization. They also have highest levels of psychosocial functioning. That is, they reported the lowest level of perceived helplessness, the highest level of functional goals (knowing what they want from life), the highest level of self-reported resilience (learning from adversities), and the highest level of intimacy (feeling very close with family and friends).

RETURNING TO A WHOLISTIC VIEW OF MENTAL HEALTH

There is increasing evidence also of the intimate connections between the physical and the mental and of the importance of good physical habits to support positive psychological well-being. One recent study found that a vegetarian diet can lead to lower levels of stress and reduced exposure to the negative mental health sequelae from exposure to stress (Varshney, Bedi, & Bhandari, 2005). Other recent research has documented the negative effects of sleep deprivation on moral judgment. One study found that two nights of sleep deprivation increases willingness of adults to agree with solutions that violate their personal normal beliefs (Kilgore et al., 2007). Another study found that after two nights of sleep deprivation, adults had difficulty in withholding an inappropriate response, even when they were able to attend to stimuli and respond accurately to stimuli (Drummond, 2006). Other research reveals that physical exercise is effective in treating depression and anxiety disorders. There appears to a dose-response relation with depression and anxiety disorders, and exercise is also associated with lower relapse rates among depressed patients (Dunn & Bettinghaus, 2006). A study of faculty at three Adventist colleges and universities found that those following good health practices reported lower levels of stress (Ashley & Cort, 2007). Thus, effective mental health interventions should be wholistic and seek more than just the recovery of illness—they should seek to promote a good life.

The Bible is clear that God wants His children to enjoy abundant health. Jesus indicated that He had come to ensure that we have an abundant life. This paper indicates that a growing body of scientific research confirms that many secrets of good mental health are found in God's revealed will in Scripture. At the same time, scientific research also indicates that distortions of God's principles can lead to untold harm, physically and mentally.

REFERENCES

American Psychological Association. (2007). Stress in America. In A. P. Association (Ed.), *Mind/body health: For a healthy mind and body, talk to a psychologist.* Washington, D.C.: American Psychological Association.

Ashley, G., & Cort, M. (2007). The effects of the practice of the Newstart health regimen on faculty stress among faculty at Seventh-day Adventist colleges and universities. *Christian Higher Education, 6*, 131–142.

Dalgalarrondo, P. L. M. (1993). Religious affiliation and psychiatric diagnosis: The influence of Christian sect membership on diagnosis distribution. *European Archives of Psychiatry and Clinical Neuroscience, 243*, 47–53.

De Sousa, A. (2005). The role of music therapy in psychiatry. *Alternative Therapy Health Medicine, 11*(6), 52–53.

Donahue, M. J. (1985). Intrinsic and extrinsic religiousness: Review and meta-analysis. *Journal of Personality and Social Psychology, 48*, 400–419.

Drumm, R., McBride, D., Hopkins, G., Thayer, J., Popescu, M., & Wrenn, J. (2006). Intimate partner violence in a conservative Christian denomination: Prevalence and types. *Social Work & Christianity, 33*, 233–251.

Drummond, S. P. (2006). Searching for the brain bases of insomnia. *Journal of Clinical Sleep Medicine, 2*, 323–324.

Dunn, A. L., & Bettinghaus, E. P. (2006). Diffusion and dissemination for increasing physical activity in world populations. *American Journal of Preventive Medicine, 31*(4 Suppl.), S94–96.

Durkheim, E. (1951). *Suicide: A Study in Sociology*. Seattle, WA: The Free Press.

Ellison, C. G., Boardman, J. D., Williams, D. R., & Jackson, J. S. (2001). Religious involvement, stress, and mental health:. *Social Forces, 80*, 215–249.

Ferraro, K. F., & Koch, J. R. (1994). Religion and health among black and white adults. *Journal for the Scientific Study of Religion, 33*, 362–375.

Freud, S. (1961). *The Future of an Illusion: Civilization and Its Discontents, and Other Works*. London: Hogarth Press and the Institute of Psycho-Analysis.

Gilkes, C. (1980). The black church as a therapeutic community. *Journal of Interdenominational Theological Center, 8*, 29–44.

Griffith, E. E. H., English, T., & Mayfield, V. (1980). Possession, prayer and testimony. *Psychiatry, 43*, 120–128.

Griffith, E. E. H., & Mathewson, M. A. (1981). Original communications: Communitas and charisma in a black church service. *Journal of the National Medical Association, 73*, 1023–1027.

Griffith, E. E. H., Young, J. L., & Smith, D. L. (1984). Therapeutic elements in a black church service. *Hospital and Community Psychiatry, 35*, 464–469.

Hummer, R. A., Rogers, R. G., Nam, C. B., & Ellison, C. G. (1999). Religious involvement and U.S. adult mortality. *Demography, 36*, 273–285.

Idler, E. L., & Kasl, S. U. (1992). Religion, disability, depression, and the timing of death. *The American Journal of Sociology, 97*, 1052–1079.

James, W. (1902). *The Varieties of Religious Experience: A Study in Human Nature*. New York: Longmans, Green and Co.

Johnson, M. E., Brems, C., & Burke, S. (2002). Recognizing comorbidity among drug users in treatment. *The American Journal of Drug Abuse and Alcohol Abuse, 28*(2), 243–261.

Kessler, R. C., et al. (2005). Lifetime prevalence and age-of-onset distributions of DSM-IV disorders in the National Comorbidity Survey replication. *Archives of General Psychiatry, 62*, 593–602.

Kessler, R. C., Chiu, W. T., Demler, O., & Walters, E. E. (2005). Prevalence, severity, and comorbidity of 12-month DSM-IV disorders in the National Comorbidity Survey replication. *Archives of General Psychiatry, 62*, 617–627.

Kessler, R. G., Gruber, M. J., Sampson, N. A., Ursano, R. J., & Wessely, S. (2008). Trends in mental illness and suicidality after Hurricane Katrina. *Journal of Molecular Psychiatry, 13*, 374–384.

Keyes, C. (2007). Promoting and protecting mental health as flourishing. *American Psychologist, 62*, 95–108.

Kilgore, W. D., Kilgore, D. B., Day, L. M., Li, C., Kamimori, G. H., & Balkin, T. J. (2007). The effects of 53 hours of sleep deprivation on moral judgment. *Sleep, 30*(3), 345–352.

Koenig, H. G., Hays, J. C., Larson, D. B., George, L. K., Cohen, H. J., McCullough, M., Meador, K., Blazer, D. G. (1999). Does religious attendance prolong survival?: A six-year follow-up study of 3,968 older adults. *Journal of Gerontology: Medical Sciences, 54A*, M370-M377.

Koenig, H. G. (2008). Concerns about measuring "spirituality" in research. *Journal of Nervous and Mental Disease, 196*, 349–355.

Larson, D. B., Pattison, E. M., Blazer, D. G., Omran, A. R., & Kaplan, B. H. (1986). Research on religious variables in four major psychiatric journals, 1978–1982. *American Journal of Psychiatry, 143*, 329–334.

Marx, K. (1844). *Deutsch-Französische Jahrbücher*, Paris, 7 & 10 February 1844. Retrieved from http://www.marxists.org/archive/marx/works/1843/critique-hpr/intro.htm

Meador, K., Koenig, H., Hughes, D., Blazer, D., Turnbull, J., & George, L. (1992). Religious affiliation and major depression. *Hospital and Community Psychiatry, 43*, 1204–1208.

Moussavi, S., Chatterji, S., Verdes, E., Tandon, A., Patel, V., & Sustun, B. (2007). Depression, chronic diseases, and decrements in health: Results from the World Health Surveys. *Lancet, 370*, 851–858.

Neighbors, H. W., Musick, M. A., & Williams, D. R. (1998). The African American minister as a source of help for serious personal crises: Bridge or barrier to mental health care? *Health Education and Behavior, 25*, 759–777.

Newport, K. G. C. (2006). *The Branch Davidians of Waco: The history and beliefs of an apocalyptic sect.* Newport, Oxford: Oxford University Press.

Office of Applied Studies. (2006). Results from the 2005 National Survey on Drug Use and Health: National Findings. *DHHS Publication No. SMA 06-4194, NSDUH Series H-30.* Rockville, MD: Substance Abuse and Mental Health Services Administration.

Ortega, S. T., Crutchfield, R. D., & Rushing, W. A. (1983). Race differences in elderly personal well-being. *Research on Aging, 5*, 101–118.

Pargament, K., et al. (1983). The psychosocial climate of religious congregations. *American Journal of Community Psychology, 11*, 351–381.

Pargament, K., Smith, B., Koenig, H., & Perez, L. (1998). Patterns of positive and negative religious coping with major life stressors. *Journal for the Scientific Study of Religion, 37*, 711–725.

Pleis, J., & Lethbridge-Cejku, M. (2005). *Summary health statistics for U.S. adults: National Health Interview Survey, 2005.* Hyattsville, MD: National Center for Health Statistics.

Powell, L. H., Shahabi, L., & Thoresen, C. E. (2003). Religion and spirituality: Linkages to physical health. *The American Psychologist, 58*, 36–52.

Rue, L. D. (1985). Our most outrageous blind spot: The academic study of religion. *The Chronicle of Higher Education, 29*, 40.

Shahabi, L., Powell, L. H., Musick, M. A., Pargament, K. I., Thoresen, C. E., Williams, D. R., et al. (2002). Correlates of self-perceptions of spirituality in American adults. *Annals of Behavioral Medicine, 24*, 59–69.

Sherrill, K. A., & Larson, D. B. (1994). The anti-tenure factors in religious research in clinical epidemiology and aging. In J. S. Levin (Ed.), *Religion in aging and health: Theoretical foundations and methodological frontiers* (pp. 149–177). Thousand Oaks, CA: SAGE Publications, Inc.

Shreve-Neiger, A. K., & Edelstein, B. A. (2004). Religion and anxiety: A critical review of the literature. *Clinical Psychological Review, 24*(4), 379–397.

Sloan, R P., Bagiella, E., & Powell, T. (2001). Without a prayer: methodological problems, ethical challenges, and misrepresentations in the study of religion, spirituality and medicine. In: T. G. Plante & A. C. Sherman, eds., *Faith and health: Psychological perspectives.* New York: Guilford Press, pp. 339–354.

Smith, T., McCullough, M. E., & Poll, J. (2003). Religiousness and depression: Evidence for a main effect and the moderating influence of stressful life events. *Psychological Bulletin, 129*, 614–636.

Stark, R., & Bainbridge, W. S. (1985). *The Future of Religion: Secularization, Revival, and Cult Formation.* Berkeley: University of California Press.

Strawbridge, W. J., Shema, S. J., Cohen, R. D., & Kaplan, G. A. (2001). Religious attendance increases survival by improving and maintaining good health behaviors, mental health, and social relationships. *Annals of Behavioral Medicine, 23*, 68–74.

Strawbridge, W. J., Shema, S. J., Cohen, R. D., Roberts, R. E., & Kaplan, G. A. (1998). Religiosity buffers effects of some stressors on depression but exacerbates others. *Journal of Gerontology, 53B*(3), S118–126.

Taylor, R. J., & Chatters, L. M. (1988). Church members as a source of informal social support. *Review of Religious Research, 30*, 193–203.

Tix, A. P., & Frazier, P. A. (1998). The use of religious coping during stressful life events. *Journal of Consulting and Clinical Psychology*, 411–422.

Trice, P., & Bjorck, J. (2006). Pentecostal perspectives on causes of depression. *Professional Psychology, 37*, 283–294.

Varshney, V. P., Bedi, M., & Bhandari, B. (2005). Effect of non-vegetarian diet on cardiovascular reactivity to mental stress in young adults. *Vascular Disease Prevention, 2*, 293–298.

Wallace, J. M., & Forman, T. A. (1998). Religion's role in promoting health and reducing risk among American youth. *Health Education & Behavior, 25*, 721–741.

Wang, P., Berglund, P., & Kessler, R. (2003). Patterns and correlates of contacting clergy for mental disorders in the United States. *Health Services Research, 38*, 647–673.

Weaver, A. J., Larson, D. B., Flannelly, K. J., Stapleton, C. L., & Koenig, H. G. (2002). Mental health issues among clergy and other religious professionals: A review of research. *Journal of Pastoral Care & Counseling, 56*, 393–403.

Williams, D. R. (1994). The concept of race in health services research: 1966 to 1990. *Health Services Research, 29*, 261–274.

Williams, D. R., Larson, D. B., Buckler, R. E., Heckmann, R. C., & Pyle, C. M. (1991). Religion and psychological distress in a community sample. *Social Science and Medicine, 32*, 1257–1262.

Williams, D. R., & Sternthal, M. (2007). Spirituality, religion and health: Evidence and research directions. *Medical Journal of Australia, 186*(10), 47–50.

Young, J. L., Griffith, E. E., & Williams, D. R. (2003). The integral role of pastoral counseling by African-American clergy in community mental health. *Psychiatric Services, 54*, 688–692.

Sabbath as a Resource for Marriage

Jana K. Boyd

Finding time to maintain marital connection through enjoyable interactions is an increasingly difficult task for couples in a society crowded with obligations and distractions. It has been argued that it is this lack of shared time and experiences that is the most significant contributor to the dissolution of marriages. The high rate of divorce and its rippling effects on larger society brings a sense of urgency to the need to find ways to protect and nourish healthy marriages.

Throughout its history, the Seventh-day Adventist church has guarded a doctrine and practice of Sabbath (Fayard, Harding, Murdoch, & Brunt, 2007) that may serve as a unique resource in helping to meet the needs of couples struggling to maintain a healthy marital relationship. Sabbath is understood here as a religious day of rest beginning at sundown Friday evening and ending sundown Saturday evening. Observing Sabbath means that one day is set aside every week for spiritual, physical, and relational rejuvenation. The religious sanction of Sabbath observance places boundaries around the hours of the Sabbath and infuses the time with particular meaning. Examples of the meaning which may be ascribed to Sabbath include the idea of the time as sacred, as set aside for rejuvenation and the deepening of relationships, as a reminder of God's work on our behalf, and as an affirmation of creaturely worth. The possible benefits examined here include greater rewarding leisure involvement and greater marital satisfaction.

There are a host of aspects of Sabbath which recommend it as a resource for marriage, such as providing a time to foster the isomorphic relationship between marital and spiritual intimacy (Shapiro & Shapiro, 1992), the relief of being able to set aside the worries and cares of the work week for one day and simply resting in Christ (White, 1976), the benefits of the corporate and family worships that tend to be a traditional part of Sabbath observance, and likely more that are better addressed elsewhere. This discussion will focus on two specific aspects of Sabbath which individually are demonstrated to contribute to marital satisfaction and in combination would seem to provide an important resource for marriages. Eugene Peterson's understanding from Scripture of the nature of Sabbath observance is that it should be an integration of *praying* and *playing* (1987). Building on Peterson's conceptualization, we can expand these terms so that *praying* refers to the act of engaging in a relationship with God, or religiosity, and *playing* to refer to enjoyable activities, or leisure. The contributions of both religiosity and leisure to marital health as demonstrated through research (Orathinkal & Vansteenwegen, 2006; Fiese & Tomcho, 2001; Lambert & Dollahite, 2006) recommend an exploration of the possible benefits when they are integrated together in the practice of Sabbath.

Before focusing more in-depth on Sabbath, first will be an exploration of these two variables, leisure and religiosity, and why they are not only relevant to a discussion of marital health but also helpful for exploring the meaning and experience of Sabbath. The theory of Symbolic Interaction (Blumer, 1986) will be utilized to assist with an understanding of how the meaning ascribed to Sabbath may influence how it is experienced and what benefits may be gained.

LEISURE AND MARRIAGE

With the industrialization of nineteenth-century Europe and North America, the worlds of husbands and wives have become increasingly separated from each other (Wynne & Wynne, 1986). Whether it is separate work environments or one spouse remaining at home while the other works, spouses have less shared activity and involvement than in the past. For this reason, leisure time has come to play a more important role in marital relationships as it is during leisure time that couples have the most opportunity for rewarding interaction. Several studies have demonstrated the positive effects of leisure time in strengthening relational bonds and enriching family relationships (Orthner & Mancini, 1990; Groves, 1989; Levy, 1987) as well as helping to neutralize the negative effects of stress on marriage (Coleman, 1993; Hoeksma, Guy, Brown, & Brady, 1993).

However, the presence of available leisure time alone does not predict improved marital satisfaction and decreased stress levels. How couples spend their leisure time significantly influences whether the leisure has a positive or negative effect on the relationship (Kaslow, Hansson, & Sundblad, 1994; Sullivan, 1996; Johnson et al., 1992). For example, time spent together in leisure has been shown to correlate with marital satisfaction whereas leisure time spent individually or with other people significantly correlated with marital distress (Smith et al., 1988). Leisure activities which promote interaction have been identified as more conducive to stress reduction and relational satisfaction than parallel activities such as watching television together (Coleman, Iso, & Seppo, 1993; Roggman, Moe, Hart, & Forthun, 1994; Pietropinto, 1985). Additionally, Hull & Michael (1995) found that leisure time spent outdoors contributed to greater stress reduction than leisure time spent at home.

At this point it may be helpful to be more specific about exactly what is meant by the term "leisure" that may help illuminate why some activities are experienced as leisure and others are not.

THE MEANING OF LEISURE

Embedded in all studies of leisure is the problem of definition. Is leisure to be equated with discretionary time? Are certain behaviors understood as leisure activities and others not? Or is leisure a subjective experience regardless of the nature of the activity? Clark, Harvey, and Shaw (1990), in a study looking at subjective and objective aspects of leisure, used time budget records and time use diaries to obtain contextual data to determine what activities were considered leisure and why. They found that the experience of leisure is highly contextual and individualized, making it difficult to classify certain activities as leisure and others as non-leisure. For example, some of the factors that were found to influence whether an individual experiences certain activities as leisure include gender of the participant, time of day/week, and location. Thus leisure is determined by the interpretation of the participant, not necessarily by the nature of the activity. These findings point to the utility of using the theory of Symbolic Interaction (Blumer, 1986) when studying leisure, as this theory deals primarily with the ascribing of meaning to situations and events as determinant of how these are experienced.

Three studies have specifically addressed the question of how leisure is differentiated from non-leisure based on subjective experience and interpretation. Shaw (1985) found that leisure could be experienced during most activities, but that the variables that most differentiated leisure from non-leisure include enjoyment, freedom of choice, relaxation, intrinsic motivation, and lack of evaluation. Tinsley and Tinsley (1986) found that in addition to the above characteristics, some types of leisure also require a sense of commitment and disciplined effort. In a later study focusing specifically on how leisure is experienced, Tinsley and Tinsley (1988) found support for their theory of leisure experience that is characterized by concentration on the ongoing experience, forgetting of self, and decreased awareness of time. Overall, leisure experiences that include the above characteristics appear to provide a rich opportunity for intrinsic satisfaction, companionship, intimacy, and renewal (Tinsley, Hinson, Hinsley, & Holt, 1993). The question is: what types of contexts are most conducive to these particular interpretations? In addition, are couples utilizing their discretionary time in ways that foster the experience of leisure? Next will be addressed trends in the availability of leisure and how leisure time is spent.

HOW LEISURE TIME IS USED

Use of leisure time has been the focus of several studies as it was observed that from the 1960s up to the present there has been a steady increase in the amount of discretionary time available (Aguiar, 2007; Bosserman & Kutcher, 1974). During the 1970s researchers became interested in how discretionary time is spent and what the implications are for individual, marital, and family well-being. It was found that discretionary time does not necessarily translate into leisure time when examining how free time is spent. In addition, the increase in individual discretionary time does not necessarily translate into shared discretionary time. A trend was identified where an increasing amount of free time was spent on personal and home upkeep rather than engaging in recreational activities, much less shared leisure (Jacobs & Gerson, 2001). These factors highlight the difficulty in marriages where the majority of time is spent separately during the work week and very little of the discretionary time is allocated to leisure activities where couples can have time to reconnect and enjoy time and activities together.

While leisure cannot be identified as a particular type of activity but is a function of the meaning assigned to an event, no studies have yet addressed what types of contexts are more conducive to interpretations of leisure and which of these contexts are most efficacious in promoting marital satisfaction. It is suggested here that Sabbath may provide such a context by offering inherent meaning to leisure time. The spirit of Sabbath observance or Sabbath rest encompasses the characteristics most conducive to the experience of leisure with an emphasis on concentration on the ongoing experience, forgetting of self, and decreased awareness of time with the added dimension of spirituality, also a contributor to marital satisfaction. For this reason, I will next examine the role of religiosity and spirituality in the marital relationship.

RELIGIOSITY AND MARRIAGE

During the late 1970s and early 1980s a number of studies were conducted which demonstrated that religiosity is a significant predictor of marital adjustment and satisfaction (Bahr & Chadwick, 1985; Glenn and Weaver, 1978; Hunt & King, 1978; Wilkinson & Tanner, 1980; Wilson & Filsinger, 1986). Other studies have focused on identifying what aspects of religiosity are contributing factors to marital satisfaction. Findings range from factors as vague as the mere presence of religion in a person's life (Schumm, Bollman, & Jurich, 1982; Snow & Compton, 1996) to things as specific as frequency of church attendance (Hansen, 1987).

As with leisure, religiosity or spirituality is difficult to operationalize and measure. However, for many, religiosity does intuitively encompass more than the specific behaviors of church membership and attendance, and something more identifiable than a dimension or presence in a person's life. Wilson and Filsinger (1986) attempted to gain a clearer picture of the specific components of religiosity which most influence marital adjustment. Using a multidimensional religiosity scale with couples from a variety of Protestant backgrounds, they were able to identify involvement in religious institutions and traditions, religious experience, and sense of morality as factors of religiosity that correlated significantly with marital adjustment. What was not addressed in this study was the motivation behind religious involvement and whether a particular orientation toward religion may influence the effect of religiosity on the marital relationship. With the movement in a large segment of mainstream Protestantism away from a "legalistic" perspective, there is greater awareness of the difference between a religiosity that is rigid and motivated either by fear or habit and a religiosity that is more open and arises out of conviction and sense of meaning. Allport and Ross (1967) contributed significantly to the study of religiosity with their theory of intrinsic and extrinsic religiosity. They viewed intrinsic religiosity as a faith oriented toward the search for meaning whereas extrinsic religiosity is oriented more toward control. Based on the variables which extrinsic religiosity has been found to correlate positively with (Allport & Ross, 1967; Hoge & Carroll, 1973; Kahoe, 1974; McConahay & Hough, 1976; Strickland & Weddell, 1972), persons with an extrinsic religious orientation are more likely to have a legalistic approach to their religious beliefs and practices. On the other hand, intrinsic religiosity has been found to correlate positively with an internal locus of control (Kahoe, 1974) and purpose in life (Crandall & Rassmussen, 1975), variables that are consistent with a religiosity oriented more toward meaning. Regarding religious practices, it would seem that persons who have an intrinsic religious orientation would be more likely to approach religious rituals and traditions from a perspective of meaning rather than as a religious duty and are thus more likely to reap positive benefits from it in their marital relationships. Stanley (1986) provided support for this notion when he found that an intrinsic religious orientation associated positively with marital satisfaction whereas an extrinsic orientation did not.

To summarize, religiosity correlates significantly with marital satisfaction. Involvement in religious rituals, religious experiences, and convictions are each factors of religiosity that have been shown to influence levels of marital satisfaction. Beyond participation in religious rituals and profession of religious convictions, the orientation and motivation toward religion is also significant in accounting for the effect of religion on one's life and one's relationships with an intrinsic orientation being more efficacious in producing positive benefits than an extrinsic one. When it comes to Sabbath observance, why a person keeps the Sabbath will likely influence how it is experienced and what effects it may have on one's marriage. Why people choose to keep the Sabbath is likely to be informed by their understanding of the meaning and significance of Sabbath. Next is an examination of Sabbath from a biblical and theological perspective.

THE SABBATH

First is an examination of the development of the concept and practice of Sabbath throughout Scripture. Next is a discussion of how Seventh-day Adventists have understood and observed Sabbath. Finally I will draw on two views of the meaning and purpose of Sabbath for modern life and marriages and look at how different understandings of Sabbath may influence how it is observed.

The word "Sabbath" is of Hebrew origin and means simply to rest or cease from work (Gaebelein, 1990). It is used in the Bible to describe the seventh day as the day God set aside for rest at creation (Gen. 2:2). He then reiterated the importance of its observance in the Ten Commandments (Ex. 20:8–11). In the creation account, one commentator points out that it is mentioned three times that God rested from His work of creating, and the reason this day is holy is because God rested. This repetition of God not working on that day seems to indicate the importance of God's example in modeling for humans how to participate in the image of God by resting (Gaebelein, 1990).

The first use of the term "Sabbath" is found in Exodus 16:23 in the account of God providing manna for the Israelites in the desert on their exodus from Egypt to Canaan. In this miracle God not only provided food for the people, but also provided for Sabbath and an understanding that all work was to be set aside, including the gathering of food.

In the Ten Commandments (Ex. 20:8–11) the observance of Sabbath is expanded to include strangers, servants, and animals. The fact that animals are included in the Sabbath rest seems to indicate that the Sabbath was not just for spiritual or religious purposes, but also for physical rejuvenation. In the instructions God gave to Moses regarding the tabernacle and governing of the people, God declares that the Sabbath is to serve as a covenant between God and God's people and desecration of the Sabbath is punishable with death (Ex. 31:12–17). Even though greater weight seems to be placed on Sabbath observance, still the only requirement is rest.

Subsequent references to Sabbath in the Old Testament point to the importance God placed on Sabbath observance for maintaining the relationship between God and God's people, and how often this relationship was desecrated through lack of Sabbath keeping (Deut. 5:12–15; Neh. 13:15–22; Isa. 56:2, 6; 58:13–14; Jer. 17:21–27; Ezek. 20:12–13).

Where Sabbath observance had been lax and unstructured before the Israelites' exile to Babylon, it became much more structured and ritualized after the return of the exiles. The Pharisees drew up thirty-nine principal forms of work with numerous minor variations that were unlawful to do on the Sabbath (Lotz, 1911).

In the New Testament we learn that the Sabbath had become more of a burden than a blessing. While Jesus upheld the sacredness of the Sabbath, He disapproved of the burdensome additions to the original law. In Matthew 12:12 Jesus declares that He is "Lord of the Sabbath" (NIV) which gave Him the authority to impart a better understanding of what Sabbath should be about. Christ did much to redefine for us the meaning of Sabbath by emphasizing that God is more pleased with kindness and love than with vain zeal for the Law (Steinmueller & Sullivan, 1950). In Matthew 12 Jesus defends His disciples relieving their hunger in the wheat field, and advocates caring for fellow humans in need as well as animals. In Luke 13:10 Jesus again defends His act of healing on the Sabbath to the Pharisees by saying that setting a person free on the Sabbath is highly appropriate. Probably the definitive statement Jesus made regarding the Sabbath is found in Mark 2:27 where He is reported as saying that "The Sabbath was made for man, not man for the Sabbath" (NIV). Rather than the Sabbath being a burden, it was meant to be a day of restoration.

By this time the Sabbath was a time for gathering in the temple—or in the synagogue in the case of the smaller towns—for religious services. During the formation of the early church the apostles would preach in the synagogues and meet with Jews to preach the gospel (Acts 13:14; 16:13; 17:2; 18:4). Eventually the day recognized as Sabbath by most Christians changed from the seventh day to the first day of the week during the rule of Constantine, a subject addressed more in-depth elsewhere (Bacchiocchi, 2000). Some commentators claim that the meaning of Sabbath became more figurative when the day of worship was transferred to the first day of the week (Leon-Durfour, 1962), while others argue that because the Sabbath was part of the creation order and included in the Ten Commandments it is still binding (Gaffin, 1988). This latter argument would support the view that the Sabbath was put in place as a means of maintaining humanity in the image of God by providing for a regular period of much needed rest.

SEVENTH-DAY ADVENTIST UNDERSTANDING OF SABBATH

The denominational name—Seventh-day Adventist (SDA)—indicates the two doctrines of the SDA church which make it most unique: an emphasis on the importance of observing the seventh-day Sabbath and a belief in the soon return of Christ in the second coming (the advent). Historically these two doctrines were closely linked with the understanding that the remnant church in the time of the end would be those who strictly observed all of the Ten Commandments. Adventists have seen the change from Saturday to Sunday Sabbath observance as a move away from following the fourth of the Ten Commandments of God. It was understood that in the end times, those who observed the seventh-day Sabbath would receive the Seal of God (Rev. 7:2–3) as a sign of complete loyalty and obedience to God (White, 1888).

More recently SDAs have begun to explore the larger meaning of Sabbath and move away from a legalistic view of Sabbath observance. Rice writes that SDAs are "in the process of moving from a doctrine of Sabbath to a more comprehensive theology of the Sabbath" (1985, p. 355). Several SDA scholars have explored the theme of Sabbath and the various theological implications that can be extracted from a deeper understanding (Andreasen, 1972, 1978a, & 1978b; Bacchiocchi, 1980; Kubo, 1978; Strand, 1982). Rice summarizes some of the more dominant themes of meaning that relate to a "theology of Sabbath." First and foremost, Sabbath is understood as a testimony to God's creative and redemptive power (Rice, 1985; White, 1989). Not only did God rest after having completed the creation of the world, but Jesus also rested after having completed the work of redemption. When we observe the Sabbath rest we are reminded of these two acts of God on our behalf. Secondly, Sabbath affirms the value of God's creation. Not only are humans commanded to rest on the Sabbath, but so also are beasts of burden. All of God's creation is of worth not for what they can do but because of their inherent value. Rice sees this as having important social implications, for when we acknowledge the inherent worth of each person we cannot help but strive for social justice. In Sabbath we are also made aware of our connection with the rest of nature. Thirdly, in Sabbath observance we not only acknowledge God's lordship over our lives, but we celebrate this sovereignty by joyfully entering into the sacred time which God asked us to observe. Finally, Sabbath has eschatological significance in the sense that it reminds us that the things that occupy us the rest of the week are only temporary concerns and that God has something better in store for us. Sabbath is an opportunity to experience some of eternity in the here and now.

Rice (1985) sees a close link between the meaning and experience of Sabbath when he writes that "A deeper understanding of what the Sabbath means can make our experience of the Sabbath richer" (p. 37). This brings us to the SDA understanding of how Sabbath is to be observed. Adventists have probably been most influenced in their understanding of Sabbath observance by the writings of Ellen G. White, viewed by many in the denomination as a prophet of God. White (1948b) writes most strongly that all secular work is to be set aside during the sacred hours from sundown Friday until sundown Saturday. The rest of the six days should be focused on preparing for the Sabbath with Friday in particular set aside as a preparation day. Yet we should not exhaust ourselves during the week so that on Sabbath we are merely recuperating so that we can return to our work.

Preparation for the Sabbath includes having clothing and food ready so they will not need to be attended to during the sacred hours. Also disagreements with family, friends, or others are to be set aside. Each moment of the Sabbath is viewed as precious and we are instructed to "jealously guard the edges of the Sabbath" (p. 356). White advises us not to overeat nor waste the hours of the Sabbath in bed. While part of the Sabbath is devoted to communal worship, White feels most of the remaining time should be spent with family, preferably out of doors (1948a). Regarding Sabbath worship, "long sermons and tedious, formal prayers" (White, 1948a, p. 583) are to be avoided. She even writes that the "church members are not to expect a sermon every Sabbath" (1948c, p. 19). Both corporate and family worship have played a significant role in the Adventist tradition of Sabbath to both positive and negative effect. As will be addressed later, when worship has been the dominant focus of Sabbath rest it has tended toward a more Puritan experience of Sabbath rather than facilitating a more wholistic experience of rest. This is not to say that both corporate and family worship cannot make significant contributions to marital and family health. White's cautions against worship dominating too much of the Sabbath hours point to the importance of not undervaluing the spiritual necessity of non-structured rest. In summary, "the Sabbath should be made so interesting to our families that its weekly return will be hailed with joy" (White, 1948a, p. 585). While Sabbath observance takes different forms among SDA individuals, there is much communality in tradition and consciousness.

SABBATH OBSERVANCE

Two authors make helpful suggestions to assist with an understanding of how to keep the Sabbath. Heschel (1951) describes the Sabbath as a "palace in time" (p. 15) that is constructed using the spiritual discipline of rest and withdrawal from the world of technology and noise. He points out that where most of the focus of modern technology and even most religions is on mastery of space and glorification of structures in space, Sabbath is a celebration of time—a cherishing of sacred moments rather than a worship of sacred places. As time cannot be saved or preserved, it must be savored in the moment. Thus Heschel views Sabbath as an opportunity to withdraw from our focus on things and achievements and to enter into sacred time where we can become aware of a God who is not limited to space and time. Heschel's approach again echoes the characteristics of the experience of leisure integrated with spirituality.

Where Heschel's view of Sabbath observance is one of abstention, Peterson (1987) proposes a proactive approach to Sabbath observance, referred to earlier, that he describes as a combination of praying and playing. Peterson points to the imagery of joyful play and prayer evident in Psalm 92, a song specifically written for Sabbath, and comments that "Puritan Sabbaths that eliminated play were a disaster. Secular sabbaths that eliminate prayer are worse" (p. 75). However, Peterson also affirms the importance of abstaining from work and resting on the Sabbath. He points out that it is only in a state of rest that we are able to appreciate ourselves and those around us for who we are rather than for what we do. This has profound implications for relationships as Sabbath allows partners to affirm each other's worth for who they are and not for what they can do for each other.

The fact that Sabbath was given religious sanction offers us the motivation we need to recognize it as important and perhaps even vital. I believe the concept of Sabbath can be useful in promoting healthy marriages by helping people understand the concept of rest and the importance of sacred time in order to assure that rest is not violated.

INTEGRATING SABBATH MEANING AND EXPERIENCE

While Sabbath-keeping has been a defining feature of Judeo-Christian history and central to the identity of Seventh-day Adventists, as stated above, most of the attention that has been paid to the Sabbath has focused on its doctrinal or theological significance rather than on how Sabbath is experienced (Rice, 1985). Perhaps in reaction to this, there has been a renewed interest in the wider culture in rediscovering Sabbath, not from a theological but from an experiential perspective (Muller, 1999; Wirzba & Berry, 2006). There is a growing recognition that the setting aside of time for spiritual, physical, and relational rejuvenation can have a host of positive benefits. One model of Sabbath observance argues for a move away from segmenting Sabbath within a specific time, but rather integrating it into one's whole life. While it seems like a good idea in principle, this approach to Sabbath is not supported in Scripture where emphasis is placed on the setting aside of a particular day. When the experience of Sabbath becomes diffuse, the meaning may also become diffuse. It is argued here that both the meaning and the experience of Sabbath be given careful consideration in order to receive maximum benefits from Sabbath observance in marriage. In the past Sabbath was made to be a burden by too much emphasis on the doctrine or theology of Sabbath and not enough on the delight or experience of Sabbath. We may again put the practice of Sabbath in danger if too much emphasis is placed on the experience of Sabbath and not enough recognition remains on its meaning. Again using the theory of symbolic interaction (Blumer, 1986), we may infer that the meaning we give to Sabbath will determine how we experience it. We can also assume that experience may inform meaning. If the experience is not what is intended, than perhaps the meaning must be reexamined.

By use of the term "meaning of Sabbath" two things are implied here: first, how a person understands the significance of Sabbath, and, second, how important that meaning is in motivating one's behaviors, both from an internal and an external locus of control. In other words, does one observe Sabbath because it is personally meaningful (intrinsic religiosity), or because of external pressures (extrinsic religiosity)? While there is not yet evidence to support which specific meanings ascribed to Sabbath produce the most benefit, research does suggest that both intrinsic and extrinsic senses of meaning are important for Sabbath observance to have a positive influence on marriages (Boyd, 1999).

SABBATH AND MARRIAGE RESEARCH

Boyd (1999) conducted a survey of 197 married Adventists recruited from SDA churches and adult Sabbath School classes in Idaho, Washington, California, and Kansas. The survey included demographic information as well as the Intrinsic/Extrinsic–Revised (I/E-R) Scale (Gorsuch & McPherson, 1989), the Inventory of Rewarding Activities (IRA; Weiss, Hops, & Patterson, 1973), the Personal Assessment of Intimacy in Relationships (PAIR; Schaefer & Olson, 1981), the Kansas Marital Satisfaction Scale (KMSS; Schumm, Bollman, & Jurich, 1982), and a Sabbath measure developed for this study (Boyd, 1999). A review of the literature did not identify an adequate measure of Sabbath attitude. A Sabbath index was constructed of eighteen items with Likert-type responses. The Sabbath items were designed to assess the participants' attitudes and beliefs about Sabbath as well as how Sabbath was experienced in the context of their marital relationship. The items were generated from an Adventist focus group and were revised based on pretest results.

The Sabbath items were factor analyzed and two scales were created. Based on correlational analysis, it was determined that the first Sabbath scale related more to intrinsic religiosity while the second to extrinsic religiosity. Thus the two scales were labeled Intrinsic Sabbath Observance and Extrinsic Sabbath Observance.

A factor analysis of the leisure items revealed a clear distinction between what might be termed traditional SDA Sabbath activities or "Sabbath Leisure" (i.e., interaction with family and friends, enjoying the outdoors, religious activities) and "Secular Leisure" (i.e., shopping, going to a movie, attending a sports event). Only the Sabbath Leisure variable was included in the path model as Secular Leisure was identified through the regression analysis as not being significantly related to the other independent and dependant variables. The results of the study are summarized in the following path model.

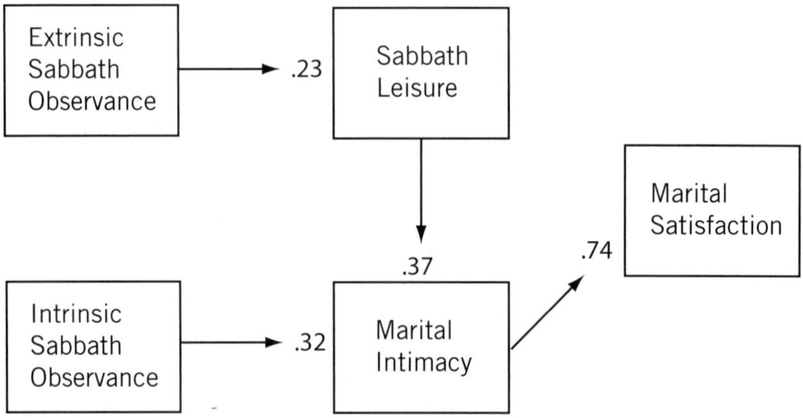

Figure 1. Results of Path Analysis

Joreskog Goodness of Fit Index (1984) = .99
Bentler-Bonett Normed Fit Index (1980) = .99
Browne-Cudeck Dross Validation Index (1990) = .12

The goal of this study was to test the theory of symbolic interaction by (1) examining how meaning was ascribed to a particular time, namely Sabbath; (2) determining how that meaning will influence how the time is spent; and (3) noting what impact is made on marital quality. While it was hypothesized that an intrinsic religious orientation in Sabbath observance would have a more positive influence on leisure involvement and marital quality than an extrinsic orientation, the results of this study suggest that both orientations make unique contributions to how SDAs practice their Sabbath and how their marriages are affected.

An intrinsic religious orientation in Sabbath observance was found to contribute directly to marital intimacy. Such an approach to Sabbath was also negatively correlated with secular leisure, a variable that had no relationship with marital intimacy or marital satisfaction. By contrast, Sabbath leisure, which was significantly associated with marital intimacy and satisfaction, is most influenced by an extrinsic religious orientation toward Sabbath observance. These results tend to support the theory of symbolic interaction by highlighting the fact that different meanings, or approaches, to Sabbath observance can have different effects on how the time is spent. Among SDAs in particular, assigning religious significance to the Sabbath hours tends to influence what kinds of leisure activities are engaged in during that period each week. Those activities that have been recognized by this community as in keeping with the spirit of Sabbath with an emphasis on prayer and play do tend to contribute to the marital intimacy and satisfaction of individuals within this community. Leisure activities that are not in keeping with the emphasis of Sabbath—such as those that involve business transactions, competition, or day-to-day preoccupations—tend not to be related to marital quality. In general, it seems that whatever the reasons or beliefs regarding Sabbath observance, marital relationships can benefit from this religious practice, suggesting that the more wholistic the approach to keeping Sabbath, the better.

These findings suggest that the relationship between intrinsic and extrinsic religiosity may not be dichotomous as previously thought, but may operate on separate continuums. The interaction of both aspects of religiosity seems to be mutually reinforcing when it comes to religious practice, specifically Sabbath observance. The circumplex model below (Figure 2) explores the interaction between these two variables in the context of Sabbath.

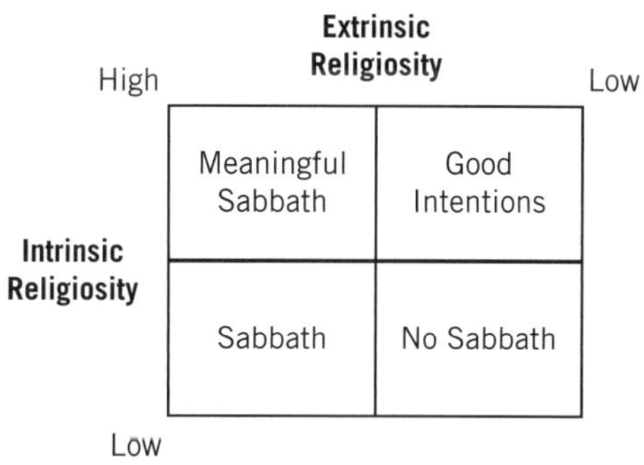

Figure 2. Intrinsic/Extrinsic Circumplex Model of Sabbath Types

It may be that persons who are high in both intrinsic and extrinsic religiosity may be oriented toward keeping Sabbath because it is personally meaningful to them, but are also influenced by external or social forces which support them in keeping the boundaries of the Sabbath (Meaningful Sabbath). Persons who observe Sabbath only because of external influences may have a tendency to be more legalistic in their Sabbath practices because they are not guided in their Sabbath observance out of internal meaning (Legalistic Sabbath). A sense of personal meaning may not be enough in many cases to enforce regular Sabbath observance (Good Intentions). It may be that an external influence is necessary for many to be able to keep Sabbath on a regular basis and not let other pressures encroach on the time. Finally, if a person has no internal or external reasons for keeping the Sabbath, it is unlikely to be observed (No Sabbath).

Peterson (1987) suggested that persons who use the Sabbath both as a time for praying and for playing will come closest to experiencing Sabbath as God intended. The results of Boyd's (1999) study examining levels of involvement in leisure activities and religiosity in Sabbath keeping suggest another way of viewing differing approaches to Sabbath using Peterson's conceptualization. While the results cannot provide conclusive support for Peterson's theory, they do point to the possibility of a continuum between high and low levels of praying (religiosity) and playing (leisure) interacting in ways that produce different types of Sabbath experiences. Figure 3 shows a circumplex model of the possible interaction of the variables of praying and playing in terms of types of Sabbaths.

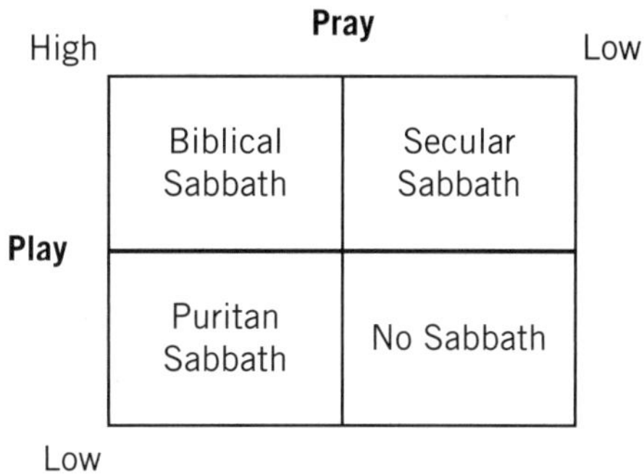

Figure 3. Pray/Play Circumplex Model of Types of Sabbaths

Peterson (1987) points out that in Psalm 92 Sabbath is described as a time for both worship and joyful play (Biblical Sabbath) where Sabbath has been interpreted in the past as a time merely for worship (Puritan Sabbath). In modern times hours that were formerly given religious significance are often seen as just part of the weekend and are used either for the pursuit of enjoyment (Secular Sabbath) or to catch up on work (No Sabbath).

To summarize, in Sabbath there is a unique opportunity for couples to experience important rest or leisure where there is opportunity for the maintenance of healthy marital connection. The religious aspect of Sabbath both provides a boundary around the time, and gives the time unique significance as sacred time—a time for valuing our connection to God and one another. It is not enough to merely decide to observe the Sabbath; how and why couples observe the Sabbath will likely influence whether or not it is beneficial for their marriage. Keeping Sabbath out of a personal or shared sense of meaning with the support of a Sabbath-keeping community is likely to provide the most benefit in contributing to marital satisfaction.

CLINICAL APPLICATION

In working in a clinical setting with couples who either come from a background of Sabbath keeping or are willing to consider integrating Sabbath keeping into their lifestyle as a resource for their marriage, it may be helpful to consider the following process. First, the meaning of Sabbath that individuals bring to their marriage will determine their experience of Sabbath as a couple. Each individual's understanding of the significance of Sabbath and his or her motivation in observing it should be explored. This may be a point of strength or conflict. Religious differences can be a source of significant strain in marriages and must be dealt with carefully. However, using a strength-based approach, the emphasis should be on finding common ground rather than emphasizing differences. Second, an examination of past experiences of Sabbath and desired experience will help to inform the next stage in the process. The goal is to assist the couple in looking for points of connection both in their experiences and in their senses of meaning in order to develop a new sense of shared meaning of Sabbath. From this sense of shared meaning they can then define and shape how they would like to experience Sabbath as a couple. Ideally this is a collaborative process with respect for the place partners come from in terms of their understanding and experience of Sabbath along with the benefit of an informed theology of Sabbath. It may be helpful for couples to do some exploration of their own into the meaning and significance of Sabbath to help foster an intrinsic motivation in their observance. Also, encouraging the couple to find a community that is supportive of Sabbath observance can help provide the extrinsic motivation to support the couple in the maintenance of Sabbath observance as a consistent part of their lifestyle.

This process may also take place through marital enrichment seminars, couples mentoring, and pre-marital and pastoral counseling. While on the surface viewing Sabbath as a tool for marital enhancement may seem to diminish the significance of Sabbath, it may also assist couples in entering into a deepening appreciation and experience of Sabbath. As Jesus clearly states, the Sabbath was made for us. What better way to use this gift for entering into the image of God than by seeking to preserve healthy marriages in our modern frenetic society?

REFERENCES

Aguiar, M., & Hurst, E. (2007). Measuring trends in leisure: The allocation of time over five decades. *Quarterly Journal of Economics, 122*, 969–1006.

Allport, G. W., & Ross, J. M. (1967). Personal religious orientation and prejudice. *Journal of Personality and Social Psychology, 5*, 432–443.

Amato, P. R., Booth, A., Johnson, D. R., & Rogers, S. J. (2007). *Alone together: How marriage in America is changing.* Cambridge: Harvard University Press.

Andreasen, N. E. (1972). *The Old Testament Sabbath: A tradition-historical investigation.* Chico, CA: Scholars Press.

Andreasen, N. E. (1978a). *The Christian use of time.* Nashville, TN: Abingdon.

Andreasen, N. E. (1978b). *Rest and redemption: A study of the biblical Sabbath.* Berrien Springs, MI: Andrews University Press.

Bacchiocchi, S. (1980). *Divine rest for human restlessness: A theological study of the good news of the Sabbath for today.* Berrien Springs, MI: Biblical Perspectives.

Bacchiocchi, S. (2000). *From Sabbath to Sunday: A historical investigation of the rise of Sunday observance in early Christianity.* Berrien Springs, MI: Biblical Perspectives.

Bahr, H. M., & Chadwick, B. A. (1985). Religion and family in middletown, USA. *Journal of Marriage and the Family, 47*, 407–414.

Bentler, P. M. & Bonett, D. G. (1980). Significance tests and goodness of fit in the analysis of covariance structures. *Psychological Bulletin, 88*, 588–606.

Blumer, H. (1986). *Symbolic interactionism.* Berkeley, CA: University of California Press.

Bosserman, B., & Kutcher, L. (1974). Leisure and the coming of post-industrial society. In M. Archer (Ed.), *Current research in sociology* (pp. 109–146). Hague, Netherlands: Mouton.

Boyd, J. K. (1999). An analysis of the relationship between Sabbath meaning and leisure, marital intimacy, and marital satisfaction among Seventh-day Adventists. *Dissertation Abstracts International: Section B: The Sciences and Engineering, 59*, 5616.

Browne, M. W., & Cudeck, R. (1990). Single sample cross-validation indices for covariance structures. *Multivariate Behavioral Research, 24*, 445–455.

Clark, M. S., & Reis, H. T. (1988). Interpersonal processes in close relationships. *Annual Review of Psychology, 39*, 609–672.

Clark, S. M., Harvey, A. S., & Shaw, S. M. (1990). Time use and leisure: Subjective and objective aspects. *Social Indicators Research, 23*, 337–352.

Coleman, D. (1993). Leisure based social support, leisure dispositions and health. *Journal of Leisure Research, 25*, 350–361.

Coleman, D., & Iso-Ahola, S. E. (1993). Leisure and health: The role of social support and self-determination. *Journal of Leisure Research, 25,* 111–128.

Crandall, J. E., & Rasmussen, R. D. (1975). Purpose in life as related to specific values. *Journal of Clinical Psychology, 31*, 483–485.

Diddams, M., Klein Surdyk, L., & Daniels, D. (2004). Rediscovering models of Sabbath keeping: Implications for psychological well-being. *Journal of Psychology & Theology, 32*, 3–11.

Fayard, C., Harding, G. I., Murdoch, W., & Brunt, J. (2007). Clinical implications for psychotherapy from the Seventh-Day Adventist tradition. *Journal of Psychology and Christianity, 26*, 207–217.

Fiese, B. H., & Tomcho, T. J. (2001). Finding meaning in religious practices: The relation between religious holiday rituals and marital satisfaction. *Journal of Family Psychology, 15*, 597–609.

Gaebelein, F. E. (Ed.). (1990). *The expositor's Bible commentary: with the New International version of the Holy Bible, Genesis–Numbers.* Grand Rapids, MI: Zondervan.

Gaffin Jr., R. (1988). Sabbath. In S. B. Ferguson & D. F. Wright (Eds.), *New dictionary of theology* (p. 606). Downers Grove, IL: InterVarsity Press.

Glenn, N., & Weaver, C. (1978). A multivariate, multisurvey study of marital happiness. *Journal of Marriage and the Family, 40*, 269–282.

Gorsuch, R. L., & McPherson, S. E. (1989). Intrinsic/extrinsic measurement: I/E-Revised and single-item scales. *Journal for the Scientific Study of Religion, 28*, 348–354.

Groves, D. L. (1989). Family leisure interactions. *Journal of Instructional Psychology, 16*(2), 98–103.

Hansen, G. L. (1987). The effect of religiosity on factors predicting marital adjustment. *Social Psychology Quarterly, 50*, 264–269.

Heschel, A. J. (1951). *The Sabbath.* New York: The Noonday Press.

Hoeksma, J. H., Guy, J. D., Brown, C. K., & Brady, J. L. (1993). The relationship between psychotherapist burnout and satisfaction with leisure activities. *Psychotherapy in Private Practice, 12*, 51–57.

Hoge, D. R., & Carroll, J. W. (1973). Religiosity and prejudice in northern and southern churches. *Journal for the Scientific Study of Religion, 12,* 181–197.

Hull, R. B., & Michael, S. E. (1995). Nature-based recreation, mood change, and stress restoration. *Leisure Sciences, 17,* 1–14.

Hunt, R. A., & King, M. B. (1978). Religiosity and marriage. *Journal for the*

Scientific Study of Religion, 17(4), 399–406.

Jacobs, J. A., & Gerson, K. (2001). Overworked individuals or overworked families? Explaining trends in work, leisure, and family time. *Work and Occupations, 28*, 40–63.

Johnson, H. A., Zabriskie, R. B., & Hill, B. (2006). The contribution of couple leisure involvement, leisure time, and leisure satisfaction to marital satisfaction. *Marriage & Family Review, 40*, 69–91.

Johnson, M. P., Huston, T. L., Gaines, S. O., & Levinger, G. (1992). Patterns of married life among young couples. Special issues: Social networks. *Journal of Social and Personal Relationships, 9*, 343–364.

Jones, W. H., & Perlman, D. (Eds.). (1991). *Advances in personal relationships* (Vol. 2). London: Jessica Kingsley.

Joreskog, K. G., & Sorbom, D. (1984). *Lisrel VI. Analysis of linear structural relationships by maximum likelihood, instrumental variables, and least squares methods.* Mooreville, IN: Scientific Software.

Kahoe, R. D. (1974). Personality and achievement correlates of intrinsic and extrinsic religious orientation. *Journal of Personality and Social Psychology, 29*, 812–818.

Kaslow, F. W., Hansson, K., & Lundblad, A. M. (1994). Long term marriages in Sweden: And some comparisons with similar couples in the United States. *Contemporary Family Therapy: An International Journal, 16*, 521–537.

Klein, D. M., & White, J. M. (1996). *Family theories: An introduction.* Thousand Oaks, CA: Sage.

Kubo, S. (1978). *God meets man: A theology of the Sabbath and second advent.* Nashville, TN: Southern Publishing Association.

Lambert, N. M., & Dollahite, D. C. (2006). How religiosity helps couples prevent, resolve, and overcome marital conflict. *Family Relations, 55*, 439–449.

Leon-Durfour, X. (Ed.). (1962). Sabbath. *Dictionary of Biblical theology* (2nd Ed. Rev.) (pp. 511–512). New York: Seabury Press.

Levy, J. (1987). Leisure and the family: Towards some conceptual clarity. *Leisure Information Quarterly, 13*, 8–9.

Lotz, W. (1911). Sabbath. In S.M. Jackson (Ed.), *The new Schaff-Herzog encyclopedia of religious knowledge* (pp. 134–136). New York: Funk & Wagnallis Co.

McConahay, J. B., & Hough, J. C. (1976). Symbolic racism. *Journal of Social Issues, 32*, 23–45.

Muller, W. (1999). *Sabbath: Restoring the sacred rhythm of rest.* New York: Bantam.

Orathinkal, J., & Vansteenwegen, A. (2006). Religiosity and marital satisfaction. *Contemporary Family Therapy: An International Journal, 28,* 497–504.

Orthner, D. K., & Mancini, J. A. (1990). Leisure impacts on family interaction and cohesion. *Journal of Leisure Research, 22,* 125–137.

Perlman, D., & Fehr, B. (1987). The development of intimate relationships. In D. Perlman & S. W. Duck (Eds.), *Intimate relationships: Development, dynamics, and deterioration* (pp. 13–42). Beverly Hills, CA: Sage.

Peterson, E. H. (1987). *Working the angles: The shape of pastoral integrity.* Grand Rapids, MI: Eerdmans.

Pietropinto, A. (1985). Recreation and the family. *Medical Aspects of Human Sexuality, 19,* 197–201.

Rice, R. (1985). *The reign of God: An introduction to Christian theology from a Seventh-day Adventist Perspective.* Berrien Springs, MI: Andrews University Press.

Roggman, L. A., Moe, S. T., Hart, A. D., & Forthun, L. F. (1994). Family leisure and social support: Relations with parenting stress and psychological well-being in Head Start parents. *Early Childhood Research Quarterly, Head Start, 9,* 463–480.

Schaefer, M. T., & Olson, D. H. (1981). Assessing intimacy: The PAIR Inventory. *Journal of Marital & Family Therapy, 7,* 47–60.

Schumm, W. R., Bollman, S. R., & Jurich, A. P. (1982). The "marital conventionalization" argument: Implications for the study of religiosity and marital satisfaction. *Journal of Psychology & Theology, 10,* 236–241.

Schumm, W., Paff-Bergen, L., Hatch, R., Obiorah, F., Copeland, J., Meens, L., & Bugaighis, M. (1986). Concurrent and discriminant validity of the Kansas Marital Satisfaction Scale. *Journal of Marriage and the Family, 48,* 381–387.

Shapiro, D. H. & Shapiro, J. F. (1992). Couples and spirituality: A Jewish perspective on exile, yearning, and return. In B. J. Brothers (Ed.), *Spirituality and couples: Heart and soul in the therapy process* (pp. 77–95). Binghamton, NY: Haworth.

Shaw, S. M. (1985). The meaning of leisure in everyday life. *Leisure Sciences, 7,* 1–24.

Smith, G. T., Snyder, D. K., Trull, T. J., & Monsma, B. R. (1988). Predicting relationship satisfaction from couples' use of leisure time. *American*

Journal of Family Therapy, 16, 3–13.

Snow, T. S., & Compton, W. C. (1996). Marital satisfaction and communication in fundamentalist Protestant marriages. *Psychological Reports, 78*, 979–985.

Stanley, S. M. (1986). *Commitment and the maintenance and enhancement of relationships.* Unpublished doctoral dissertation, University of Denver.

Steinmueller, J. & K. Sullivan (1950*). Catholic Biblical encyclopedia: NT* (pp. 558–559). New York: Joseph F. Wagner.

Strand, K. A. (ed.) (1982). *The Sabbath in Scripture and history.* Washington, DC: Review & Herald Publishing.

Strickland, B. R., & Weddell, S. C. (1972). Religious orientation, racial prejudice, and dogmatism: A study of Baptists and Unitarians. *Journal for the Scientific Study of Religion, 11*, 395–399.

Sullivan, O. (1996). The enjoyment of activities: Do couples affect each others' well-being? *Social Indicators Research, 38*, 81–102.

Tinsley, H. E., Hinson, J. A., Tinsley, D. J., & Holt, M. S. (1993). Attributes of leisure and work experiences. *Journal of Counseling Psychology, 40*, 447–455.

Tinsley, H. E. A., & Tinsley, D. J. (1986). A theory of the attributes, benefits and causes of leisure experiences. *Leisure Sciences, 8*, 1–45.

Tinsley, H. E. A., & Tinsley, D. J. (1988). An expanded context for the study of career decision making, development, and maturity. In W. B. Walsh & S. H. Osipow (Eds.), *Career decision making* (pp. 213–264). Hillsdale, NK: Erlbaum.

Weiss, R. L., Hops, H., & Patterson, G. R. (1973). A framework for conceptualizing marital conflict, a technology for altering it, some data for evaluating it. In F. W. Clark & L. A. Hamerlynck (Eds.), *Critical issues in research and practice: Proceedings of the Fourth Banff International Conference on Behavior Modification* (pp. 309–342). Champaign, IL: Research Press.

White, E. G. (1888). *The great controversy.* Mountain View, CA: Pacific Press.

White, E. G. (1948a). *Testimonies for the church, vol. 2.* Mountain View, CA: Pacific Press.

White, E. G. (1948b). *Testimonies for the church, vol. 6.* Mountain View, CA: Pacific Press.

White, E. G. (1948c). *Testimonies for the church, vol. 7.* Mountain View, CA: Pacific Press.

White, E. G. (1976). *Steps to Christ.* Washington, D.C.: Review & Herald.

White, E. G. (1989). *The Desire of Ages.* Mountain View, CA: Pacific Press.

Wilkinson, M. L. & Tanner, W. C. (1980). The influence of family size, interaction, and religiosity on family affection in Mormon sample. *Journal of Marriage and the Family, 42*, 297–304.

Wilson, M. R., & Filsinger, E. E. (1986). Religiosity and marital adjustment: Multidimensional interrelationships. *Journal of Marriage and the Family, 48*, 147–151.

Wirzba, N., & Berry, W. (2006). *Living the Sabbath: Discovering the rhythms of rest and delight.* Grand Rapids, MI: Brazos Press.

Wynne, L. C., & Wynne, A. R. (1986). The quest for intimacy. *Journal of Marital and Family Therapy, 12*, 383–394.

Children's Perceptions of God's Role in Their Families: An Exploratory Study

Barbara Couden Hernandez and Jamie D. Aten

The recent revival of interest in religious beliefs as a mental health resource has prompted researchers and clinicians to re-examine the potential benefits of incorporating and addressing religion in the therapeutic process (Miller & Delaney, 2004; Richards & Bergin, 2003). Religion is distinct from spirituality in that it involves a corporate, organized system of beliefs about God, moral expectations for adherents, and affiliation with a faith community (Walsh, 1999) while spirituality often refers to a highly individualistic and personal guiding philosophy of meaning and way of being in the world (Miller & Thoresen, 1999). Doherty (1999) noted that there is insufficient attention given to religious beliefs and practices in the study of families, and Miller (1999) underscored the need for more empirical literature on both religion and spirituality as mental health variables.

Seventh-day Adventists (SDAs) have long taught that parental practices are associated with their children's view of God. "Great is the honor and the responsibility placed on fathers and mothers in that they are to stand in the place of God to their children" (White, 1942, p. 375). The Bible makes numerous references to the parental qualities of God (Ps. 103:13; Hosea 11:1; Matt. 6:6; Rom. 8:15), and anecdotal evidence indicates that this idea is a common theme in sermons. In her book, *The Adventist Home* (1952), early church leader Ellen White wrote, "Every mother should have time to give her children....little endearments which are so essential during infancy and childhood.... She is to them what God is to us" (p. 197).

Christian authors report that one's attachment to faith communities and even to God are highly influenced by one's family of origin (Carder, Henslin, Townsend, Cloud, & Brawand 1991). Griffith (1999) reported that a number of her clients likened God to various family members such as "an exasperated mother," "a strict old grandfather," and "a nursing mama" (p. 214). In his research regarding the moral and spiritual experience of children, Coles (1990; 1997) used drawings as vehicles for communication of religious beliefs such as the person of God, eschatology, expectations for righteous living, and the depiction of events from Scripture. Several cases were cited in his work in which drawings and descriptions of God paralleled relationships the child had with a parent or guardian figure. Thus, it seems that children spontaneously make this connection.

Much of the religiously oriented literature on childrearing and family life addresses the theological ramifications of family relationships and goal behaviors. However, no explanation exists regarding how God or belief in God facilitates behaviors of parents or children in order to reach those goals. Given that religious instruction for SDA children repeatedly references the importance of asking Jesus to help them obey, to help their parents, and to get along with their siblings, there is potential for children to view the role of God in the family in numerous ways. However, very few studies in the field include children as chief reporters, particularly in terms of spiritual issues.

KINETIC FAMILY DRAWINGS

Projective drawings in eliciting family process have been used as a nonthreatening way to move therapy toward issues which need family attention (Zilbach, 1986). Therapists and health care workers have effectively used drawings to assist children in expressing concerns which may be too difficult or complex to verbalize, such as (1) divorce sequella (Cohen & Ronen, 1999; Spigelman, Spigelman, & Englesson, 1992), (2) adoption (Black & Kaczmarek, 1992), (3) oppositional defiant behavior (Carlson, 1997), (4) child abuse (La Roche, 1994; Manning, 1987; Oaklander, 1978), (5) attachment to pets (Kidd & Kidd, 1995), (6) aging (Falchikov, 1990), and (7) physical illness (Clunies-Ross & Lansdown, 1988; Stefanatou & Bowler, 1997).

The Kinetic Family Drawing (KFD) is a well-established projective device used to elicit children's perceptions of familial relationships, self-concept, and gender roles of family members (DiLeo, 1983). Children are given a sheet of paper and instructed, "Draw a picture of everyone in your family, including you, everyone doing something. Try to draw whole people, not cartoons or stick people. Make everyone doing something—some kind of action" (Burns & Kaufman, 1970, p. 5). No time limit is imposed and children are encouraged to depict family members in whatever way they choose. After the child indicates she or he has completed the drawing, the examiner asks the child to identify figures and clarify the activities portrayed.

As with many projective tests, the KFD is best understood in conjunction with an interview or clinical observations and should not be interpreted outside such a context. Care is taken to avoid "over-interpretation" of drawings, as a high level of subjectivity inherent in such interpretation may promote false conclusions. Hence, general impressions of the drawings are combined with interpretation of obvious indicators if supported by interview responses (Handler & Habenicht, 1994).

Some critics of the KFD believe that the drawings reflect a child's mood state at the time of drawing rather than long-term family trends (Mostkoff & Lazarus, 1983). College students have been found to depict desired feelings of closeness and interaction in the KFD rather than actual interpersonal dynamics (Holtz, Brannigan, & Schofield, 1980). Reliability and validity of the KFD as a definitive diagnostic adjunct is controversial with contradicting studies and indications (e.g., Hibbard & Hartman, 1990; LaRoche, 1994). However, the KFD continues to be commonly used in practice (Stein, 2001) to generate hypotheses and describe feeling states (Ogdon, 1988), and as a research instrument (Packman et al., 2008).

DEVELOPMENT OF GOD IMAGE

Pitts (1976) posited that children's view of God develops between the ages of two and six years. His study of children's depictions of God indicates that differences in anthropomorphism (drawing God as a person in a body) varies across the range of religious affiliation according to theology of the person of God, with more person-like representations corresponding to increased religious education and integration of religion into daily life of the denomination.

Fowler (1984) outlined seven stages of faith and moral development over the course of one's lifetime. Children between the ages of 6 and 12 are at the *mythic-literal* stage during which they readily and concretely describe the beliefs of the community into which they have been socialized. Responses from these children, therefore, were expected to be rich in interpretation of their faith, perspectives, and ideas about the actions of God.

To the best of our knowledge, there is no study that surveys children's perceptions of the influence of God or Higher Power on the family. Children are seldom the chief respondents in family research, nor are children's religious beliefs often studied. Additionally, little is known about how to work in therapy with children whose religious beliefs impact their view of family dynamics.

PURPOSE STATEMENT

This phenomenological qualitative study was conducted in order to examine the ways in which children think about God's role in their families' everyday life. The Kinetic Family Drawing (KFD) device and semi-structured interviews were used to explore the following research questions: (1) Do SDA children think that God influences the way family members get along with one another? (2) To what family-related phenomena do SDA children attribute the direct or indirect influence of God? (3) Do SDA children's beliefs about the role of God in influencing family function impact the way they interpret behaviors or events within their families? and (4) What are SDA children's perceptions of God?

METHOD

PHILOSOPHICAL PARADIGM

This study was conducted from a post-positivistic philosophical paradigm. Five primary assumptions underscore this perspective: (1) The nature of reality and the way that people perceive reality is highly subjective; (2) perceptions and personal experience have a direct impact on how people interpret reality; (3) these can vary greatly from person to person; (4) interpretations of reality are not static and may alter with time; and (5) people construct knowledge contextually (McGrath & Johnson, 2003).

RESEARCHER-AS-INSTRUMENT

The primary investigator is a Caucasian female associate professor at Loma Linda University who is a life-long Adventist. She has actively participated in the education of children and adults regarding family life education and religious instruction in a variety of contexts. She also has therapeutic experience with abused children in faith-affiliated families. She teaches doctoral coursework on the integration of religion and spirituality in therapy. The secondary investigator is a Caucasian male associate professor at a Christian university in the Midwest. He completed a pre-doctoral internship at a Christian training site affiliated with an Evangelical graduate school that emphasized the integration of psychology and Christianity. He has also counseled children in faith-affiliated families in a variety of outpatient settings. The secondary investigator grew up in an Evangelical Christian family, raised in the Church of Christ. A former youth pastor and campus ministry intern, he is currently active in a large non-denominational community church.

PARTICIPANTS

This study was conducted in a southern California SDA K-10 school with a strong religious education curriculum. Consent was obtained for thirty-five children between the ages of eight and ten years of age. The majority of students were third graders with a mean age of nine years. Racial diversity of the sample is represented in Table 1. Three students were excluded due to either non-Christian or no religious affiliation. The majority of participants were from SDA families (97%), with one Catholic family (3%). Three children were not able to participate due to illness, leaving a final sample of twenty-nine children of whom nineteen were female and ten were male.

Table 1. Racial diversity of children

	%	n
African American	10%	3
Asian	10%	3
Middle Eastern	3%	1
Latino	14%	4
Caucasian	62%	18
		n = 29

PROCEDURES

A large SDA elementary school in southern California was selected as the data collection site. Research procedures were explained to the principal who agreed to endorse the study and solicit parental consent for participants. A letter from the vice-principal was sent to parents of forty third- and thirty-seven fourth graders explaining the purpose of this study along with consent forms for the participation of their child. Consent was obtained from thirty-five (45%) parents. Interviews were conducted over the course of five days within a two-week period of time. Teachers released children from class and sent them to an empty adjacent classroom to meet with the first author at scheduled times. Verbal consent was obtained for participation from each child. Data collection for each child required an average of thirty minutes, ranging from eleven minutes to two hours.

MEASURES

In order to explore the perceived interplay between God and the family, an adaptation of the Kinetic Family Drawing, developed by Burns and Kaufman (1970), was used as the data collection tool. This instrument was designed to identify areas for further investigation, not to diagnose participants. Children were instructed, "Draw everyone in your family, and God, everybody doing some activity. Do not draw stick people or cartoons." Pencils and unlined white paper were used for the drawings.

Following the drawings, semi-structured interviews were tape-recorded and transcribed. The interview questions explored each child's beliefs about God, how or if God influenced the family, as well as the child's experience as a member of the family. Examples of the questions included on the interview protocol were:

> Explain what is happening in your picture.
> Does God do anything in your family? How do you know?
> What is it like if God doesn't do anything in your family?

Field notes were taken over the duration of and after each interview with the children. Each child's drawing demeanor, salient behavioral features, and comments were documented in the field notes.

DATA ANALYSIS

Analysis consisted of a four-step process that most closely followed phenomenological methods of qualitative research (Kvale, 1996). Drawings were first given a cursory analysis without reading the child's corresponding interview transcript. The interpretive guidelines used were those of Burns and Kaufman (1972) based on their analysis of some 10,000 KFD drawings obtained in clinical settings. Other considerations for interpretation were taken from studies of drawing trends across ranges of ages, cultures, household structures, and in diverse populations of children (Andersson, 1995; Payne, 1996). Additional resources were the human figure drawing and House-Tree-Person drawing interpretation guidelines for enigmatic human figure depictions (Ogdon, 1988; Wenck,

1970). The most evocative feature of each picture was noted and potential interpretations made. Menacing facial features, indications of despair or isolation, the transcendence of God, and family relationship dynamic portrayals were particularly salient during the first step of analysis. Pictures were sorted according to indicators which reflected the following emerging themes: (1) family relationship quality, (2) features of parents reflected in depictions of God, (3) indicators of stress and trauma, (4) family structure variations, (5) family dynamics, and (6) depictions of God interacting with family members.

Each transcript was then read without consideration of the corresponding drawing to develop an overall sense of each child's belief, family dynamic, and emotional content. After a second reading of transcripts, the most dominant theme of each interview was noted in terms of the child's beliefs, experiences, perceptions of family and God, or emotional indicators. Drawings were then interpreted in light of the most salient features identified in each corresponding interview transcript. Drawing devices that were corroborated by interview data and field notes were then interpreted according to the research questions.

EVALUATIVE CRITERIA

According to Lincoln and Guba (1985), qualitative research should be judged by the following evaluative criteria: (1) credibility, (2) transferability, (3) dependability, and (4) confirmability. A number of rigor-enhancing strategies were utilized during this study to attend to Lincoln and Guba's evaluative criteria: (1) field notes, (2) thick descriptions, (3) memos, (4) triangulation, (5) outside auditors, and (6) reflexivity practices (i.e., discussing potential researcher biases).

RESULTS

This exploratory study yielded several recurring themes in both interview responses and drawings which warrant further investigation. Each major theme will be briefly described, followed by participant narratives. It should be noted that it was not uncommon to find indicators of more than one theme when considering the combined drawing-interview-field note data.

PERCEPTIONS OF GOD

God was depicted as Jesus by fourteen (48%) of the twenty-nine participants, consistent with SDA Trinitarian beliefs. Children depicted God and the family involved in interactive activities such as playing sports, helping the family, or giving instruction in nine drawings (31%). God was shown in an elevated position surrounded by clouds ("in heaven") in eleven pictures (38%) and performing omnipotent acts such as healing the sick or creating the world in ten pictures (34%). God was drawn with human bodily features by 97% of the participants. In ten (34%) cases, God was portrayed without visible function or connection to the family. Proximity-distance, an indicator of interaction, between God and the family approximated the degree of distance among family members in twenty-four (83%) of the pictures.

BELIEF IN GOD AS AN EMOTIONAL RESOURCE

God was described or depicted by nine (31%) of the children as an emotional resource for them as individuals. These children often spoke of stressful family, school, or social situations in which the guidance and support they needed was not forthcoming. Children cited limitations in their parents' abilities to resolve crises, such as illness, potential loss of a job, or dangerous work conditions. However, they seemed to believe that God would provide material help or solutions such as in providing protection, healing, imparting needed information, or through fortuitous events.

Julie (all identifiers have been changed) is an eight-year-old child. She drew herself, her brother, and stepfather on a couch watching television (see Figure 1). Her mother, cooking in the kitchen, was partitioned off from the rest of the family by three lines, suggesting emotional unavailability. The family dog, Milton, is shown at her feet. Julie's father and his fiancé are seen joining the family in the living room. This child presented an

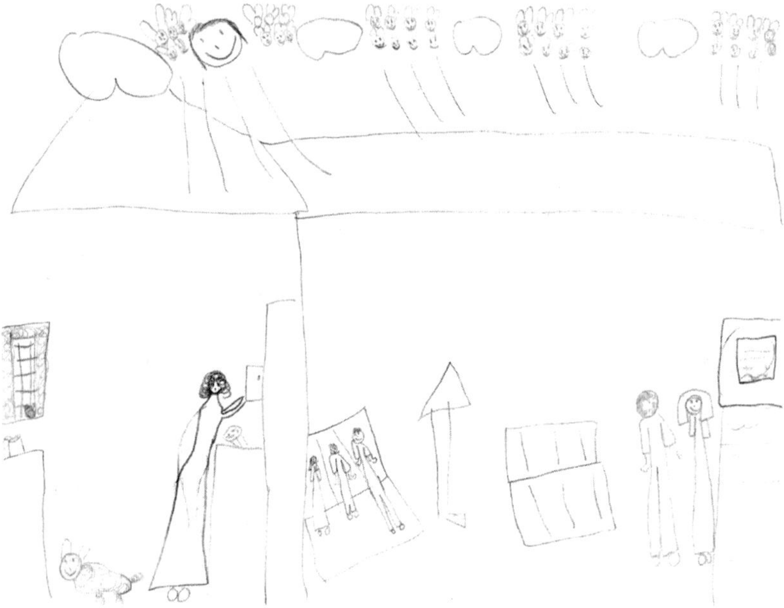

Figure 1. Julie's mother and dog, Milton, are seen in the kitchen. Julie, her brother, and stepfather are watching television, with Julie's father and girlfriend "coming for a visit." God, angels, and "something like lights" are seen above the horizon line.

impressive list of concerns in her life beginning with the adjustment to the altered family structure by the addition of a new step-father. "I don't get along well with [step-father]. He told me I'll have to stay in my room all week. I wish my mom and dad would get back together." She stated that she had to decide which parent to live with, expressing dismay and anxiety about this choice. She feared that her diabetic brother would not get to the hospital in time during his next hypoglycemic episode. She described the recent death of her uncle in a car accident as being particularly traumatizing. Several times in the interview Julie discussed the importance of prayer in dealing with her fears about the family:

> We pray about my mom not dying after she has her baby, and about Milton because he has a bad back.…I prayed about Milton and he

> seems to be doing fine....God's making him able to play and stuff. We pray about my dad's business and hope it runs well...and that it's not going to be too much stress with all the bills....and that the marriage is going to go well.

Julie's drawing includes thirty-five angels along with God, emanating "something like lights" (downward lines) toward the family. The notion that light indicates a need for warmth and love (Burns & Kaufman, 1972) seems to fit well with the narrative of multiple stressors in this child's life. Children in threatening home environments often externalize both aggression and fear by filling the sky of their drawings with signs of inclement weather (Manning, 1987). It is possible that Julie attempted to compensate for her fears by depicting a large number of "resources" in the form of angels in her drawing. Perhaps a child's belief of an omnipotent God or guardian angels acts to counterbalance fear or stress in situations that are disenfranchising, or during times in which help does not appear forthcoming.

A second illustration of this emerged in the drawing completed by Sam, a nine-year-old boy (see Figure 2). He drew a family in which no interaction occurred between members. His sister was encapsulated by the figure of a tree (emotional distance) and was rotated in such a way that she could not see Sam, while the father sat with his back to both children. Sam's figure seemed to move toward the father in a menacing way. "I'm practicing martial arts," he said. The mother figure not only had her back to the rest of the family, but was encapsulated in a box shape and was separated from them by four vertical lines in addition to the television set. Sam reported that she is a student and also has a full-time job. He revealed that his parents attend different churches because of their stylistic preference. Sam and his parents do not get along well. A larger-than-life smiling God appears at the top of the drawing. To the left of God is "the family angel. He looks over our family." Notice again warmth indicated by the light emanating from both God and the angel. A striking feature of the picture of God is the exaggerated size

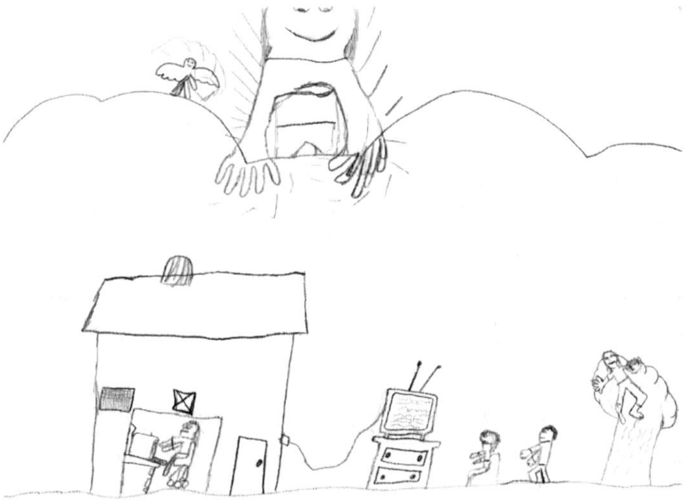

Figure 2. Sam's family. The family angel is to the left of God in this picture.

of the arms and hands, an indication of power and activity (Wenck, 1977). It may be that this child views God as a source of warmth and positive power in this setting of emotional disconnection.

ASSOCIATION BETWEEN DEPICTIONS OF FAMILY INTERACTION STYLE AND PERCEPTION OF GOD

In ten (34%) of the drawings, the family interaction styles and behaviors, along with interpersonal distances, were comparable. Some families were shown engaged in solitary activities such as reading or swinging, while God was portrayed in solitary activity, such as creating the world, protecting the family, or sitting on a throne. Similarly, a number of these pictures showed God drawn on the same plane as the family, involved in games, conversation, or church activities. The degree of involvement between God and the family often mirrored the level of involvement among family members. This was particularly evident in John's drawing. John is the eldest of two brothers living with his mother and stepfather. His biological father lives 1,000 miles away. The most salient impression I (BCH) had was John's presentation: sad expression, disheveled clothing, enthusiasm as he spoke of visiting his father, and his obvious delight in having my full attention. The latter was evident as he engaged me in conversation right up to the time he closed the door behind him as he left the test site. I was struck by his obvious effort to obtain my attention and approval and by the sadness I felt as I listened to him talk about his life. John began his picture by portraying himself as the catcher at a baseball game (see Figure 3). His mother was drawn to the left in a small barred compartment, "watching me." He stopped drawing after completing these two figures. When questioned about God and other family members, he drew God watching the game from a cloud at the other end of the baseball field, and added two other friends who are team members. "...[my brother] doesn't want to go [to my games] because he says they give him headaches and plus, there's nothing to do. My dad doesn't come because he works at night." He explained that he worries about his stepfather who works as a fire fighter. Because his stepfather sleeps during the day and works during the evening, John spends very little time with him. With the exception of the two eyes on the representation of himself, none of the figures had facial features, giving the impression of incidental attachment and the absence of meaningful identity. When I (BCH) reflected that God seemed far away from where John was in the picture, he said:

> Okay...when my parents stopped seeing each other and then they separated and said they wanted a divorce, ...it put me through a really bad time because I had to keep going back and forth and I didn't like that...and it was very hard and it seemed that He [God] wasn't close at all. I tell [God] to help me get over [my problems] and just forget them so life can go on.

John explained that he and his brother spend summers with his father but have little time with him because of his father's late work hours. He described frequently waiting for his father to come home so they could "do something." "I think [God] would say [to my father], 'Have a lot of fun with your boys when they come up to see you. Try to do more

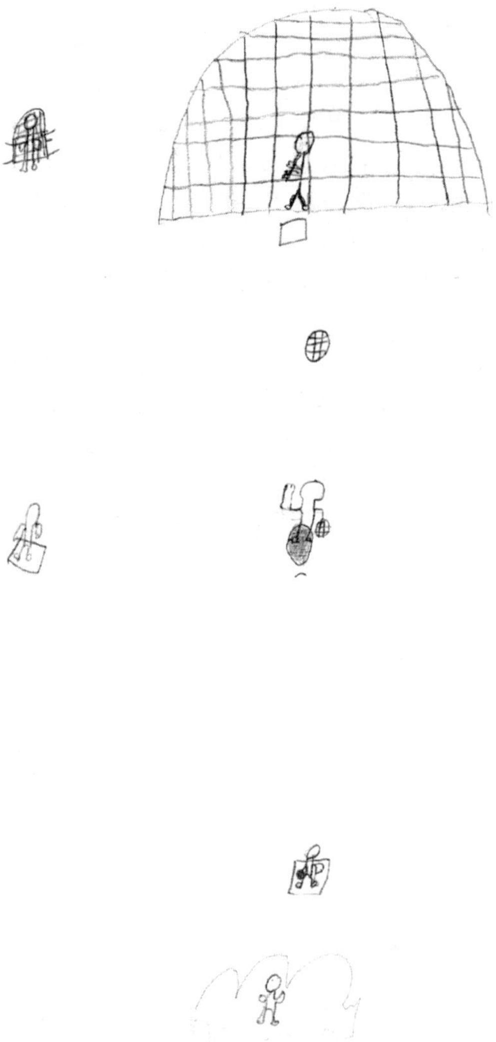

Figure 3. John playing baseball. God is drawn in the foreground on a cloud.

things with them.'" The general tone of the picture indicates distance and John's feelings of separation from his family. He and his mother both are encapsulated in jail-like enclosures, indicative of emotional isolation. Everyone seems disconnected from meaningful interaction.

The unusually small sizes of the figures possibly reflect John's sense of insignificance in the larger scheme of things. It is interesting to note that God is depicted as small, distant, encapsulated, and generally featureless.

GOD WITH PARENTAL FEATURES

Seven of the twenty-nine drawings (24%) included parallel activities or qualities between at least one parent and God. Scott, age eight, drew his family of four and Jesus on the same plane and of similar size (see Figure 4). He depicted himself throwing a ball at his sister, and displayed rapid speech, difficulties staying on topic, and constant motor movement. The father is a businessman and is shown holding his briefcase. Scott states that his mother, who is a physician, has a chronic debilitating disease:

> My mother is very sick....the doctors can't do anything about it and...my mom feels like she is gonna' die. Her chest is like, [makes a stridorous inhalation sound] and she can barely move and she can't do things....she has a lot of pain.

When asked what God might say to his mother he responded, "He'd compliment her because she's done real good things. I wouldn't be surprised if suddenly she comes up with a cure of the AIDS virus!"

Notice that Scott depicted Jesus in a parallel role to that of his

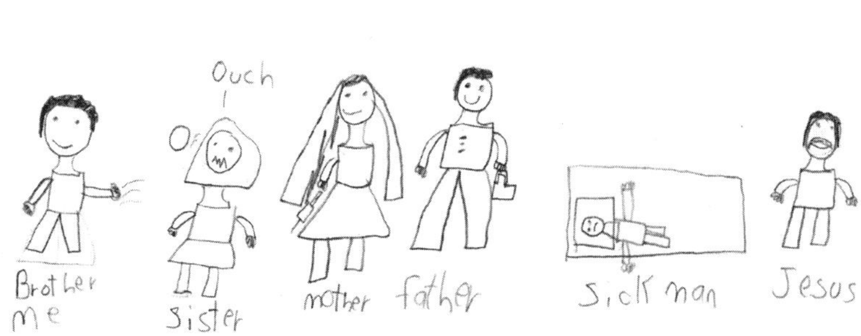

Figure 4. Scott's family: Scott throwing a ball at his sister, mother with a syringe in her hand, father with a briefcase, "sick man," and Jesus.

mother, offering glowing comments about God's approval of her skills as a healer. In addition to highlighting her God-like characteristics, this may reflect his unstated wish for divine healing of his mother.

Sandy, a child of ten, drew her father reading a book, her mother cooking, her sister talking on the telephone, and herself roller-blading (see Figure 5). Depictions of cooking in KFD's are considered to be indicators of nurturance and warmth (Burns & Kaufman, 1972). She viewed her mother as having strong ties to God: "…someone who is very close to God. I see my mother pray a lot. She reads the Bible all the time..." Sandy also commented about God's activity in the drawing: "God is watching a cooking show with Julia Child on TV. He likes cooking.…God is really, *really* kind. If He decided to talk to someone in the family it would be my mom." This mutual interest of God and Sandy's mother could be an indication of God's special approval of her mother, or perhaps that God is some type of extension or parallel identity to her mother.

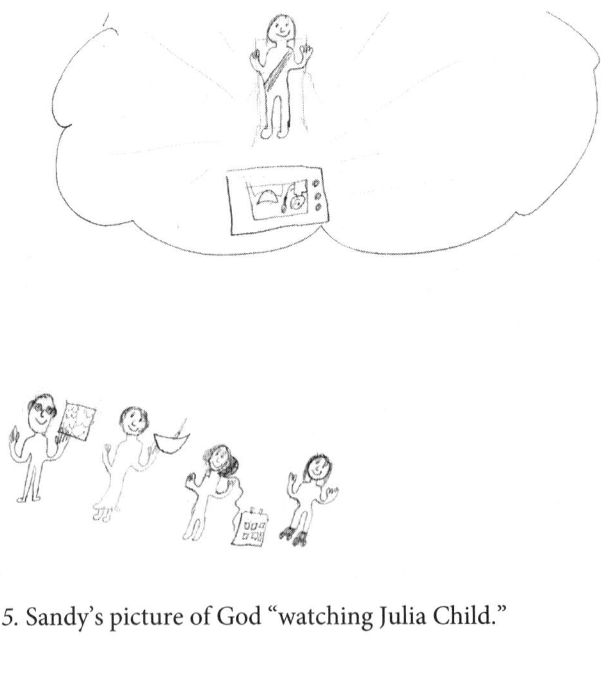

Figure 5. Sandy's picture of God "watching Julia Child."

HOW GOD HELPS THE FAMILY

Closely tied to the notion of belief in God as an emotional resource was the belief that God's presence had positive effects on the family. This was a salient theme in eight (28%) of the drawings. Material gains, decreased sibling or parental fighting, prevention of natural disasters, and protection were described as indicators of God's intervention or presence in the family. Fifteen (52%) children reported prayer made them worry less by assuring them of their family's well-being. Many of these children explained that God's absence or being "far away" seemed to impact the family negatively. When asked what happens when God is not "close" to the family, Mike, age nine replied:

> ...sometimes when He's not with our family we don't get along very much....sometimes we just get in arguments and then He's not there anymore or something....No...it's almost like He tries to stop us from fighting.

As noted earlier, children pray about the health of their families, financial concerns, and protection for family members. These requests for specific, tangible things are consistent with the concrete thinking typical of this developmental stage. However, a number of children reported praying about the quality of family relationships. For instance, Mary, age nine, stated, "If God is not in our family I'd get in lots of trouble. We would always be fighting."

Children also indicated an association between good behavior and closeness to God. John, age nine, described an instance in which he believed God was "close" to him:

> There's a way I can feel that [God was close to me]...my brother was bugging me because my mom...left me in charge to go to bed at 8:30 and my brother was saying, "Let's go to bed at 9:00, please?" And I said, "No"...when we went to bed at 8:30 it seemed that God was talking to me because I felt like...happy inside me....And it seemed that Jesus was saying, "Good boy! You did just what your mom said."

Protection of family members and their relationships was a common topic of children's reported prayers, as depicted by Samantha, age nine:

> Well, I talk to [God] about taking care of my family…and to help my family…um…have peace to one another…and that my gramma, that my grampa won't die…and that my aunt and uncle won't break up.

Asked if God made reply to her requests, she stated, "Well, He says it will be all right. That whatever happens, it will be okay."

Prayer also seemed to help children cope with challenging personal situations. "I pray a lot because of my fatness.…it really helps.…I get teased by my brothers all the time because I can't do math.…it hurts my feelings.…and being fat. I know Jesus helps me."

DISCUSSION

This sample of children made frequent references to their perceptions of God's influence in the family. Such intervention was often obtained through prayer or through efforts to fulfill God's expectation for "good" behavior. Unsolicited providential intervention was also cited in cases of near drowning, catastrophic earthquake, and conflict with friends. Thus, it is possible that a child's belief in God may serve as an emotional resource and enhance individual resiliency. Belief that God loves and cares for them emotionally and materially may be a protective factor for children living with multiple family stressors.

Anthony and Cohler (1987) described resilient children who, in the midst of chaotic or otherwise challenging family settings, were able to find stability in their religious beliefs. These beliefs "…brought meaning, order, and dedication into their lives…and developed a wide range of coping skills" (p. 173). Rutter (1999) described "neutralizing effects" that environmental and peer influences play on children in emotionally disadvantaged circumstances. Brokaw and Edwards (1994) found that internalizations of a gracious and loving God in young adults are positively correlated with healthy ego functions. Belief in God may act as such a neutralizing effect in children from stressed homes. As of yet we do not fully understand the mechanism whereby religious beliefs enhance resilience in children, though children in this study frequently expressed confidence in their perception of an all-knowing, powerful, and empowering force when speaking of God. It remains unclear whether a child's view of God as a resource is an independent, transcendent notion; a projection of existing family relationships; or a combination of both. There is evidence in this data that some children perceive God as having the same relationship properties as their family members. This was depicted by the use of parallel artistic devices when drawing family members and drawing God, such as distance, partitioning, and physical features. However, it is interesting to note that in an integration of attachment theory and neuroaffective neuroscience, Noffke & Hall (2007) demonstrated that the relationship with one's parent figure creates an experiential sense of relating to God and forms the template for interactions with others. Pitts (1976) earlier stated that as children move from Piaget's preoperational to operational stage of development, their concept of God is augmented by their ability to create representations of God through artistic means and verbal articulation. He further described the sense of awe children have for their parents and how this can become incorporated into the child's perspective of what God is like. Coles (1990) discussed similarities in behavior and character attributions children make about God in his discussion of a child who believed that God might "get pale and pass out, too" (p. 56) just like his grandfather looks like he will do when he is angry. Coles describes another child whose description of God's judgment procedures paralleled that of her uncle's "fierce admonishment" (p. 47).

The belief in God of these children with strong faith affiliation seemed to be integral to their sense of family identity. Throughout the data, the idea that God wants families to be harmonious through courtesy, respect, and obedience was evident. Therefore it was not surprising to hear participants express their belief that God is actively involved in family dynamics and events. The belief that God contributes to family function and individual relationship integrity is a salient feature of many SDA books and media programs. Many of my adult clients (BCH) have discussed their expectations that God would improve their relationships with difficult in-laws, special needs children, or conflictual marital relationships. Children also struggle to find connection between their belief in a God who is interested in the well-being of their family and the reality of family challenges.

Several limitations exist in the interpretation of this study. The high degree of subjectivity required to interpret drawings allowed only tentative assertions of conclusiveness. The reliability of the KFD instrument may have been influenced by the children's mood at the time of administration. Therefore, a full understanding of family traits or the trend of family behavior cannot be assumed by interpretation of drawings alone.

This study took place two weeks after a magnitude eight earthquake occurred in this region. Increased anxiety may have been reflected in children's responses, as several of them spoke about their reactions to the earthquake either during or before beginning their drawings.

The efficacy of the KFD with the inclusion of a depiction of God to portray God and family interactions has not been previously explored. Results obtained by use of this instrument must therefore be interpreted cautiously. A more detailed interview would also be helpful to gain specific insight into these children's family dynamics, faith beliefs, and notions of God's interaction in the family.

Because the sample consisted of only SDA children, this study has limited generalizability. Study results could be considerably different in samples of children from Catholic, Mormon, Unitarian, or non-Christian religious groups. This study could not be replicated in faith communities in which attempts to depict God may be considered inappropriate or even blasphemous.

IMPLICATIONS

A number of implications naturally follow the findings of this exploratory study pertaining to therapy situations in which children wish to discuss their religious beliefs. Therapists may not recognize the important role of a child's spiritual beliefs and minimize the need for exploration by implicit discouragement of discussion. This may occur if the clinician is fearful of acting in a leading manner, somehow changing the child's beliefs by inadvertently or intrusively presenting their own beliefs for emulation.

Children's ways of knowing are often undervalued, as their knowledge is assumed to be faulty and incomplete due to their level of cognitive development. Adults frequently fall into a teaching role without assessing what children believe, how they arrived at their beliefs, and the significance of their beliefs in everyday life. Religious affiliation and spiritual beliefs provide a framework for meaning and cohesiveness of life events for many individuals. Failure to explore and respect this matrix of behavior, attitudes, and beliefs removes therapeutic intervention from such a client's relevant context and can privilege the therapist's biases and agenda. While clinicians may not know exactly how to include a child's beliefs in therapy, the findings of this study indicate that it is not therapeutically prudent to ignore them.

Ethical practice requires therapists to become spiritually literate by learning about multiple religious groups in order to become familiar with the context, language, and norms of the child's belief system (Haug, 1998). In populations such as this sample, it is important to recognize that all SDA children may not have the same beliefs, practices, or family experiences, all of which influence their ideas about God's role in their formative relationships. Inquiring about a child's belief in God's influence on the family may provide a useful background against which to formulate therapeutic interventions.

CONCLUSION

This exploratory study yielded four primary themes about children's perceptions of God and family. Children believed that God was an emotional resource for the family. Many turned to God for emotional support to cope with stressful situations and to find reassurance. There was also an association between children's depictions of their families' interaction style and their perception of God. Similarly, children depicted God with parental features. For instance, a child who thought of his mother as standoffish and emotionally unavailable superimposed this image onto God, thereby attributing similar characteristics to God. A number of ways that children believe God helps the family were also identified—that God could provide material help or healing, for instance. On the whole, children conceptualized God with human qualities and held perceptions of God that were consistent with SDA Trinitarian beliefs.

There is still a need for more research in this area of study, as very little literature is currently available regarding the incorporation of children's spiritual beliefs in therapy. Further study is needed regarding the possibility that children experience a sense of security and well-being as they attribute improving family relationships, assisting family decisions, and preserving the family to how well they fit into Divine and parental expectations of behavior. Utilizing more reliable methods of data collection, children's beliefs about SDA doctrines such as soul sleep after death, Sabbath observance, and end-time eschatology need to be investigated. Given children's changing cognitive capabilities across developmental stages, the way in which children form their belief about the influence of God on the family needs to be explored further as do the developmental transitions into adult beliefs.

A comparative survey of children from a wide range of religious groups may provide a broader base of understanding the way children's perspectives of God develop, and its relevance to family function, while controlling for doctrinal differences. Likewise, longitudinal measures may provide insight about how children's views of God's intervention as well as depiction ability develop over time. This brief glimpse into SDA children's perceptions of how God influences families indicates that both awareness and further study are needed to address the spiritual, religious, and family realities of children.

REFERENCES

Andersson, S. B. (1995). Social scaling in children's family drawings: A comparative study in three cultures. *Child Study Journal 25,* 97–121.

Anthony, E. J., & Cohler, B. J. (1987). *The invulnerable child.* New York: Guilford Press.

Black, C. A., & Kaczmarek, M. A. (1992). Projective drawings in the treatment and evaluation of a late-adopted child. *American Journal of Art Therapy, 31,* 10–16.

Brokaw, B. F., & Edwards, K. J. (1994). The relationship of God image to level of object relations development. *Journal of Psychology & Theology, 22*(4), 352–371.

Burns, R. C., & Kaufman, S. H. (1970). *Kinetic Family Drawings (K-F-D): An introduction to understanding children through Kinetic Drawings.* New York: Brunner/Mazel.

Burns, R. C., & Kaufman, S. H. (1972). *Actions, styles and symbols in Kinetic Family Drawings (K-F-D): An interpretive manual.* New York: Brunner/Mazel.

Carder, D., Henslin, E., Townsend, J., Cloud, H., & Brawand, A. (1991). *Secrets of your family tree.* Chicago: Moody Bible Institute of Chicago.

Carlson, T. D. (1997). Using art in narrative therapy: Enhancing therapeutic possibilities. *American Journal of Family Therapy, 25,* 271–283.

Clunies-Ross, C., & Lansdown, R. (1988). Concepts of death, illness and isolation found in children with leukaemia. *Child: Care, health and development, 14,* 373–386.

Cohen, O., & Ronen, T. (1999). Young children's adjustment to their parents' divorce as reflected in their drawings. *Journal of Divorce & Remarriage, 30,* 47–70.

Coles, R. (1990). *The spiritual life of children.* Boston: Houghton Mifflin Company.

Coles, R. (1998). *The moral intelligences of children: How to raise a moral child.* New York: Plume.

DiLeo, J. H. (1983). *Interpreting children's drawings.* New York: Brunner/

Mazel Pub.

Doherty, W. J. (1999). Morality and spirituality in therapy. In F. Walsh (Ed.), *Spiritual resources in family therapy* (pp. 179–192). New York: The Guilford Press.

Falchikov, N. (1990). Youthful ideas about old age: An analysis of children's drawings. *International Journal of Aging and Human Development, 31,* 79–99.

Fowler, J. W. (1984). *Becoming adult, becoming Christian: Adult development and Christian faith.* San Francisco: Harper & Row.

Giorgi, A. (1994). A phenomenological perspective on certain qualitative research methods. *Journal of Phenomenological Psychology, 25,* 190–220.

Griffith, M. E. (1999). Opening therapy to conversations with a personal God. In F. Walsh (Ed.), *Spiritual resources in family therapy* (pp. 209–222). New York: The Guilford Press.

Handler, L., & Habenicht, D. (1994). The Kinetic Family Drawing technique: A review of the literature. *Journal of Personality Assessment, 62*(3), 440–464.

Haug, I. E. (1998). Including a spiritual dimension in family therapy: Ethical considerations. *Contemporary Family Therapy, 20,* 181–194.

Hibbard, R. A., & Hartman, G. L. (1990). Emotional indicators in human figure drawings of sexually victimized and nonabused children. *Journal of Clinical Psychology, 46,* 211–219.

Holtz, R., Brannigan, G. G., & Schofield, J. J. (1980). The Kinetic Family Drawing as a measure of interpersonal distance. *Journal of Genetic Psychology, 137,* 307–308.

Kidd, A. H., & Kidd, R. M. (1995). Children's drawings and attachment to pets. *Psychological Reports, 77,* 235–241.

Kvale, S. (1996). *InterViews: An introduction to qualitative research interviewing.* Thousand Oaks, CA: Sage Publications.

La Roche, L. (1994). Emotional indicators identified in the drawings of sexually abused children. *American Journal of Art Therapy, 33,* 45–51.

Lincoln, Y. S., & Guba, E. G. (1985). *Naturalistic inquiry.* Beverly Hills, CA: Sage Publications.

Manning, T. M. (1987). Aggression depicted in abused children's drawings. *The Arts in Psychotherapy, 14,* 15–24.

McGrath, J. E. & Johnson, B. A. (2003). Methodology makes meaning: How both qualitative and quantitative paradigms shape evidence and its interpretation. In: P. M. Camic, J. E. Rhodes, & L. Yardley (Eds.), *Qualitative research in psychology: Expanding perspectives in methodology and design.* Washington, D.C.: American Psychological Association, 2003, pp. 31–48.

Miller, W. R. (1999). Diversity training in spiritual and religious issues. In W. R. Miller (Ed.), *Integrating spirituality into treatment: Resources for practitioners* (pp. 253–263). Washington, D.C.: American Psychological Association.

Miller, W. R., & Delaney, H. D. (2004). *Judeo-Christian perspectives on psychology: Human nature, motivation, and change.* Washington, D.C.: American Psychological Association.

Miller, W. R., & Thoresen, C. E. (1999). Spirituality and health. In W. R. Miller (Ed.), *Integrating spirituality into treatment: Resources for practitioners* (pp. 3–18). Washington, D.C.: American Psychological Association.

Mostkoff, D. L., & Lazarus, P. J. (1983). The Kinetic Family Drawing: The reliability of an objective scoring system. *Psychology in the schools, 20,* 16–20.

Noffke, J. L., & Hall, T. W. (2007). Chapter 4: Attachment psychotherapy and God image. *Journal of Spirituality in Mental Health, 9*(3/4), 57–78.

Oaklander, V. (1978). *Windows to our children: A Gestalt therapy approach to children and adolescents.* Moab, UT: Real People Press.

Ogdon, D. P. (1988). *Psychodiagnostics and personality assessment: A handbook* (2nd ed.). Los Angeles: Western Psychological Services.

Packman, W., Mazaheri, M., Sporri, L., Long, J. K., Chesterman, B., Fine, J., et al. (2008). Projective drawings as measures of psychosocial functioning in siblings of pediatric cancer patients from the Camp Okizu study. *Journal of Pediatric Oncology Nursing, 25*(1), 44–55.

Payne, M. A. (1996). Some effects of sex, age, and household structure on family drawings of Barbadian children. *Journal of Social Psychology, 136,* 567–578.

Pitts, V. P. (1976). Drawing the invisible: Children's conceptualizations of God. *Union College Character Potential: A Record of Research, 8,* 12–24.

Richards, P. S., & Bergin, A. E. (2003). *Casebook for a spiritual strategy in counseling and psychotherapy.* Washington, D.C.: American Psychological Association.

Rutter, M. (1999). Resilience concepts and findings: Implications for family therapy. *Journal of Family Therapy, 21,* 119–144.

Spigelman, G., Spigelman, A., & Englesson, I. (1992). Analysis of family drawings: A comparison between children from divorce and non-divorce families. *Journal of Divorce & Remarriage, 18,* 31–54.

Stefanatou, A., & Bowler, D. (1997). Depiction of pain in the self-drawings of children with sickle cell disease. *Child: Care, health and development, 23,* 135–155.

Stein, M. T. (2001). The use of family drawings by children in pediatric practice. *Journal of Development and Behavior, 22*(2), S49–S54.

Walsh, F. (1999). Religion and spirituality: Wellsprings for healing and resilience. In F. Walsh (Ed.), *Spiritual resources in family therapy* (pp. 3–27). New York: The Guilford Press.

Wenck, L. S. (1970). *House-Tree-Person Drawings: An illustrated diagnostic handbook.* Los Angeles: Western Psychological Services.

White, E. G. (1942). *The Ministry of healing.* Mountain View, CA: Pacific Press.

White, E. G. (1952). *The Adventist home.* Nashville, TN: Southern Publishing Association.

Zilbach, J. J. (1986). *Young children in family therapy.* New York: Brunner/Mazel.

Section 4

Clinical Applications

Clinical Implications for the Practice of Psychotherapy from the Seventh-day Adventist Tradition: A Summary

Carlos Fayard

When asked to participate in an interfaith panel at the Fourth World Psychotherapy Congress (Fayard, 2005), I was challenged to reflect upon the ways in which my Adventist faith and experience informed my work, particularly in the area of psychotherapy. Two sources were invaluable in organizing my ideas. One came from psychoanalyst Anna-Maria Rizzuto (2004) who wrote an evocative piece containing a personal account as to how her experience as a Catholic shaped her clinical work and theory. The second came from philosopher Nancey Murphy's (2005) rigorous ideas exploring and articulating how a Christian worldview informs, provides a foundation for, and weaves its way through psychological theory and research. Like Rizzuto (2004), I will speak from my experience as an Adventist psychologist, and how that informs my work. Thus, the aim of this article is not to present clear or distinctive theorizing, but to mimic what happens in psychotherapy. I will portray a set of ideas that are helpful to guide the conversation, but could never in its search for precision encapsulate all that needs to be said as it seeks to remain close to the ground of human experience.

Following Murphy (2005), it is my view that one of the most important contributions which theology provides to psychotherapy resides in biblical anthropology. Biblical anthropology speaks to dimensions of human experience that lie beyond the reach of psychology's self-imposed boundaries by virtue of its declared allegiance to naturalistic explanations. In doing so, the manner of integrating biblical anthropology into psychotherapy is closer to what Robert C. Roberts states:

> We are unabashed about bringing theology right into the heart of psychological reflection and research, not as an afterthought, to be

> "integrated", but as a basic guiding commitment; and not merely as supplying "control beliefs" that set limits to what we can accept from twentieth-century psychology, but as contributing substantively to our conceptualization of the human person. (Roberts & Talbot, 1997, p. 8)

The dimensions of human nature that I will summarize are not intended to be complete or thorough. There may be others that are as important or more distinctive to Adventism, as in fact many categories would be recognizable by other Christians and many non-Christians. The intent is to highlight the dimensions that appear significant to the practice of psychotherapy, as informed by my (limited) understanding of Seventh-day Adventist theology and practice. The anthropological dimensions constitute the foundational worldview, upon which I will lay psychological theory and research that contribute to forming a scientific understanding for each dimension. It will be followed by the implications for the practice of psychotherapy that can be derived from these ideas.

To borrow Ludwig Wittgenstein's phrase, a worldview is part of the riverbed that channels one's thinking. There are ten dimensions of human nature that are "part of the riverbed that channels" my clinical thinking: a holistic concept of the person, spirituality as a core component of being, intrinsic relational motivation, love as an organizer of psychological experience, values and Imago Dei, agency, the experience of sin or disordered love, self-regulation (temperance), temporal consciousness, and transformation.

I will now turn to briefly discuss the clinical implications for the practice of psychotherapy from each of the ten anthropological dimensions. For the sake of brevity, a full theological discussion will not be included, and only the biblical themes and language that have potential evocative power are incorporated (see Appelbaum, 2000, for a discussion and relevant research), followed by references from contemporary behavioral science and clinical applications.

DIMENSIONS IN BIBLICAL ANTHROPOLOGY

The notions of human nature as informed by the Bible that are potentially relevant to the practice of psychotherapy include a holistic concept of the person—human psychology does not function independent of the body, nor away from spiritual stirrings. Thus, spirituality has to be conceived as a core and indivisible component of being. The challenge of the Christian clinicians is to discover spiritual activity when the client may not be using religious language. Humans are created to relate to each other and to God. Thus, the Bible suggests that we have an intrinsic motivation to relate. Any relationship will either thrive or be injured depending on how love is experienced. The Bible suggests that love is an organizer of psychological experience. It asserts that love is more than an emotion. Love is informed by values that protect it and that protect interpersonal relationships. These values are normative in that they promote emotional health and reflect the *Imago Dei* in our humanity. Even though these values may represent a psychological ideal, they are not imposed and automatic. Human agency is ultimately involved. Many factors contribute to human freedom, and the biblical notion of temperance or self-regulation is one of the most relevant. The Bible is filled with narratives that reflect how emotional health can be derailed by poor choices. It is not blind to the fact that it is part of our condition to struggle with negative forces from within, reflecting the falleness brought about by sin. But the Bible also teaches us that there is hope. As humans, our hope is anchored in Christ: not only the Christ on the cross, but also the Christ who arose from the dead and is coming again. Humans live in the consciousness of time, related to the promises or worries of the future, and the accomplishments or burdens from the past. The Seventh-day Adventist community is particularly keen on the experience of time. The hope of the second coming brings us to the future; the cycle of the week marked by the rest found on the seventh day creates an awareness of time informed by hope in the future, and the sacredness of the present as a foretaste of the future. Finally, hope is not only looking to the future for fulfillment. It can also be savored in the present, as change and even transformation are possible through God's grace and power.

What follows describes each one of these dimensions of human nature, provides a rather succinct review of relevant research, and offers some suggestions as to how these ideas can benefit the psychotherapeutic process.

1. HOLISTIC CONCEPT OF THE PERSON

Adventists have long held a holistic perspective on being human, which is seemingly gathering some consensus in the theological community in this regard (Beck & Demarest, 2005; Murphy & Brown, 2007). Ellen White (1905) applies it to a clinical context in this way: "Many illnesses that affect humanity have their origin in the mind and only can be cured when the mind is cured." "The body is a very important means through which the soul and the mind contribute to character development" (p. 242). Biblical terminology reflects God's indivisible care for our whole being. The term *Shalom* conveys a sense of peace, prosperity, health, intrapsychic and interpersonal harmony, and wholeness.

Theory, Research, and Clinical Applications

While the advent of modern neurobiology has been dealt what some consider a fatal blow to dualistic perspectives on human nature (Gibbs, 2006), epidemiological research has demonstrated the close connection between health, mental health, and religious practices (Miller & Thoresen, 2003). Potential mechanisms detailing the connection of psychological, neurobiological, endocrine, immunological, and social elements to spirituality and religion have been summarized by Koenig and Cohen (2002) and Seybold (2007).

The applications to the practice of psychotherapy are multiple. Every clinical assessment should include psychological, social, physical, and spiritual parameters. Just as psychological distress can result from emotional conflict, as well as physical and spiritual sources, so psychotherapeutic interventions should seek to enhance emotional, physical, and spiritual well-being (Rizzuto, 2005). Spiritual interventions can also enhance emotional and physical well-being (Pargament, Murray-Swank, & Tarakeshwar, 2005; Reed & Enright, 2006; Oman, Hedberg, & Thoresen, 2006; Seybold, 2007).

McCullough, Kuhn, Andrews, Kaplan, Wolf, and Hurley (2003; see also Greenberg & Watson, 2006) suggest a clear application of a holistic, embodied approach to psychotherapy: "learning [in psychotherapy] means more than cognitive book learning, declarative knowledge, or intellectual insight. For behavior change, patients must experience procedural learning, or learning by doing. Patient's feelings, thoughts, and behaviors must be grounded in physically felt, bodily experience" (p. 16). A holistic approach would then reflect neurobiological, cognitive, affective, behavioral, relational, social, and spiritual aspects, with a theory of technique that will track felt experience as foundational to understanding the Self (Fayard, Pereau, & Ciovica, 2009).

2. SPIRITUALITY AS A CORE (AND INSEPARABLE) COMPONENT OF BEING

Christianity teaches that human beings are created to relate to God (Neh. 9:6; Eccles. 3:11; Col. 1:16), and the Psalmist sees it as a need as basic as thirst: "As the deer longs for flowing streams of water, so my soul longs for you, O God. My soul thirsts for God, for the living God" (Ps. 42:1–2, GW). Every human being has experienced what it means to be spiritual in some way.

In my view, the Apostle John offers parameters for a Christian spirituality that lend themselves well to the practice of psychotherapy when quoting Jesus: "On the last and greatest day of the feast, Jesus stood and said in a loud voice, 'If anyone is *thirsty,* let him *come to me* and drink. Whoever *believes in me, as the Scripture has said,* streams of living water will flow from within him" (John 7:37–38, NIV, italics added). At least three components emerge from Jesus' invitation. First, the notion of thirsting seems to refer to a psychophysical sense of basic need and longing. Second, this longing has a relational dimension: connecting humanity to Christ. Third, there is a belief system organized around the life, teachings, and person of Jesus as informed by Scripture. These features—a spiritual longing, a relational dimension to the human experience, and a belief system—seem to transcend cultural differences and be common to the human race. In turn, these components may reflect basic brain organizations (the Seeking, Attachment, and Theory-of-Mind systems), which could serve as a basic template for experiencing God (Fayard, Pereau, & Ciovica, 2009), and, I suggest, a way of mapping the spiritual stirrings of our patients.

Theory, Research, and Clinical Applications

A wholistic anthropology sees the spiritual dimension of being as always present in human experience, and thus in the therapeutic context, be it in explicit (i.e., "God talk") or implicit ways (Tan, 1996), regardless of the religious self-definition of the individual. It is intrinsic to being human, and because it reflects the imprint of the Creator, it has contours that transcend cultural experience, finding its full expression in accordance to its Designer.

I suggest that our clients' spirituality will be most powerfully intertwined in what they really love or worship (Matt. 6:21), that is, in what is activated by the Seeking system (Panksepp, 1998). How our clients experience and conceive God (or their own definition of the transcendent) will be informed just as much by the Attachment system (Beck, 2005) as by the doctrines they profess to believe (Theory-of-the-Mind of God). Discerning the spiritual in the psychological becomes an unavoidable task for the therapist (Benner, 1998).

Thus, spirituality should be a part of every formal evaluation, and thoughtfully incorporated into therapeutic interventions (Richards & Bergin, 1997). Explicit inclusion of spiritual considerations can be crucial for healing (e.g., addictions; May, 1992), or be a part of the problem (Pargament, Murray-Swank, & Tarakeshwar, 2005), and therefore in need of examination. Resolving spiritual concerns can significantly add to overall mental health gains (Murray-Swank & Pargament, 2005). I propose an approach (Fayard 2007; Fayard, in preparation; Fayard, Harding, Murdoch, & Brunt, 2007; Fayard, Pereau, & Ciovica, 2009) grounded on a wholistic biblical anthropology, informed by developmental and cognitive psychology, as well as recent developments in neurobiology. It remains sensitive to overt as well as implicit manifestations of spirituality in the clinical context and therefore it does not solely rely on the patient's "God talk," religious beliefs, or explicit spiritual understanding. Discerning the spiritual in the psychological is eased by recognizing the anthropological themes developed below.

3. INTRINSIC RELATIONAL MOTIVATION

The Bible uses multiple metaphors to describe the relational drive inherent to being human. For instance, it refers to God as Father and Mother, the creatures as children, and the relationship between Jesus and the church as a marriage. The relational motive also includes a vertical dimension (John 17:21, 23). Both interpersonal and vertical relations require that trust be developed for its healthy psychological and spiritual fulfillment (Pss. 20:7; 25:2; 31:14; Isa. 12:2; Zeph. 3:2; John 14:1; Rom. 15:13; Heb. 2:13; Roberts & Talbot, 1997).

Theory, Research, and Clinical Applications

John Bowlby's (1990) seminal work on attachment theory, the research of Mary Ainsworth (1978) and her students, and the neuroaffective developmental work of Alan Schore (2003) have demonstrated that the relational drive is a motivational system in its own right. The type of relational pattern established early on literally sculpts the brain (Schore, 2003) and generates implicit expectations about the Self and others and about how relationships unfold.

The centrality of the therapeutic relationship and the therapeutic alliance is one of the more consistent findings in psychotherapy research (Hubble, Duncan, & Miller, 1999), to the point that in an era of evidence-based practices, the field of psychotherapy can speak of an "evidence-based relationship." This accounts for a substantial amount of the variance in psychotherapy outcome research (Duncan & Miller, 2006). Emotional attunement and contingent responding in the context of the therapeutic relationship is considered to be crucial to emotional healing, just as relationships also play a crucial role in the formation and maintenance of emotional maladjustment (Stolorow, Atwood, & Brandchaft, 1994). Therapeutic interventions that focus on attachment processes that guide the restoration of relational breakdown show considerable promise, particularly when considered in a systemic context (Johnson, 2004).

4. LOVE AS AN ORGANIZER OF PSYCHOLOGICAL EXPERIENCE

The Bible states that "God is love." The character, motivation, and essence of the Divine is love. The Apostle Paul indicates that *any* experience devoid of love is meaningless (1 Cor. 13). God's nature and identity as manifested in the created world and Jesus' life are organized by love; thus, love has a grounding significance for the understanding of reality, including human nature (White, 1892; Exod. 33:18; John 1:18).

There are several dimensions of love that are relevant for the practice of psychotherapy. The parable of the Good Samaritan (Luke 10:30–37) exemplifies the compassion that results from Godly love, as well as the need for self care or love for self. Don Browning (2006) summarizes it: "we are entitled to love ourselves with the same seriousness that we are commanded to love the other" (p. 143). Love as "agape" connotes more than the absence of selfishness, as it includes social, mutual, even intimate experiences of love that not only focus on the good of the recipient, but perhaps, most importantly, focus on God working through the giver. Perhaps for that very reason, it seems unable to divorce the affective from the ethical; it is altruistic but it seems unable to only affirm the moral contours without also affirming the individuals involved in a compassionate way (Clough, 2006).

Theory, Research, and Clinical Applications

Psychology's interest in love as a meaningful human experience has been described as neglected (Marazziti, 2005), odd (Tjeltveit, 2006), and relegated to the poets (Weis, 2006). Recently, comprehensive models of the neurobiology of love are being developed (Zeki, 2007). The impact of feeling loved on brain activity is thought to activate limbic structures responsible for emotion, attention, motivation, and memory, which in turn control the autonomic nervous system inducing a state of decreased anxiety and increased pleasure tone that is bound to result in better health and mental health (Esch & Stefano, 2005). The absence, intermittence, or unpredictability of the experience of feeling loved can cause significant neurobiological dysfunction (van der Kolk, 2006).

The impact of feeling loved by God has been researched by measuring the type of attachment to God, and the relevance of loving God through intrinsic religiousness. A secure attachment to God has been associated with lower levels of distress in community samples (Bradshaw & Ellison, 2010; Bradshaw, Ellison, & Flannelly, 2008; Bradshaw, Ellison, & Marcum, 2010; Flannelly, Koenig, Galek, & Ellison, 2007), whereas experimental paradigms have shown a more nuanced manner in which an individual's attachment to God contributes to emotional self-regulation. While individuals securely attached to their parents show a secure attachment to God, insecurely attached individuals may also develop a secure attachment to God, a process described as compensation, resulting in improved emotional processing (Granqvist, 2006).

A series of studies conducted by Koenig (1998a; 1998b; Koenig, Pargament, & Nielsen, 1998) documented the correlations present between intrinsic religiosity and depression in a large sample of hospitalized elderly individuals. He found that increased church attendance and reliance on religious coping were associated with lower levels of depression. Intrinsic religiosity was associated with fewer hospitalization days and improved remission rates from depression.

Recent scholarship is explicitly discussing the proper role of love in the context of the patient-psychotherapist relationships (Cohen, 2006; Natterson, 2003). A Christian perspective needs to reflect the compassionate attitude of its founder. A compassionate attitude moves beyond sympathy (an awareness of the other's psychological situation), pity (aware of someone's pain but seeing it a sign of weakness), and empathy (the ability to recognize the emotions of others). Compassion moves the caregiver to get involved in alleviating the pain (Wachholtz & Pearce, 2007). An attuned tracking of attachment-based emotional experience provides the roadmap to understanding love and its injuries (Johnson, 2004), and guides therapeutic engagement in a compassionate manner.

Forgiveness intervention (Enright & Fitzgibbons, 2000; Worthington, 2001) may not only restore interpersonal conflict, but it may also restore a fragmented sense of self. A more explicitly Christian frame of reference links forgiveness with altruistic love and moral reasoning. The acknowledgement of justice motives along with moral virtues informed by the life of Jesus bring the notion of love as a principle (as a complex affective/cognitive/spiritual experience) to the clinical context of psychotherapy in a comprehensive way, perhaps one that is more effective than secular approaches (Worthington & Sharp, 2006).

In the Christian faith, love also can take the form of correction (Post, 2003). A loving attitude may also require that a therapist point out arrogance, self-serving behaviors, and other features that are contrary to an ethic of love in the patient's world. A Christian understanding of love does not stop at recognizing its interpersonal importance. It asserts that love makes a difference, that God's love is personal and powerful, and therefore that it is active in our lives (Chartier, 2007).

5. VALUES AND IMAGO DEI

Adventist Christians assume a moral order that reflects the image of the Creator in the creature. They believe the Decalogue found in Exodus 20 to be the expression of eternal values that regulate interpersonal expectations with God and with other humans (Veloso, 2000), which I call boundary values. Love understood as the ground for moral obligation rests on the belief that God's commands are not arbitrary or pointless, but designed to increase that which is good for humanity, given His motivation towards His creatures, and His superior knowledge about human nature as Creator (Evans, 2006).

The other set of values relevant to psychotherapy is expressed in Galatians 5:22–25, which reflect the core of a Christian character (love, joy, peace, patience, kindness, goodness, faithfulness, gentleness, and self-control) as embodied in the person and life of Jesus Christ. These virtues represent not only ethical ideals, but emotion-informed, concern-based construals (Roberts, 2007). Issues of character disposition, motivation, goals, moral emotions, moral judgment, behavior, and relationships in the context of communities and society are frequently found in therapeutic dialogue, although not necessarily recognized as such (Fowers, 2005). A Christian view on values also includes the experiential sense of moral stirrings as indicative of Divine activity through the Holy Spirit.

Theory, Research, and Clinical Applications

"Values are an inevitable and almost omnipresent part of the therapeutic process" (Bergin, 1980; p. 95). Research has provided evidence that a therapist's values influence every phase of psychotherapy. This can be seen in the theories of personality and therapeutic change, assessment strategies, goals of treatment, the design and selection of interventions, and evaluations of therapy outcome. Patients are influenced by a therapist's values, often adopting their health, moral, and religious values (Miller, 1999). In fact, it may well be said that in the absence of a "values-free" enterprise, any psychotherapy dialogue will be a moral process, among other things (Evans, 1989), despite its silence (or deprecation) witnessed in clinical theory and professional training (Fowers, 2005). Since psychotherapy cannot claim value neutrality, the question of *which* values are to be considered important and *which* are to be considered negative remains open from a scientific perspective. If secular therapists were to be epistemologically congruent with their naturalistic assumptions, their conclusion would mirror Nietzche's: "To be natural is to dare to be as immoral as nature is" (Nietzche, 1901/1967, p. 73).

Vigorous research in positive psychology (Peterson & Seligman, 2004), moral psychology and moral neurobiology (Moll, de Oliveira-Souza, Garrido, Bramati, Caparelli-Daquer, Paiva, Zahn, & Grafman, 2007) show that virtues and morality have distinct cognitive and neurobiological signatures, and that their proper recognition could enhance the lives of psychotherapy patients in several ways. One is the consideration that moral issues are unavoidable and need to be recognized as such. Doherty (1996) has contributed a most helpful set of guiding principles in this regard. Second, the cultivation of human virtue and character may contribute to the betterment of mental health. Third, moral emotions and cognitions (including those with clear spiritual and religious connotations), and the dilemmas that come with them, may be more fruitfully understood as ethical, just as well as psychological issues. Fourth, if reactions that involve moral issues are downgraded to unpleasant emotions, inadequate therapeutic work may result. For instance, a view on the experience of contrition informed by a Christian perspective (Roberts, 2007) will allow the sense of moral failure (for instance, betraying a spouse) to resonate emotionally in the person, not just as embarrassment (feeling bad about getting caught), nor solely as guilt (feeling responsible for the betrayal) or shame (feeling tainted and unworthy in every respect), but as an experience that also includes one's relationship to God (that is, His grace is always present). Furthermore, the Decalogue provides a moral compass in regards to boundary values in a context of personal and social justice, and the fruits of the Spirit a set of core values that may optimize intra as well as interpersonal health. Sorenson's (2004) study with student therapists clearly shows the clinical impact of taking religion seriously in the course of psychotherapy in regard to how values are encouraged or ignored.

6. AGENCY

The creation account indicates that the original order of things not only had moral implications, but was sustained by the freedom humans had to choose between "good and evil" (Gen. 2:17). Eric L. Johnson (1997) provides a helpful discussion of the biblical features of agency. First, agency is bound by the body. Both decision-making capacities and action are limited or enhanced by the integrity of the body (naturally, including the brain). Second, human actions tend to be the result of co-agents. As exemplified in the healing of the man with paralysis (Luke 5), his decision to seek Jesus was assisted by those who brought him down to the Savior through the roof, and the divine restoration of spiritual and physical wholeness. Third, intentionality and motivation have a non-linear relationship to self-activated behavior (Mark 7:21–22; 1 Cor. 13:3). Fourth, agency goes beyond choice; it also "moves" the individual in ways that have moral implications (Rom. 6:13; 8:5–7; Gal. 5:16, 25; Col. 3). Finally, if one can choose, then one is responsible for the consequences of one's choices (Gen. 2).

Theory, Research, and Clinical Applications

Beyond the long debate in philosophy and theology on the nature of human free will and determinism (Moreland & Craig, 2003), an Adventist perspective has to deal with the complex issues arising from a non-dualist anthropology—what Murphy and Brown (2007) call moral agency without "the soul." Recent developments in neuropsychology (i.e., Arnsten & Li, 2005) have provided evidence for the vital role played by the brain's executive functions, the supervisory system—the meta-comparator and meta-organizer of top-down brain activity (Murphy & Brown, 2007). These include: self-regulation, self-determination, self-control, self-management, self-direction, and maturation. Interestingly, executive functions which organize action, thought, and emotion are not determined by immediate environmental factors, and not by body states or immediate impulse, nor are they determined by the control of others.

Two areas related to human agency have recently been researched: a comprehensive, neurocognitive model of the decision-making process (Ernst & Paulus, 2005; Farrer, Franck, Georgieff, Frith, Decety, & Jeannerod, 2003), and its relation to moral sensitivity (Moll, de Oliveira-Souza, Garrido, Bramati, Caparelli-Daquer, Paiva, Zahn, & Grafman, 2007). Second is the role of willpower for task completion (Baumeister, 2005), which can be morally compromised when an individual has a dim view on human agency (Shariff, Schooler, & Vohs, 2008).

The power to choose is essential to any change, psychological or spiritual. In fact, psychotherapy would not be possible under a deterministic viewpoint without it (Miller, 2004). It is thus important to strengthen a patient's decision-making capacities and the development of responsibility for one's own actions, as Yalom (1980) has pointed out and provided helpful therapeutic indications. Improved agency can be accomplished as implicit negative behavioral patterns are recognized and interpreted. It may be significant to identify what the primary and secondary gains for the patient might be, and to recognize that feelings of guilt or regret should not be dismissed without a clear analysis, as these emotions contribute to controlling undesired preferences (Connolly & Reb, 2005). Strengthening positive choices made can be aided when linked to values held in high regard by the individual (Ainslie, 2005).

Specific interventions, such as motivational interviewing, can help the clinician guide the patient from indifference to contemplation and eventual enactment of positive behaviors (Miller & Rollnick, 2002). The process is strengthened by self-regulation strategies (e.g., self-monitoring, avoiding or altering sources of temptation). Cue-driven reminders may be needed to prompt a different course of action, as well as interruptions and rewards for alternative, healthier behaviors. Finally, Miller (Miller & Atencio, 2008) highlights the role of integrity and faithfulness to values as a resource to override negative temptation and increase adherence to rule-governed behaviors.

The Adventist tradition has been critical of the use of approaches that reduce or compromise personal agency such as the misuse of psychotropic drugs, excessive dependency on a therapist, and hypnosis (Provonsha, 1977). Adventist ethicist Jack Provonsha quoted Ellen White's (1903) perspective: "every human being, created in the image of God, is endowed with a power akin to that of the Creator—individuality, power to think and do" (p. 199), concluding that "whatever diminishes that image is wrong" (p. 201).

7. DISORDERED LOVE (INNER CONFLICT)

The biblical terminology for sin involves relational as well as moral language that has an ontological status in its anthropology. It is disordered love because it involves a loss of basic trust (e.g., idolatry) and infliction of harm (Chartier, 2007). "It is faithlessness, lawlessness, Godlessness" (Plantinga, 1997, p. 248).The language used in the Bible resonates clearly with the one heard in the office of a psychotherapist: "missing a target" or expectation (Lev. 5:5; Rom. 5:12–13), "deception or wrongful intention" (Ps. 36:3; Isa. 41:29), "willful rebellion" (Job 34:7), "restlessness" (Isa. 57:20), "unwillingness to listen" (Rom. 5:19; 2 Cor. 10:6), "transgression" or passing beyond to forbidden territory (Rom. 4:15, 25; Gal. 3:19), a sense of injustice or "unrighteousness" (Rom. 1:18–19), and "wrongdoing" (2 Pet. 2:15; 1 John 5:17). Certainly, many of us can identify with the Apostle Paul's description of inner conflict (Rom. 7:15–25).

There are at least four notions of sin potentially useful for the practice of psychotherapy. First, sin as a state. The apostle Paul summarized it thus: "The desires of the flesh are against the Spirit, and the desires of the Spirit are against the flesh" (Gal. 5:17, ESV). Second, sin as a broken relationship (vertically and horizontally) that generates emotional distress (Isa. 59:2). Third, sin as a chosen rebellion against God that has moral overtones (Isa. 14:14). Fourth, the Bible continuously speaks of God's faithfulness, mercy, and grace for the sinner. Christian therapists would do well in heeding Kierkegaard's (1844/1980) observation: "When sin is treated in a place other than its own, it is altered by being subjected to a nonessential refraction of reflection. The concept is altered, and thereby the mood that properly corresponds to the correct concept is also disturbed" (p. 14).

Overall, a distinction between sin and evil might be helpful. Sin may be seen as a condition, the way we tend to approach life. It is a complex of inclinations, attitudes, and behaviors that arise from self-importance and attachment. Its recognition may bring one to an awareness of fallibility and repentance. Evil has a more basic quality: it appears as a force that impels or compels away—it fragments within and without, eroding the human heart from longing. Acts that arise from revenge, envy, or other purely destructive motivations are evil.

Theory, Research, and Clinical Applications

Since the early days of psychotherapy, internal conflict between constructive and destructive tendencies has occupied a central place in clinical theory (Freud, 1923/1989; Jung, 1959), and was confirmed by Zimbardo's (2004) classical "prison experiment." Research with clinical populations (e.g., Hare, 1999) using brain imaging techniques (Kiehl, 2008; Raine & Yang, 2006) and on non-clinical samples (Young, Cushman, Hauser, & Saxe, 2007) document the neurocognitive features in the spectrum of destructive tendencies, ranging from those resulting from brain injuries to the ones showing absence of adequate moral reasoning.

What language then, shall the Christian psychotherapist utilize to address issues of disordered love? Should she reflect the field's tendency to avoid the moral and existential dimensions of evil (Spinelli, 2000)? Should she use the language of psychopathology and dysfunction, or the moral language of Scripture (Yarhouse, Butman, & McRay, 2005)? The Christian psychotherapist is challenged to discern, in the midst of a patient's pain, the possible marks and traces left by deliberate choices made, remain clear about the fallen state of the individual in front of him or her, and yet never forget first and foremost that dealing with sin and its consequences is preceded and guided by God's faithfulness, mercy, and grace (McMinn, 2008). Perhaps a holistic perspective in clinical context may not be as concerned with sharply differentiating notions of "sin, crime, disease, folly, and immorality" (Plantinga, 1997, p. 245), but rather in recognizing that any or all of these components may be intertwined in causing a condition, as their conceptual counterparts (e.g., grace, responsibility, health, emotional balance, and morality) can be integrated in their healing as Shalom.

8. TEMPERANCE (SELF-REGULATION)

The Bible connects the idea of a fallen human nature and human struggles to redemption and the saving grace of God. God's love is expressed in the preservation of human agency so that each individual's response to Him is born out of love, and not as the result of coercion or manipulation (Charthier, 2007). Growth in love—that is, growth into the likeness of God's character—requires that the strength of human agency be enhanced. The Bible speaks of the importance of developing self-control to facilitate this process. Self-control is one of the fruits of the Spirit that frequently is presented in the context of temptation and the subjective power of psychobiological forces (i.e., "passions and desires," Gal. 5:24; Titus 2:11; 1 Pet. 1:13). The Apostle Peter (1 Pet. 2:3–6) seems to suggest that any such development will have to begin with faith, that is, trust in God as its foundation, upon which goodness and knowledge (moral discernment) can flourish, leading to self-control. Self-control is a link in this chain that leads, with perseverance, to personal integrity (godliness), interpersonal well-being (brotherly kindness), and finally the reflection of God's character (love).

Theory, Research, and Clinical Applications

The idea that temperance can be translated into psychological terminology as self-regulation implies that temperance is the master key (Geyer & Baumeister, 2005) that undergirds the capacity to restrain and override negative tendencies, particularly those associated with moral choices (Gramzow, Sedikides, Panter, Sathy, Harris, & Insko, 2004). Developmental theories emphasize the central role of early interactive mother-infant relations in sculpting the brain's ability to self-regulate (Schore, 1994; Schore, 2003; Schore & Schore, 2008). Cognitive (Geyer & Baumeister, 2005) and neurocognitive (Beauregard, 2007) models of self-regulation have been advanced, mapping the processes involved.

Optimal self-regulation in the context of psychotherapy may be attained by the implicit relational systems that operate in the patient-psychotherapist relationship (Schore, 2003; Schore & Schore, 2008). The therapist will also encourage participation in social milieus like Twelve Step groups and/or spiritual communities that will provide standards, accountability, and a context of grace to prevent or repair unregulated self states. A Christian therapist may also teach self-regulation approaches with specific Christian content such as guided imagery, meditation on Scriptural passages, and prayer. Finally, a Christian perspective may also involve a discernment of moral expectations, clarification of moral emotions as engines that can lead to appropriate corrective action, an explicit sense of trust in the availability of grace, and the power of the Holy Spirit to sustain, cleanse, and deliver. Finally, the Christian discipline of abstinence (Foster, 1988) can be particularly helpful in fostering an increased awareness of one's own "passions and desires." Solitude and silence promote a confrontation with the individual's internal cacophony and competing demands. Fasting, perhaps like no other discipline, confronts the person with his own bodily-based urges. A Christian discipline has as its goal not only to increase self-awareness through experience, but to open oneself up to God as the source that can satisfy humanity's deepest longings (May, 1992).

9. TEMPORAL CONSCIOUSNESS

The Bible appears to suggest that temporality is constitutive of being human (Eccles. 3:1–8; Anderson, 2006). Time consciousness is at the heart of Adventist identity: the seventh-day Sabbath and the anticipation of the second advent of Christ in the near future. Furthermore, the Adventist understanding of the state of the dead sharpens the focus of human existence in the here and now, as there is a distinct differentiation of the times and manner of living for those who are alive in contrast to those who have died.

The Bible links the hope of the advent with the psychological state of those awaiting it. "Why are you downcast, O my soul? Why so disturbed within me? Put your hope in God, for I will yet praise him, my Savior and my God" (Ps. 43:5, NIV). "Hope" is a key word in the Adventist psyche: "While we *wait* for the *blessed hope*—the glorious appearing of our great God and Savior, Jesus Christ" (Titus 2:13, NIV). There is no "wait" that is not embedded in a notion of temporality (Lain Entralgo, 1962).

Whereas a trusting hope anchors our sight in the future transforming the present, the Sabbath as a commandment from God (Exod. 20:8–10) transforms the present by facilitating an encounter with the sacred and providing a glimpse of the future. The Sabbath connects the present moment with eternity, the mundane with the sacred. According to Minkowski (1970), death is the most distant horizon where hope is challenged. As death looms, threatening notions of ultimacy and meaning are developed in the human mind. Supplication or prayer is the existential position where the most distant future moves to the present. Rest, meditation, and prayer bring glimpses of eternity to the present moment and transform it, thus challenging the power of death. The sacredness of the Sabbath allows the time to engage in these worshipful activities.

Clinically relevant features associated with temporal consciousness, namely hope, and meditative practices will be reviewed below.

Theory, Research, and Clinical Applications

Hope has long been recognized as a vital element in healing and has been operationalized in a variety of ways which capture aspects of the concept, including optimism (primarily a personality disposition), the placebo effect (a sense of trusting), remembered wellness (safe past experiences are summoned to anticipate like-manner future experiences), and positive expectancies (Yahne & Miller, 1999). Comprehensive cognitive models of hope have been developed (Snyder, 1994), and neurocognitive approaches for optimism and placebo effects advanced (Beauregard, 2007). Religious beliefs often provide a worldview that is both optimistic and hopeful, infusing difficult or traumatic life events with purpose and meaning (Bradshaw & Ellison, 2010; Flannelly, Koenig, Galek, & , 2008; Ellison, 2002).

Evoking hope for the hopeless is one of the most difficult challenges we face as clinicians. William Miller (Yahne & Miller, 1999) provides a most helpful summary of the ways in which hope can be enhanced in the context of psychotherapy. Echoing Martin Buber, he states: "On our clearest days, we bring to these encounters a vision of God-in-the-other, a deep and numinous respect for that center that is whole and holy in the person sitting next to us" (p. 228), making therapists not only "helpers" but also "hopers."

Although Eastern forms of meditation are widely used in clinical contexts (e.g., Kabat-Zinn, 1990), the utilization of Christian-based meditative practice applied to medicine or psychotherapy is only now being empirically explored (Oman, Hedberg, & Thoresen, 2006). Meditative practices deepen the experience of the present moment and provide a foretaste of the most distant existential horizon, thus promoting hopefulness. In my clinical practice, I have used guided imagery that calls on Christ to be present in a given situation, thus facilitating healing.

10. TRANSFORMATION

The Apostle Paul sees the Christian journey as one in which personal change is expected: "Do not conform any longer to the pattern of this world, but be transformed by the renewing of your mind" (Rom. 12:2, NIV). The Bible reports on sudden changes or quantum transformations such as the apostle Paul's, and also gradual growth as experienced by the apostle Peter. Christian writers have conceptualized the process of transformation through centuries as involving three steps. The first one is "purgative," in which old life patterns are perceived in negative ways, giving way to the painful process of awakening or "illumination" and culminating in a sense of "union" with God, where God is sought for His own sake and not for the favors a believer might receive (May, 1987). An interesting alternative to the "classical" description of spiritual transformation involves the identification of spiritual motives that could promote it. Theologian F. LeRon Shults (Shults & Sandage, 2006) states that seeking wisdom in a spiritual relational context (knowing and being known), longing for justice, and longing for freedom (from the oppression of evil and for a hopeful existence) can be discerned as scripturally based forces that generate a desire for change. Longing for wisdom, justice, and freedom are themes that emerge in the context of psychotherapy, if not necessarily or clearly couched in spiritual terms. If understood in this manner, it might be harnessed to help a patient move beyond symptom reduction and into transformation.

Theory, Research, and Clinical Applications

Change is not only part of life, but arguably the main goal of any psychotherapy. Change that is the result of nongenetic factors—such as beliefs, hopes, and expectations—or shifts that are the result from psychotherapy (Beutel & Huber, 2008) or any other human endeavor must be feasible because the brain changes (Beauregard, 2007). Without pretending to provide a full explanation for spiritual transformation, some authors are beginning to speculate about the neurobiological such as neural plasticity and neurogenesis (Newberg, 2006; Spezio, 2006).

An influential, contemporary approach to psychotherapy argues that transformation should be the end point of psychotherapy, not merely symptom relief (Fosha, 2006; 2008a; 2008b), by focusing on and amplifying themes of hope, resilience, joy, and gratitude. Furthermore, Christian psychotherapists (Leffel, 2007a; Shults & Sandage, 2006) advocate the "via negativa" as a pathway to spiritual transformation in order to gain the depth described in the Bible. In this, the believer holds on to an attachment to God even though at the same time God's presence is not experienced as close or soothing. Leffel (2007a,

b) argues that unless the patterns of behavior cultivated through a lifetime are weakened, there is no real possibility for durable change. The twenty-third psalm would not be as powerful if the reader only focused on the image of the Good Shepherd without an experiential focus on the "valley of death." In the same way, the "valley of death" is not survivable without the presence of the Good Shepherd. Finally, the longing for wisdom or truth, the longing for freedom, and the longing for justice could be harnessed even when presented in non-spiritual language, and not necessarily with the level of definitional clarity that Shults and Sandage (2006) describe.

CONCLUSION

Good ideas, even the correct ideas, however helpful, are insufficient. An Adventist Christian psychotherapist, in my view, ought to have a "Spirit friendly" approach—that is, someone who is open to the direction of the Spirit of God while conducting psychotherapy and who is also friendly to the voice of the Spirit as it might be perceived by the patient. Moreover, an Adventist psychotherapist should conduct psychotherapy from a perspective of "informed compassion," thus reflecting the heart of God.

Ellen White (1905) articulates the Adventist perspective and describes this ideal as a "Ministry of Healing." She states: "Our Lord Jesus Christ came to this world as the unwearied servant of man's necessity. He 'took our infirmities, and bore our sicknesses,' that He might minister to every need of humanity (Matthew 8:17)....It was His mission to bring to men *complete restoration*; He came to give them *health* and *peace*" (p. 11, italics added). "During His ministry, Jesus devoted more time to healing the sick than to preaching" (p. 12). "The Savior made each work of healing an occasion for *implanting* divine principles in the mind and soul. This was the purpose of His work. He imparted earthly blessings, that He might *incline* the hearts of men to receive the gospel of His grace" (p. 13, italics added). "Gracious, tenderhearted, pitiful, He went about lifting up the bowed-down and comforting the sorrowful. Wherever He went, He carried blessing.... Christ recognized no distinction of nationality or rank or creed" (p. 15). "He passed by no human being as worthless, but sought to apply the healing remedy to every soul" (p. 16). Psychotherapy interventions emerging out of this relational matrix should always have an awareness of implicit spiritual themes that potentially may elicit evocative stirrings in the patient's experience, and occasional, appropriate, patient-centered explicit spiritual and religious themes.

In summary, a "Spirit friendly, informed, and compassionate" Adventist psychotherapist will have, as a goal, complete restoration (physical, psychological, social, and spiritual). She will spend more time devoted to healing than to preaching, and will show the true compassion and radical acceptance embodied by Christ.

REFERENCES

Ainslie, G. (2005). Precis of breakdown of will. *Behavioral and Brain Sciences, 28*, 635–650.

Ainsworth, M. (1978). *Patterns of attachment: A psychological study of the strange situation*. Chicago: Lawrence Earlbaum.

Anderson, R. (2006). *Explorations into God: Sermonic meditations on the book of Ecclesiastes*. Pasadena, CA: Fuller Theological Seminary.

Appelbaum, S. (2000). *Evocativeness: Moving and persuasive interventions in psychotherapy*. New York: Jason Aronson.

Arnsten, A., & Li, B. (2005). Neurobiology of executive functions. *Biological Psychiatry, 57*, 1377–1384.

Baumeister, R. (2005). Self and volition. In W. Miller & H. Delaney (Eds.), *Judeo-Christian perspectives on psychology: Human nature, motivation, and change*. Washington, D.C.: American Psychological Association.

Beauregard, M. (2007). Mind does really matter: Evidence from neuroimaging studies of emotional self-regulation, psychotherapy, and placebo effect. *Progress in Neurobiology, 81*, 218–236.

Beck, J. & Demarest, B. (2005). *The human person in theology and psychology: A biblical anthropology for the twenty-first century*. Grand Rapids, MI: Kregel Academic & Professional.

Benner, D. (1998). *Care of souls: Revisioning Christian nature and counsel.* Grand Rapids, MI: Baker Book House.

Bergin, A. (1980). Psychotherapy and religious values. *Journal of Consulting and Clinical Psychology, 48,* 95–105.

Beutel, M. & Huber, M. (2008). Functional neuroimaging—can it contribute to our understanding of processes of change? *Neuropsychoanalysis, 10,* 5–16.

Bowlby, J. (1990). *A secure base: Parent-child attachment and healthy human development.* New York: Basic Books.

Bradshaw, M., & Ellison, C. (2010). Financial hardship and psychological distress: Exploring the buffering effects of religion. *Social Science & Medicine, 71(1),* 196–204.

Bradshaw, M., Ellison, C. G., and Flannelley, K. J. (2008). Prayer, God imagery, and symptoms of psychopathology. *Journal for the Scientific Study of Religion, 47*(4), 644–659.

Bradshaw, M., Ellison, C., & Marcum, J. (2010). Attachment to God, images of God, and psychological distress in a nationwide sample of Presbyterians. *International Journal for the Psychology of Religion, 20*(2), 130–147.

Browning, D. (2006). *Christian ethics and the moral psychologies.* Grand Rapids, MI: Eerdmans.

Chartier, G. (2007). *The analogy of love: Divine and human love at the center of Christian theology.* Devon, UK: Imprint Academic.

Clough, W. (2006). To be loved and to love. *Journal of Psychology and Theology, 34,* 23–31.

Cohen, Y. (2006). Loving the patient as the basis for treatment. *The American Journal of Psychoanalysis, 66,* 139–155.

Connolly, T., & Reb, J. (2005). Regret and the control of temporary preferences. *Behavioral and Brain Sciences, 28,* 653–654.

Doherty, W. (1996). *Soul searching: Why psychotherapy must promote moral responsibility.* New York: Basic Books.

Duncan, B., & Miller, S. (2006). Treatment manuals do not improve outcome. In J. Norcross, R. Levante, & L. Beautire (Eds.), *Evidence-based practices in mental health.* Washington, D.C.: American Psychological Association.

Enright, R., & Fitzgibbons, J. (2000). *Helping clients forgive.* Washington, D.C.: American Psychological Association.

Ernst, M., & Paulus, M. (2005). Neurobiology of decision making. *Biological Psychiatry, 58,* 597–604.

Esch, T., & Stefano, G. (2005). The neurobiology of love. *Neuroendocrinology Letters, 26,* 175–192.

Evans, C. (1989). *Wisdom and humanness in psychology: Prospects for a Christian psychology.* Grand Rapids, MI: Baker Book House.

Evans, C. (2006). Is there a basis for loving all people? *Journal of Psychology and Theology, 34,* 78–90.

Farrer, C., Franck, N., Georgieff, N., Frith, C., Decety, J., & Jeannerod, M. (2003). Modulating the experience of agency. *Neuroimage, 18,* 324–333.

Fayard, C. (2005). Cristianismo y Psicoterapia. Invited presentation, IV World Psychotherapy Congress, Buenos Aires, Argentina.

Fayard, C. (2007). Case Presentation: A Failed Spiritual Marriage. Grand Rounds, Loma Linda University School of Medicine, Department of Psychiatry.

Fayard, C. (2008). *A neuro-psycho-spiritual approach to psychotherapy: Western spirituality meets neuroscience in clinical practice.* Manuscript in preparation.

Fayard, C., Harding, G. I., Murdoch, W., & Brunt, J. (2007). Clinical implications for psychotherapy from the Seventh-day Adventist tradition. *Journal of Psychology and Christianity, 26,* 207–217.

Fayard, C., Pereau, M., & Ciovica, A. (2009). "Love the Lord with all your mind": The neurobiology of the experience of God. *Journal of Psychology and Christianity, 28*(2), 567–580.

Flannelly, K. J., Koenig, H. G., Galek, K., & Ellison, C. G. (2007). Beliefs about God, psychiatric symptoms and evolutionary psychiatry. *Journal of Nervous and Mental Disease, 195*(12), 996–1003.

Fosha, D. (2006). Quantum transformation in trauma and treatment: Traversing the crisis of healing change. *Journal of Clinical Psychology, 62,* 569–583.

Fosha, D. (2008a). Transformation of affect and core state in AEDP: The emergence and consolidation of joy, hope, gratitude and confidence in (the solid goodness) of the self. *Journal of Psychotherapy Integration, 18*(2), 167–190.

Fosha, D. (2008b). Transformance, recognition of self by self, and effective action. In Schneider, K. (Ed.), *Existential-integrative psychotherapy: Guideposts to the core of practice.* New York: Routledge.

Foster, R. (1998). *Celebration of discipline: The path to spiritual growth.* San Francisco: HarperOne.

Fowers, B. (2005). *Virtue and psychology: Pursuing excellence in ordinary practices.* Washington, D.C.: American Psychological Association.

Freud, S. (1923/1989). *The ego and the id.* New York: W. W. Norton and Company.

Geyer, A. & Baumeister, R. (2005). Religion, morality, and self-control: Values, virtues, and vices. In R. Paloutzian & C. Park (Eds.), *Handbook of the psychology of religion and spirituality*. New York: Guilford Press.

Gibbs, R. (2006). *Embodiment and cognitive science*. Cambridge: Cambridge University Press.

Gramzow, R., Sedikides, C., Panter, A., Sathy, V., Harris, J., & Insko, C. (2004). Patterns of self-regulation and the Big Five. *European Journal of Personality, 18*, 367–385.

Granqvist, P. (2006). Religion as a by-product of evolved psychology: The case of attachment and implications for brain and religion research. In P. McNamara (Ed.), *Where God and science meet: How brain and evolutionary studies alter our understanding of religion*. Westport, CT: Praeger.

Greenberg, L., & Watson, J. (2006). *Emotion-focused therapy for depression*. Washington, D.C.: American Psychological Association.

Hare, R. D. (1999). Psychopathy as a risk factor for violence. *Psychiatric Quarterly, 70*(3), 181–197.

Hubble, M., Duncan, B., & Miller, S. (1999). *The heart and soul of change: What works in therapy*. Washington, D.C.: American Psychological Association.

Johnson, E. (1997). Human agency and its social formation. In R. Roberts & M. Talbot (Eds.), *Limning the psyche: Explorations in Christian psychology*. Grand Rapids, MI: Eerdmans.

Johnson, S. (2004). *The practice of emotionally focused marital therapy*. New York: Guilford.

Jung, C. (1959). *The undiscovered self*. New York: Signet.

Kabat-Zinn, J. (1990). *Full catastrophe living: Using the wisdom of your body and mind to face stress, pain and illness*. New York: Delta.

Kiehl, K. (2008). Without morals: The cognitive neuroscience of criminal psychopaths. In W. Sinnot-Armstron (Ed.), *Moral psychology, Volume 3, The neuroscience of morality: Emotion, brain disorders, and development*. Cambridge: The MIT Press.

Kierkegaard, S. (1844/1980). *The concept of anxiety: A simple psychologically orienting deliberation on the dogmatic issue of hereditary sin*. Princeton: Princeton University Press.

Koenig, H. (1998a). *Handbook of religion and mental health*. New York: Academic Press.

Koenig, H. (1998b). Religiosity and remission of depression in medically ill older patients. *American Journal of Psychiatry, 155*, 536–542.

Koenig, H. G. (2002). An 83-year-old woman with chronic illness and strong religious beliefs. *Journal of the American Medical Association 288*(4): 487–493.

Koenig, H., & Cohen, H. (2002). *The link between religion and health: Psychoneuroimmunology and the faith factor.* Oxford: Oxford University Press.

Koenig, H., Pargament, K., & Nielsen, J. (1998). Religious coping and health status in medically ill hospitalized older adults. *Journal of Nervous & Mental Disease, 186*, 513–521.

Lain Entralgo, P. (1962). *La espera y la esperanza: Historia y teoria del esperar humano.* Madrid: Revista de Occidente.

Leffel, G. (2007a). Emotion and transformation in the relational spirituality paradigm (Part 2): Implicit morality and "minimal prosociality." *Journal of Psychology and Theology, 35*, 281–297.

Leffel, G. (2007b). Emotion and transformation in the relational spirituality paradigm (Part 3): A moral motive analysis. *Journal of Psychology and Theology, 35*, 298–316.

May, G. (1987). *Will and spirit: A contemplative psychology.* San Francisco: Harper One.

May, G. (1992). *Addiction and grace.* San Francisco: Harper One.

Marazziti, D. (2005). The neurobiology of love. *Current Psychiatry Reviews, 1*, 331–335.

McCullough, L., Kuhn, N., Andrews, S., Kaplan, A., Wolf, J., & Hurley, C. (2003). *Treating affect phobia: A manual for short-term dynamic psychotherapy.* New York: Guilford Press.

McMinn, M. (2008). *Sin and grace in Christian counseling.* Downers Grove, IL: IVP Academic.

Miller, R. (2004). *Facing human suffering: Psychology and psychotherapy as moral engagement.* Washington, D.C.: American Psychological Association.

Miller, W. (1999). Diversity training in spiritual and religious issues. In W. Miller (Ed.), *Integrating spirituality into treatment.* Washington, D.C.: American Psychological Association.

Miller, W., & Atencio, D. (2008). Free will as a proportion of variance. In J. Baer, J. Kaufman, & R. Baumeister (Eds.), *Are we free? Psychology and free will.* Oxford: Oxford University Press.

Miller, W., & Rollnick, S. (2002). *Motivational interviewing: Preparing people to change addictive behavior.* New York: Guilford Press.

Miller, W., & Thoresen, C. (2003). Spirituality, religion and health: An emergent field. *American Psychologist, 58*, 1–24.

Minkowski, E. (1970). *Lived time: Phenomenological and psychopathological studies.* Chicago: Northwestern University Press.

Moll, J., de Oliveira-Souza, R., Garrido, G., Bramati, I., Caparelli-Daquer, E., Paiva, M., Zahn, R., & Grafman, J. (2007). The self as a moral agent. *Social Neuroscience, 2*, 336–352.

Moreland, J., & Craig, W. (2003). *Philosophical foundations for a Christian worldview*. Downers Grove, IL: InterVarsity Press.

Murphy, N. (2005). Integration from a radical-reformation perspective. In A. Duek & C. Lee (Eds.), *Why psychology needs theology: A radical-reformation perspective*. New York: Eerdmans.

Murphy, N., & Brown, W. (2007). *Did my neurons make me do it? Philosophical and neurobiological perspectives on moral responsibility and free will.* Oxford: Oxford University Press.

Murray-Swank, N., & Pargament, K. (2005). God, where are you? Evaluating a spiritually-integrated intervention for sexual abuse. *Mental Health, Religion & Culture, 8*, 191–203.

Natterson, J. (2003). Love in psychotherapy. *Psychoanalytic Psychology, 20*, 509–521.

Newberg, A. (2006). The neurobiology of spiritual transformation. In J. Koss-Chioino & P. Hefner (Eds.), *Spiritual transformation and healing: Anthropological, theological, neuroscientific, and clinical perspectives.* Lanham, MD: Altamira Press.

Nietzche, F. (1901/1967). *The Will to power*. New York: Random House

Oman, D., Hedberg, J., & Thoresen, C. (2006). Passage meditation reduces perceived stress in health professionals: A randomized, controlled trial. *Journal of Consulting and Clinical Psychology, 74*, 714–719.

Panksepp, J. (1998). *Affective neuroscience: The foundation of human and animal emotions*. New York: Oxford University Press.

Pargament, K., Murray-Swank, N., & Tarakeshwar, N. (2005). An empirically based rationale for a spiritually-integrated psychotherapy. *Mental Health, Religion & Culture, 8*, 155–165.

Peterson, C., & Seligman, M. (2004). *Character strengths and virtues: A handbook and classification.* Oxford: Oxford University Press.

Plantinga, C. (1997). Sin and addiction. In R. Roberts & M. Talbot (Eds.), *Limning the psyche: Explorations in Christian psychology.* Grand Rapids, MI: Eerdmans.

Post, S. (2003). *Unlimited love: Altruism, compassion, and service.* Philadelphia: Templeton Foundation Press.

Provonsha, J. (1977). Mind manipulation: a Christian ethical analysis. In General Conference Department of Education (Ed.), *An Adventist approach to psychology*. Washington, D.C.: General Conference Department of Education.

Raine, A., & Yang, Y. (2006). Neural foundations to moral reasoning and antisocial behavior. *Social Cognitive and Affective Neurosciences, 1*, 203–213.

Reed, G., & Enright, R. (2006). The effects of forgiveness therapy on depression, anxiety, and posttraumatic stress for women after spousal emotional abuse. *Journal of Consulting and Clinical Psychology, 74*, 920–929.

Richards, P., & Bergin, A. (1997). *A spiritual strategy for counseling and psychotherapy*. Washington, D.C.: American Psychological Association.

Rizzuto, A. (2004). Roman Catholic background and psychoanalysis. *Psychoanalytic Psychology, 21*, 436–441.

Rizzuto, A. (2005). Psychoanalytic considerations about spiritually oriented psychotherapy. In L. Sperry & E. Shafranske (Eds.), *Spiritually oriented psychotherapy*. Washington, D.C.: American Psychological Association.

Roberts, R. (2007). *Spiritual emotions: A psychology of Christian virtues*. Grand Rapids, MI: Eerdmans.

Roberts, R., & Talbot, M. (Eds.). (1997). *Limning the psyche: Explorations in Christian psychology*. Grand Rapids, MI: Eerdmans.

Schore, A. (1994). *Affect regulation and the origin of the self: The neurobiology of emotional development*. Hillsdale, MI: Lawrence Erlbaum Associates.

Schore, A. (2003). *Affect regulation and the repair of the self*. New York: W. W. Norton.

Schore, J., & Schore, A. (2008). Modern attachment theory: The central role of affect regulation in development and treatment. *Clinical Social Work Journal, 36*, 9–20.

Seybold, K. (2007). Physiological mechanisms involved in religiosity/spirituality and health. *Journal of Behavioral Medicine, 30*, 303–309.

Shariff, A., Schooler, J., & Vohs, K. (2008). The hazards of claiming to have solved the hard problem of free will. In J. Baer, J. Kaufman, & R. Baumeister (Eds.), *Are we free? Psychology and free will*. Oxford: Oxford University Press.

Shults, F., & Sandage, S. (2006). *Transforming spirituality: Integrating theology and psychology*. Grand Rapids, MI: Baker Academic.

Snyder, C. (1994). *The psychology of hope*. New York: The Free Press.

Sorenson, R. (2004). *Minding Spirituality*. New York: Analytic Press.

Spezio, M. (2006). Narrative in holistic healing: Empathy, sympathy, and simulation theory. In J. Koss-Chioino & P. Hefner (Eds.), *Spiritual transformation and healing: Anthropological, theological, neuroscientific, and clinical perspectives*. Lanham, MD: Altamira Press.

Spinelli, E. (2000). Therapy and the challenge of evil. *British Journal of*

Guidance and Counseling, 28, 561–567.

Stolorow, R., Atwood, G., & Brandchaft, B. (1994). *The intersubjective perspective*. New York: Jason Aronson.

Tan, S. (1996). Religion in clinical practice: Implicit and explicit integration. In E. Shafranske (Ed.), *Religion and the clinical practice of psychology*. Washington, D.C.: American Psychological Association.

Tjeltveit, A. (2006). Psychology's love-hate relationship with love. *Journal of Psychology and Theology, 34*, 8–22.

van der Kolk, B. (2006). Clinical implications of neuroscience research in PTSD. *New York Academy of Sciences, 1196*, 1–17.

Veloso, M. (2000). The law of God. In R. Dederen (Ed.), *Handbook of Seventh-day Adventist theology*. Hagerstown, MD: Review and Herald.

Wachholtz, A., & Pearce, M. (2007). Compassion and health. In T. Plante & C. Thoresen (Eds.), *Spirit, science, and health: How the spiritual mind fuels physical wellness*. Westport, CT: Praeger.

Weis, K. (2006). Introduction. In R. Sternberg & K. Weis (Eds.), *The new psychology of love*. New Haven, CT: Yale University Press.

White, E. (1892). *Steps to Christ*. Hagerstown, MD: Review and Herald.

White, E. (1903). *Education*. Nampa, ID: Pacific Press.

White, E. (1905). *The ministry of healing*. Hagerstown, MD: Review and Herald.

Wittgenstein, L. (1969). *On certainty*. Oxford: Oxford University Press

Worthington, E. (2001). *Five steps to forgiveness: The art and science of forgiving*. New York: Crown Publishers.

Worthington, E., & Sharp, J. (2006). Interpersonal forgiveness as an example of loving one's enemies. *Journal of Psychology and Theology, 34*, 32–42.

Yahne, C., & Miller, W. (1999). Evoking hope. In W. Miller (Ed.), *Integrating spirituality into treatment*. Washington, D.C.: American Psychological Association.

Yalom, I. (1980). *Existential psychotherapy*. New York: Basic Books.

Yarhouse, M., Butman, R., & McRay, B. (2005). *Modern psychopathologies: A comprehensive Christian appraisal*. Downers Grove, IL: InterVarsity Press.

Young, L., Cushman, F., Hauser, M., & Saxe, R. (2007). The neural basis of the interaction between theory of mind and moral judgment. *Proceedings of the National Academy of Sciences, 104*, 8235–8240.

Zeki, S. (2007). The neurobiology of love. *FEBS Letters, 581*, 2575–2579.

Zimbardo, P. (2004). A situationist perspective on the psychology of evil. In A. Miller (Ed.), *The social psychology of good and evil*. New York: Guilford.

The Science of Forgiveness: Implications for Christian Faith

Henry H. Lamberton and Antonia Ciovica

Theologian Lewis Smedes cites Hanna Arendt's assertion that the two "most persistent challenges of human existence" are that we are created with the ability to remember the past but with the "powerlessness to change it," and that we have the capacity to imagine the future but the "powerlessness to control it" (as cited by Smedes, 1998, p. 341). Based on this premise, Arendt concluded that "the only effective response to the first challenge was to use the faculty of forgiveness, and the only effective response to the second challenge was the ability to make and keep promises" (p. 341). Smedes emphasizes the necessity of practicing forgiveness and keeping promises if we are to cope with a past that cannot be changed and a future we cannot control. He contends that the only viable way of moving from the past to the future is by way of the journey from forgiveness to hope.

The current paper is the study of such a journey, from a past with an experience of hurt and injustice to a destination of healing and hope. We will focus on a path or road for getting to this destination that is of recent construction—namely the road developed by social scientists who have been studying the benefits of forgiveness and have identified ways to help facilitate it. There are, of course, other roads by which to begin this journey. The most widely known are the older, pre-existing ways that have been marked out by the world's major religions.

An important question is how the newer road of social science compares or relates to the religious roads that pre-exist it. This paper is concerned with one particular dimension of this larger question: namely how the phenomenon of forgiveness in the social science literature compares with its place and function in the religion of Christianity. Is this more recent road parallel and complementary to forgiveness as it is imbedded in Christian theology? Is the practical effect of its addition analogous to what happens today when a road is widened and an extra lane added? Or do the two roads take their travelers through very different terrain and perhaps to different destinations? The short answer, we believe, is that it all depends. But we will work toward the development of a longer answer that we hope will be more useful.

The paper begins with a brief overview of the biblical view of forgiveness. This is followed by a more extended description of the work that social scientists have accomplished in the area of forgiveness research. We have tried to write the section on the scientific study of forgiveness in a way that will be useful its own right for students who are studying the social sciences and are not acquainted with this field of concentration. In the next section of the paper we discuss questions that may arise when the two paths to forgiveness are integrated. In the process we focus on the way that insights and interventions from the field of psychology can enhance the mission of the church and how they may be used to distort and impede that mission.

BIBLICAL VIEW OF FORGIVENESS

Rice (2000) makes the following observation about the centrality of forgiveness in the teaching and practice of religious systems:

> Forgiveness is not only a religious concern; it is one of religion's central concerns. In fact, forgiveness is arguably what religion is all about. Given our inevitable moral failures, what is to become of us? That is one way to express the central human predicament. With our lives plagued by failures, by transgression, broken promises, unfulfilled obligations, etc., is there any hope for us? This is the fundamental question that every religion addresses, each in its own way.

What Rice says about the centrality of forgiveness for religions in general certainly applies to Christianity (see Rye et al., 2000, for a comparison of perspectives on forgiveness given by leaders from within each of the major world religions).

A biblical theology of forgiveness is based on the fact that a readiness to forgive is an identifying aspect of God's character and His relationship with humanity. When the Lord met Moses on Mt. Sinai and gave him the law, He described Himself with these words: "The LORD, the compassionate and gracious God, slow to anger, abounding in love and faithfulness, maintaining love to thousands, and forgiving wickedness, rebellion and sin" (Exod. 34: 6–7, NIV).

The Bible teaches that as human beings we were created in the image of God. The image of God included the innate ability and disposition to love unselfishly and consistently and to live in harmonious relationships with God and others. Through sin we became separated from God, each other, and ourselves. A description of God's initiatives to heal this severance and restore the broken relationships that resulted from it is the central theme of the Bible. Sin rendered us powerless to undo its effects and to change the direction of our future. Restoration could only be accomplished through Divine forgiveness, something which God is shown to exercise repeatedly throughout Scripture and which He provided and revealed with finality through the death and resurrection of Christ.

The sanctuary services which were instituted at the beginning of Israel's history as a nation illustrated the pivotal role of forgiveness in the worship of Israel. The ark of the covenant was located in the sanctuary's most holy place and was the focal point of the daily and yearly services. The ark contained the Ten Commandments, but over the commandments was the mercy seat. Thus the central lesson of the sanctuary is this: God's law is a holy revelation of how we are meant to live, and the law is covered with mercy. The message of the sanctuary service, when distilled to its basic essence, is one of righteousness and forgiveness.

Turning to the New Testament, we continue to see God as eager to forgive and to restore His relationship with His children. Nowhere is this eagerness more clearly illustrated than in the parable of the prodigal son whose father saw him when he was a great distance from home and ran to greet him (Luke 15:11–32). The prodigal did nothing to earn or obligate the father to forgive. The father's forgiveness was an act of mercy. Yet as Guthrie (1981) observes, the parable also shows that there is a link between forgiveness and penitence.

This connection between repentance, confession, and forgiveness is taught throughout Scripture (e.g., Ps. 23:1–6; Acts 2:37–38; 1 John 1:9). The connection does not mean, however, that those who treat us more unjustly must repent and acknowledge their wrong as a precondition of our readiness to forgive them. This point is most clearly illustrated in the prayer of Jesus for those who were crucifying him: "Father, forgive them; for they do not know what they are doing" (Luke 23:34, NRSV). A theme of the Bible is that the example of Christ toward those who harmed Him is a model for His followers. Jesus said, "Love your enemies, do good to those who hate you, bless those who curse you, pray for those who abuse you" (Luke 6:27–28, RSV; see also Exod. 23:4–5; Prov. 25:21; 1 Cor. 4:12).

As we shall see, the importance of making a distinction between forgiveness and repentance is emphasized in the psychological literature on forgiveness. Another element of a biblical theology of forgiveness which is also congruent with current psychological conceptions is that the act of forgiving is not to be confused with condoning, minimizing, or indulging sin. Rice (2000) makes this point clearly:

> It is true that those who forgive are guided by motives other than revenge. But this hardly means that they ignore justice. From a Christian perspective, the cross of Christ is a towering monument to the cost of forgiveness. The fact that God forgives freely does not mean that God forgives casually. As many theologians now interpret Christ's work, the cross means that God takes into God's own life the suffering human evil creates. So, judgment is not set aside. Instead, the judge is judged in our place, to quote Karl Barth (p. 8).

A further emphasis in Scripture that is relevant for this paper is that forgiveness does not necessarily remove the consequences of evil. God will bring justice on those who do not repent for destroying the earth and its people (e.g., Rev. 11:17–18ff.). This has practical significance. Knowing that God has said, "Vengeance is mine, I will repay" (Rom. 12:19, ESV) provides a reason on an individual level not to repay evil for evil but, instead, to live a life of peacemaking (Rom 12:17–21). A backdrop of the biblical view of forgiveness is that governments and the church have a legitimate responsibility to impose discipline on the unjust in order to protect those who would fall victim to evil (Matt. 18:15–17; Rom. 13:1–7). This teaching of Scripture removes a possible conclusion that practicing forgiveness the way the New Testament teaches would overlook evil and bring anarchy upon a society.

Before concluding this discussion we need to highlight a point which is central to a biblical theology of forgiveness. To again quote Rice, "The most important thing Christianity contributes to an understanding of forgiveness is its emphasis on the priority of being forgiven. Being forgiven obligates and enables us to forgive" (2000, p. 8).

The corollary of the fact that God forgives is that those who experience God's forgiveness will themselves be forgiving (Eph. 4:32). This link between having been forgiven and forgiving is made repeatedly in Scripture, including the words of what Christians commonly refer to as the *Lord's Prayer*: "Forgive us our debts as we also have forgiven our debtors" (Matt. 6:12, NIV). But it is even more clearly made when Jesus said in His most famous sermon, "Your heavenly Father will forgive you if you forgive those who sin against you; but if you refuse to forgive them, He will not forgive you" (Matt. 6:14–15, LB). This could be taken to mean that we merit or earn God's forgiveness when we forgive others. But such a conclusion would run counter to the overall message of Scripture and to what we have already noted about God's nature and His eagerness to forgive. What this verse and others like it are meant to teach is that practicing forgiveness is not optional or peripheral for those who follow Christ (Rice, 2000). From a Christian perspective, readiness to forgive is a consequence of having been forgiven and a confirmation that one is in communion with the God who forgives.

Morales-Gudmundsson (2007) noted that the two words most often translated as "forgiveness" in the New Testament are *charizomai* and *aphiemi*. *Charizomai* is used in reference to God's forgiveness in Christ and is understood as granting "a favor gratuitously out of kindness, not from any worthiness on the part of the receiver[;] it implies rescuing or delivering someone from certain danger or death" (p. 51). *Aphiemi* is a "horizontal process of forgiveness that calls for self-analysis, acknowledgment of sin, repentance, and confession from the sinner/offender in order to remain in a right relationship with God and his fellow human" (p. 52). Based on the *charizomai* and the relationship that God provides through Christ, we become able to live a life of purification from unrighteousness, ourselves striving to represent *aphiemi*. This process is characterized by "a mutual collaboration in which we are "educated" into the character of God through the habits of forgiveness" (Morales-Gudmundsson, 2007, p. 52).

We have so far attempted to describe the place of forgiveness in Christian theology and experience. We will now turn to the contributions of contemporary social scientists on the topic of forgiveness.

THE STUDY OF FORGIVENESS BY SOCIAL SCIENTISTS

THE INTEREST OF SOCIAL SCIENTISTS IN THE TOPIC OF FORGIVENESS

Prior to the mid 1980s there were no scientific studies of forgiveness published in scholarly literature. The few articles that did exist consisted of case studies, personal reflections of mental health professionals, and a model of forgiveness based on the work of Elizabeth Kubler-Ross (Enright & Fitzgibbons, 2000). Several researchers credit Lewis Smedes's (1984) groundbreaking book on interpersonal forgiveness with creating an interest in the topic of forgiveness in the psychological community. Among these is Robert Enright, from the University of Wisconsin, Madison, who pioneered research in this field in the late 1980s. A significant impetus to the study of this topic came in 1998 when the John Tempelton Foundation began offering competitive grants for research in issues related to forgiveness. A result was that the number of empirical studies on the topic of forgiveness quadrupled between the years of 1997 and 2004 (McCullough et al., 1998; Worthington & Scherer, 2004).

The processes and benefits of forgiving others, forgiving oneself, seeking forgiveness, granting forgiveness, and being forgiven became topics of interest in various research laboratories. However, most of the available empirical research to date, and clinical outcome research, concentrates on helping injured persons develop a spirit of forgiveness when they have been hurt by someone else. This research has demonstrated that there are significant psychological and physical benefits from practicing forgiveness in contrast to holding onto feelings of anger, bitterness, and resentment. In terms of psychological well-being, research has demonstrated a positive association between forgiveness and success in overcoming addictions and in feeling comforted when upset (Wuthnow, 2000). Other studies found that forgiveness was inversely related to psychological distress (Toussaint et al., 2001), psychopathology (Mauger et al., 1992), and, more specifically, depression (Tangey, Fee, Reinsmith, Boone, & Lee, 1999), anxicty (Subkoviak et al., 1995), and anger (Freedman & Enright, 1996). In another study, a clinical intervention to help increase one's ability to forgive was found to result in improved existential well-being (Rye & Pargament, 2002).

Physical health benefits have also been documented, although less frequently. Findings indicate that forgiveness is positively associated with physical health, particularly when a readiness to forgive is a stable dispositional trait rather than a temporary state (Lawler-Row, Karremans, Scott, Edlis-Matityahou, & Edwards, 2008; Lawler et al., 2003; Maltby, Macaskill, & Day, 2001; Seybold, Hill, Neumann, & Chi, 2001; Toussaint, Williams, Musick, & Everson, 2001; Witvliet, Ludwig, & Van der Laan, 2001; Witvliet, Phipps, Feldman, & Beckham, 2004). Forgiveness is believed to influence physical health through a number of direct or indirect pathways, including the overall effects on the body of reduced stress as measured by cortisol levels (Berry & Worthington, 2001); reduced hostility, which is a risk factor for heart disease (Miller, Smith, Turner, Guijarro, & Hallett, 1996); increased social support (e.g., where forgiveness resulted in mending or improving relationships); and an increase in health promoting behaviors and spiritual well-being (Thoresen et al., 2000).

THE PSYCHOLOGY OF FORGIVENESS: CONCEPTUAL ISSUES

Before a phenomenon such as forgiveness can be scientifically investigated, it must be defined in a manner that can be operationalized. When it came to developing a model of the complex process of forgiveness, researchers found it easier to arrive at a consensus on what forgiveness *was not* rather than on what it *was* (Enright & Coyle, 1998). There was relatively early agreement that forgiveness should not be equated with pardoning, which implies a legal context; condoning, which denies the wrongfulness; excusing, which provides a rationalization for the offense; forgetting, or failing to remember the offense; or denying, which is refusal to acknowledge an offense. A final point of agreement was that forgiveness is not synonymous with reconciliation, although it was noted that it often can lead to reconciliation (Enright & Coyle, 1998; McCullough, Pargament, & Thoresen, 2000).

Establishing a common operational definition of forgiveness to use in developing testable hypotheses is complicated by the fact that theoretical and theological perspectives influence the way one understands forgiveness (Worthington, Sandage, & Berry, 2000). Not surprisingly, a review of the initial literature on forgiveness reveals a variety of definitions (e.g., DiBlasio, 1998; Enright, Eastin, Golden, Sarinopoulos, & Freedman, 1992; Enright & The Human Development Study Group, 1996; Enright & Zell, 1989; Luskin, 2002; McCullough, Worthington, & Rachal, 1997; Thompson et al., 2005; Wade & Worthington, 2002).

However, by 2005 Worthington could conclude in the *Handbook of Forgiveness* that a general agreement had been reached among researchers on several core concepts related to forgiveness and its operationalization. First, forgiveness was commonly understood as the process of reducing, or even eliminating, unforgiveness, which consists of the chronic, negative thoughts and emotions which result from being victimized (Worthington, Sandage, & Berry, 2000; Worthington & Scherer, 2004; Worthington & Wade, 1999). Second, forgiveness involved an increase in positive emotions such as compassion and love, cognitions (empathy), and motivations to give the altruistic gift of forgiveness to the offender (Enright & Coyle, 1998; Enright & Fitzgibbons, 2000; McCullough, Fincham, & Tsang, 2003; Worthington, 2005; Worthington & Wade, 1999). Third, while an aspect of forgiveness involved giving an altruistic gift of beneficent thoughts, feelings, or behaviors to an offender, forgiveness greatly benefits the forgiver. Hence, forgiveness involves both inter- and intra-personal dynamics.

In sum, current definitions of forgiveness include acknowledging that an injustice has been perpetrated, while focusing on the process of healing taking place in the forgiver, a process which involves offering the offender the paradoxical gift of not responding in kind. Through this process—a decrease in anger and fear—the healing of emotions occurs; through a decrease in ruminations, cognitions are healed; and through the removal of the need to actively seek revenge, cognitive healing is fostered. In turn, this process engenders a sense of psychological well-being and improved interpersonal interactions. Some researchers explicitly identify a spiritual dimension in this process while others merely imply it, and yet others disregard or dismiss such a dimension. One of the most influential definitions of forgiveness states is this:

> People, upon rationally determining that they have been unfairly treated, forgive when they willfully abandon resentment and related responses (to which they have a right), and endeavor to respond to the wrongdoer based on the moral principle of benevolence, which may include compassion, unconditional worth, generosity, and moral love (to which the wrongdoer, by nature of the hurtful act or acts, has no right). (Enright & Fitzgibbons, 2000, p. 24)

While this definition provides a generally agreed upon framework for understanding the concept of forgiveness, differences in points of focus and emphasis remain. Worthington (2005) observed that researchers who study forgiveness primarily within the context of continuing relationships, such as intimate relationships between married couples or between parents and children, tend to emphasize the replacement of negative emotions, cognitions, and behaviors with positive ones. On the other hand, researchers who study the application of forgiveness to cases of victimization by strangers or those in non-continuing relationships tend to simply focus on reducing or eliminating unforgiveness.

A second point of divergence can be seen in the degree of emphasis given to an emotional, versus decisional, understanding of forgiveness (Worthington & Scherer, 2004). The core of this divergence is the philosophical as well as pragmatic issue of whether forgiveness is an ongoing intra- and inter-personal process, or a once-and-for-all personal decision that is both spontaneous and decisive. In practical terms, this is seen as either the decision to control one's behaviors (decisional forgiveness) or the transactional process leading to transformed emotions, cognitions, and motivations (emotional forgiveness). These two differing views can be seen in the work done by researchers represented by two prominent scholars in the area of the scientific study of forgiveness, namely, Worthington and DiBlasio.

Worthington emphasizes the experience of emotional transformation inherent in the process of forgiveness and describes his approach as an "emotion focused copying strategy" (Worthington & Scherer, 2004).

Emotional forgiveness—the experience of forgiveness, as distinguished from decisional forgiveness—is defined as the emotional juxtaposition of positive other-oriented emotions such as empathy, sympathy, compassion, altruistic love, or romantic love over the negative emotions of unforgiveness (Worthington & Wade, 1999).

> As unforgiveness and the positive emotion collide, the intensity

> of unforgiveness is reduced. If forgiveness is complete, the person might experience, at worst, neutral emotion toward the perpetrator and, at best, residual positive emotion toward the perpetrator. Regardless of how forgiveness is initiated (e.g., cognitively, behaviorally, decisionally, socially, or spiritually), the process of forgiveness involves neutralization of negative emotions with more positive emotions. (Worthington, Mazzeo, & Canter, 2005, p. 239)

DiBlasio (1998), on the other hand, has argued that forgiveness is a decision-based process, a cognitive exercise of "letting go of resentment and bitterness and need for vengeance" (p. 78). While the cognitive process of letting go "is not always the end to emotional pain and hurt," the forgiver in this perspective is greatly empowered, as he or she is actively engaged in an "act of the will" (p. 78).

> Forgiveness here is viewed as an act of the will, a choice, to let go or to hold on. People can separate their thoughts of resentment and bitterness from their feeling of hurt. In fact, such negative thoughts often prevent healing, as cognitive and emotional energy are misdirected into bitterness.... The approach here takes a different path, where victims become empowered when they make cognitive choices that promote harmony in their relationships, peace within themselves and, for believing clients, serenity with God. (DiBlasio, 1998, pp. 78–79)

DiBlasio's emphasis on the cognitive aspects of forgiveness is easily distinguished from one that conceptualizes forgiveness as a process primarily involving changes in affective states. DiBlasio questions Enright's assertion (e.g., Enright & Human Developmental Study Group, 1991) that "forgiveness is a process that takes time and emotional readiness," and argues for a "way to accelerate the process" in therapy (DiBlasio, 1998, p. 78).

A third notable dimension was highlighted by McCullough, Worthington, and Rachal (1997) as they introduced the notion of a close relationship between motivation and the act of forgiveness. They suggested that an understanding of forgiveness should include the concept of a pro-social change in *motivation*, whereby the motivation to retaliate against the offender decreases while the motivation to reconcile and act benevolently towards the offender increases. Forgiveness is thus viewed as a reduction in negative motivations and an increase in positive ones.

Conceptual differences in the way social scientists understand and define forgiveness remain. While forgiveness is generally defined as the process of decreasing negative emotions, cognitions, and motivations that resulted from being the victim of an act of injustice, and increasing or replacing these negative experiences with positive ones, various researchers highlight different pathways in this process such as suggesting that emotions, cognitions, or motivations may take primacy in achieving the desired outcome. Gorsuch and Hao (1993) contend that a truly comprehensive definition of forgiveness would necessarily integrate a spiritual aspect along with the above mentioned cognitive, affective, and behavioral components. Thus, while there is general agreement that forgiveness can be a powerful therapeutic intervention, the diversity of views regarding conceptual matters has made the development of one single authoritative approach to fostering forgiveness difficult.

THERAPEUTIC FORGIVENESS

Once the benefits of forgiveness have been identified—including those pertaining to psychological, physical, social, and spiritual arenas—and conceptual considerations have been reconciled, the question of how to effectively facilitate the attainment of forgiveness remains. There are currently two prevailing models of forgiveness interventions: a decision model and a process model. Baskin and Enright (2004) trace these models to two different philosophical underpinnings. One, which is based on the thought of the philosopher William R. Neblett (1974), sees forgiveness as taking place the moment the decision to forgive is made. The other, which is drawn from the writings of Joanna North (1987, as cited in Baskin & Enright, 2004), understands forgiveness as a process that develops through a series of steps or phases. The process starts with acknowledging and attending to the resentment and hurt experienced and continues to a conscious choice to let go of this resentment and to attempt to foster benevolence towards the perpetrator. It progresses further by remaining engaged in the difficult process of searching for love, grace, and justice.

PROCESS-BASED FORGIVENESS INTERVENTIONS

To date, two models of process-based interventions have predominated the research. One is the model developed by Enright and colleagues (Enright & Fitzgibbons, 2000), and the second is by Worthington and colleagues (2001, 2006). However, other less influential models have also been created and tested (e.g., DiBlasio, 2000; Harris et al., 2006).

THE ENRIGHT MODEL

Enright and the Human Development Study Group (1991; Enright & Fitzgibbons, 2000) have developed an intervention that delineates four phases of treatment (see Appendix A). These four phases are made up of twenty units which provide a "map" for the journey of forgiveness. These phases include guideposts and reminders that help one examine various offenses suffered, gain a new understanding of the offender, let go of anger, and finally make a moral response of goodness toward the offender. This is a process that may require many months or even years—one in which everyone may not go through the individual phases and units in the same way or at the same speed.

The first phase is called the *Uncovering* phase during which the therapist's role is to assist the injured person in the process of gaining insight into how the injustice affected his or her life. This phase can include a particularly painful "pit stop" that requires an examination of the possible use of defenses such as denial, repression, and displacement as a means of managing hurt. It also includes confronting anger, admitting shame, and becoming aware of the negative effects of depleted emotional energy and cognitive ruminations. The offended person also comes to acknowledge that without forgiveness he or she faces the possibility of living with a permanent emotional/spiritual injury and a more pessimistic philosophy of life.

The *Decision* phase involves developing an accurate understanding of what forgiveness is and is not. This understanding then creates a basis for making a conscious and well-informed decision to forgive. The tasks during the third or *Work* phase include coming to a new understanding of the offender through reframing, exhibiting empathy and compassion for the offender, and thus offering him or her a moral gift of forgiveness. The final *Deepening* phase involves coming to embrace hope and meaning in suffering. By realizing that each of us has required, and will continue to require, the forgiveness of others, one comes to experience a renewed purpose in life and an experience of greater connection with others (Enright & Fitzgibbons, 2000).

THE WORTHINGTON MODEL

Worthington and colleagues developed the Pyramid Model, a five-step model known by the acronym REACH. This approach seeks to "induce states of empathy and humility (including a recognition of one's own guilt, gratitude for having been forgiven in the past, and the decision to give a gift of forgiveness)" (Worthington, 1998, p. 112). The five REACH steps, which Worthington notes are not always followed in an invariant order, are: *R*ecalling the hurt, *E*mpathizing with the one who committed the offense, giving the *A*ltruistic gift of forgiveness, making a *C*ommitment to forgive, and *H*olding on to forgiveness.

The first step of R*ecalling the hurt* is based on the belief that fully facing, rather than avoiding or denying, the cognitive and emotional aspects of an injury is an important pre-condition for healing. As such, it has points of similarity with the first phase of the Enright model. This step takes place in a supportive and safe atmosphere

(McCullough & Worthington, 1995; McCullough, Worthington, & Rachal, 1997) which helps the re-experiencing of the hurt to become increasingly less associated with the pain of the original offense. The state of unforgiveness, which is viewed as fear-based, is diminished by "creating cognitive and emotional conditions that activate other emotional systems" (Worthington, 1998, p. 118). These include the emotional system of empathy. *Empathy towards the offender* is developed by imagining oneself in the place of the offender and speculating what he or she might have been thinking or feeling during the hurtful event. Increased empathy is accompanied by an increase in humility and gratitude. Humility is developed by gaining an accurate appreciation of one's own wrongdoings and experiencing one's own guilt. Gratitude comes from realizing the forgiveness that one has received for his or her own transgressions. The combination of empathy, humility, and gratitude is seen to create an aroused motivational state in which the person becomes ready to take the third step. Up to this point in the process, forgiveness has largely been dealt with in an emotional manner; however, by making the cognitive and rational decision and commitment to forgive, Worthington and colleagues argue that a stronger sense of forgiveness is instilled through various processes, such as underscoring cognitive dissonance and commitment theory.

The third step in Worthington's model is a decision to offer an *altruistic gift of forgiveness* to the offender while the fourth step is *making a commitment to forgive*. The commitment step is typically accompanied by a ceremonial action such as writing out a certificate of forgiveness which solidifies the reality of the commitment. The distinction between the third and fourth steps would in the Christian religion be analogous to a decision to become a follower of Jesus and the formalizing of that decision in the act of baptism. The first steps in the REACH model promote forgiveness in a manner that heavily targets the emotional components of unforgiveness. However, by making the cognitive and rational decision and commitment to forgive,

Worthington and colleagues argue that a stronger sense of forgiveness is instilled. Finally, during the fifth step, the forgiver is equipped, through psycho-education and emotion-management techniques, with ways of maintaining the gains achieved, or *holding on to forgiveness.*

In Worthington's model, the emotional juxtaposition of positive, other-oriented, emotions against negative unforgiveness is believed to eventually result in the replacement of negative emotions with positive emotions, or at the very least their neutralization (Worthington & Scherer, 2004).

DECISION-BASED THERAPY MODELS

Decision-based forgiveness is the cognitive letting go of resentment, bitterness, and the need for vengeance. DiBlasio (1998) and McCullough and Worthington (1995) developed brief, decision-based forgiveness interventions with a goal of encouraging people to arrive at the decision to forgive (see Appendix B). Specifically, McCullough and Worthington (1995) developed a one-hour psycho-educational intervention to promote forgiveness which included didactic material and individual exercises and discussion. The intervention included a focus on building empathy toward the offender, developing new perspectives on the experience of having been victimized, and recalling one's own needs to be forgiven.

DiBlasio (1998) proposed a more intense decision-based model which was designed to address old hurts between an adult child and a parent. The six-hour intervention began by focusing on both the child's and the parent's perception of their past family life and moved to a discussion of the usefulness of forgiveness. Specific goals of the intervention included bringing the parent and child to a thorough understanding of the offense and the hurt and pain that it caused while assisting them in the development of a plan to stop or prevent the offensive behavior from recurring. The intervention ended with the participants formally requesting forgiveness and participating in a ceremonial act to represent forgiveness.

THE EFFICACY OF FORGIVENESS INTERVENTIONS

The best available evidence about the effectiveness of interventions to promote forgiveness comes from two published meta-analyses. The first, which was conducted by Baskin and Enright (2004), included all available published studies that used quantitative treatment measures. The authors identified nine such studies which involved a total of 330 participants with a variety of forgiveness interventions. Participants in one study were elderly women (mean age 74.5) who were self-identified as having been emotionally hurt by a specific individual and who were not going through a grieving process. Another study examined results of forgiveness therapy with female incest survivors, and yet another study involved men who had been hurt by the decision of their partner to have an abortion. Three of the studies used subjects who were college students in introductory psychology classes and whose goals included their hope to forgive parents or others who had hurt or betrayed them. Each of the nine studies used an experimental method that included random assignment into control and treatment groups.

The authors of this meta-analysis categorized the studies into three types, depending on the characteristics of the intervention that was used: (1) decision-based forgiveness interventions, (2) process-based forgiveness interventions delivered in a group format, and (3) process-based forgiveness interventions delivered in an individual format. Four of the nine studies encompassing a total of 188 participants used short–term, decision-based interventions that consisted of either a single session, four one-hour group sessions, six one-hour sessions, or, in one case, eight one-hour sessions conducted over a single weekend. The meta-analysis failed to demonstrate any measurable treatment effects in promoting forgiveness for these short-term, decision-based interventions (the mean effect size was $d = -0.04$; 95% confidence interval [CI]: -0.24 to 0.16). These may in fact have produced iatrogenic effects.

However, the analysis did demonstrate a significant increase in the indicators of forgiveness in both the individual and in the group format interventions which were process based. The process-based group interventions (a total of three interventions with 120 participants) demonstrated a large effect size (d = 0.82; 95% CI: 0.43 to 1.21). In other words, the average person in the intervention group did as well as or better than 75% of the control group. An even greater effect size was observed in the individually delivered process-based interventions which consisted of two studies and twenty-two participants. Outcomes revealed that the average person in the intervention group did as well as or better than 95% of the control group (d = 1.66; 95% CI: 0.68 to 2.64).

When the effects of forgiveness interventions on emotional health—such as changes in self-esteem, state- and trait-anxiety, depression, hope, state anger, and grief—were considered as the dependent variables, there was, again, no significant improvement between decision-based interventions (n = 102) and control groups (d = 0.16; 95% CI: -0.16 to 0.48). However, the participants in the process-based group and individual interventions demonstrated a significant positive change, with medium to large effect sizes. Specifically, process-based group interventions (three interventions, total n = 120) demonstrated a medium-effect size (d = 0.50; 95% CI: 0.28 to 0.90) while process-based individual interventions (two interventions, n = 22) demonstrated a large-effect size (d = 1.42; 95% CI: 0.66 to 2.18). Thus, process-based forgiveness interventions were found to be effective in improving emotional health. The average person who participated in process-based group treatment did as well as, or better than, 65% of the control group while the average person who participated in the process-based individual treatment did as well as or better than 92% of the control group. The authors concluded that their analysis showed that process-based therapy is not only efficacious in facilitating forgiveness, but that it also showed a clear link between forgiveness and mental health.

A second meta-analysis (Lundahl et al., 2008) augmented the study done by Baskin and Enright (2004) by investigating additional outcome studies which had become available after the first study was conducted. Because Baskin and Enright did not find decision-based forgiveness models to be efficacious, Lundahl and colleagues focused their analysis solely on studies that were processed-based. The range of situations for which forgiveness therapy had been applied in studies they analyzed included adolescents adjusting to parental divorce, issues of an inpatient substance-dependent population, college students dealing with a hurtful break in a romantic relationship, therapeutic groups on forgiving an ex-spouse, and a forgiveness exercise to promote character development in students at a Christian college. The larger number of studies the authors had available (N = 15) allowed them to examine a number of moderating variables that they hypothesized might influence outcomes, described as follows:

> Five characteristics of participants were coded: level of distress prior to entering treatment..., participant age and status of college involvement....the duration of the offense for which participants sought relief [i.e., specific insult, ongoing, mixture], the percentage of the sample that was female, and the percentage of the sample that was minority. Six characteristics of forgiveness intervention programs were coded: comparison group type [i.e., alternative treatment, and control group], delivery mode [i.e., group and individual], inclusion of the perpetrator in treatment [i.e., not included, and included], the intervention model used [i.e., Enright model, REACH (Worthington), and Other], the number of sessions, and the amount of time spent in forgiveness intervention. (Lundahl et al., 2008, p. 468)

In terms of the immediate outcome of the process-based forgiveness intervention, the populations who received the interventions showed a statistically significant increase in forgiveness (g = 0.82, CI: 0.51 to 1.13), an increase in positive affect (g = 0.81, CI: 0.33 to 1.30), a decrease in negative affect (g = 0.54, CI: 0.32 to 0.77), and an increase in self-esteem (g = 0.60, CI: 0.14 to 1.06) when compared to the control groups. Outcome measures revealed improvement in three variables across time. These were forgiveness (g = 1.23, CI: 0.60 to 1.85), negative affect (g = 0.98, CI: 0.48 to 1.48), and self-esteem (g = 1.47, CI: 1.03 to 1.91). In summary, process-based forgiveness interventions demonstrated a long-term effect not only in maintaining an attitude of forgiveness, but also by decreasing negative affect and increasing self-esteem.

Several findings within this meta-analysis seem particularly relevant for mental health clinicians, teachers, and clergy when they are called upon to assist others in the process of forgiveness. First, results indicated that process-based forgiveness therapy increased positive affect and self-esteem and decreased negative affect both in the short- and long-term. Second, the length of time in treatment and the number of treatment sessions were positively related to better outcomes. Third, individually applied programs were associated with better results. They were, in fact, four times more effective than the group programs based upon the outcome measures used. Fourth, the effectiveness of the interventions did not seem to be dependent upon age (results were positive for both adolescents and the elderly), life status, gender, or being a member of a minority group. Fifth, participants who entered treatment with clinically elevated distress demonstrated better outcomes than those with more moderate distress, both immediately following treatment and at follow-up periods. Measurable outcomes were almost two standard deviations higher in the treatment groups as compared with control groups. Sixth, results from the eight studies that conducted post-treatment follow-up assessments revealed that the lapse of time between the end of treatment and the follow-up assessment was positively correlated with improvement in outcomes. This finding supports the idea that actualizing forgiveness takes time. The authors end their article with this description of the existing evidence:

> Overall, process-based forgiveness interventions show promise in achieving clinical treatment goals. Individuals exposed to such interventions, compared to those in alternate treatment or wait list groups, were much more likely to forgive past insults. Moreover, expressions of negative emotions, such as depression and anxiety, were significantly lower, whereas expressions of positive emotions such as hope, were significantly higher for participants in the intervention

> programs. Importantly, those desirable outcomes tended to be durable for as long as 4 months beyond treatment....The forgiveness model of therapy holds substantial hope for an evidence-based model of practice that can be used in clinical practice. (Lundahl et al., 2008, pp. 477–478)

ISSUES FOR THE INTEGRATION OF THERAPEUTIC FORGIVENESS WITH CHRISTIAN FAITH AND PRACTICE FROM AN ADVENTIST PERSPECTIVE

We chose to write on the topic of forgiveness because of its direct relevance to the lives of students and clients with whom we work, as well as the significance in our own lives. We also chose this topic because it leads to a consideration of many of the fundamental issues that arise when the relationship between Christianity and psychology are considered. One such issue, for example, is what happens when religious language is translated into a psychological framework. When we attempt to define a complex religious concept such as forgiveness, in an effort to make it fit the mold of our scientific methods so that it can be studied quantitatively, do we lose something important in the process? Or do we end up better off for having sharpened our thinking and making our language more precise?

I (HL) include a module on forgiveness in a class I teach to first-year medical students on the topic of personal growth and wholeness. The students read an article from *Christianity Today* (Thomas, 2000) that gives an overview of the work of Smedes, Enright, and others who point out the personal benefits of forgiveness and describe ways to help people experience it. Students generally find the article to be intellectually stimulating and practically relevant to their lives. Sometimes, it leads them to write openly about painful personal experiences and their own struggles to forgive those who have hurt them. But it is not uncommon for some to express discomfort with the emphasis given to pursuing forgiveness as a means of increasing the forgiver's health and happiness, and with the apparent removing of forgiveness from its religious context. An example of such a response was written by a thoughtful young woman in the class, who gave me permission to quote what follows. After acknowledging some positive aspects to the psychological study of forgiveness, she went on to voice these concerns:

> It seemed that the article was saying that forgiveness at its root is selfish, but if that were the case, then we would be saying that God, in forgiving us, is selfish. Another point that I struggled with was simply having a discussion of forgiveness in a clinical setting. It seems as though it should be something discussed in a church instead of a clinic. The steps for reaching forgiveness I found particularly intriguing. The first step, according to the article was to confront anger, then consider forgiveness as an option, accept the pain, and finally recognize a need to be forgiven in the past. It sounded like such a recipe that is used in so many other areas of life such as AA or anger management. A discussion of forgiveness from a psychological view originally seemed foreign and unscientific to me, but then, after reading the article, it seemed more like a procedure that we would order rather than a conviction that must be experienced. Can forgiveness just be prescribed and counseled into existence? Somehow, leaving God out of the discussion of forgiveness just really did not fit into my worldview at all. Any suggestions?

I responded by writing that I found her comments thoughtful and important and encouraged her to bring them up in our class discussion. I also added the following:

> As far as the selfishness issue is concerned, I understand how the idea of forgiving for our own sake may seem self-serving. At the same time, when I reflect on this, it seems that there are a number of areas of life where we, as Christians, often speak of the benefits to self that come from healthy behaviors. If someone had a drug problem, or was overweight, and we appealed to their self-interest as well as God's plan for their life as a motive for change, would it seem less objectionable?

POINTS OF AGREEMENT BETWEEN THERAPEUTIC AND CHRISTIAN PERSPECTIVES

Teachers, like therapists, who receive multi-faceted comments such as the one above may choose to respond in a number of ways. One would be to use the student's comment as an opportunity to make the argument that the Bible teaches universal principles for how to live in ways that are for our best good as well as the good of others. In her book, *Thoughts from the Mount of Blessing*, Ellen White (1900, 1928) articulated this belief as she wrote, "There is not one commandment of the law that is not for the good and happiness of man, both in this life and in the life to come" (p. 67).

Christian psychologists Henry Cloud and John Townsend (2001) also emphasize the idea that following God's revelation for how we should live is beneficial. "All growth is spiritual growth" is a phrase they use repeatedly in their book, *How People Grow: What the Bible Reveals about Personal Growth,* to reflect their conviction that all genuine growth comes from God. Individuals whose lives follow the principles of growth taught in Scripture still benefit, whether or not they know God personally or fully understand the source of the principles they are following. This is a significant belief not only for what it says about God's revelation (i.e., that truth about God and His creation can be available in nature, reason, and experience in addition to Scripture, as Wesley taught), but also because it affirms that God loves us, and that His rules for living are not arbitrary. Thus, helping people forgive because it will be good for them may be no different than appealing to individuals to stop smoking or drinking or to start following a healthy diet because it will help them feel better and live longer. An Adventist Christian appeal says more than this, of course. Adventists have emphasized that practicing good health and living a moral life are ways to "glorify God in our bodies" (1 Cor. 6:20, 21st Century KJV).

DO PSYCHOLOGICAL RESEARCH FINDINGS AID SPIRITUAL DEVELOPMENT?

In addition to concerns about appeals to self interest as motivation to forgive, the student whose comments we have been addressing expressed discomfort with the prescribed, or seemingly formulaic, quality of the psychologically based methods for facilitating forgiveness. Hers is a significant and valid question which may be motivated by a number of more basic questions that are significant for integration of psychology and spirituality. One such question relates to the extent to which human cognitive and emotional processes follow laws or patterns which can in turn make them generally predictable. If this was not assumed to be the case, the effort to identify standardized, repeatable interventions would be futile. A second question may reflect discomfort that the seemingly secular discipline of psychology, which has often been critical of religion, would add something of value to the process of growth in a realm that has been thought of as predominately spiritual.

As teachers we could respond to the student's question by observing that scientifically derived knowledge facilitates physical healing: Should we not expect that knowledge gained from the social sciences can facilitate psychological health? Furthermore, is there not a body of knowledge to be learned that can promote spiritual health and wholeness? The Seventh-day Adventist church has built schools of medicine and nursing, and developed programs in psychology in addition to theology to equip students to, as stated in Loma Linda University's mission statement, for example, "continue the healing and teaching ministry of Jesus Christ" (Loma Linda University, p. 35). Just as we study the science of physical health, should we not study the science of the mind as aids to developing psychological health and more Christ-like characters?

A specific instance of how the scientific study of forgiveness may help with psychological and spiritual growth arises from Jesus' teaching that we must not only refrain from murdering or insulting our brother, but we must not be angry with him either (Matt. 5:21–25). Likewise, the parable of the unforgiving servant ends with a dire warning of judgment to come for his listeners if they fail to "forgive your brother or sister from the heart" (Matt. 18:35, NRSV). We may obey by refraining from murdering or verbally insulting our brother or sister, but to be commanded to forgive from the heart is another matter. How, if we are serious about sanctification, can we accomplish such a seemingly impossible task?

Psychological research has identified models to help us forgive emotionally as well as volitionally in a way that corresponds with what biblical scholars indicate Jesus meant by the Greek word *kardia,* which is translated as "heart." According to Danker (2001), *kardia* refers to the core of thinking, feeling, and behavior. The research on the efficacy of process models compared with decision-based models supports the importance of attending to the emotional as well as the strictly volitional aspects of forgiveness. It may be good to pause at this point of the argument to emphasize the statement that psychological research has *identified* processes by which the heart can be changed. This is not the same as saying that psychological research has invented or developed ways of modifying emotions that are foreign to how God created us or that are foreign to Scripture. Procedures by which feelings are modified are natural processes that, once identified and found to be effective, can then be taught and used (see Appendix C).

A practical illustration that relates to the point just made comes from the work of a recent study (Hernandez, et al., 2011) which employed forgiveness education workshops specifically designed for Seventh-day Adventists. The researchers reported preliminary observations that participants were surprised to find out about physiological and emotional facets of forgiveness, as they had previously believed that "...forgiveness is a solely spiritual endeavor" (p. 22). The researchers noted that they saw "a collective sigh of relief" when they explained what forgiveness is and is not to this self-identified religiously committed population. The authors stated, "It would seem prudent to provide Seventh-day Adventist clergy with tools to assist individuals and families move through forgiveness in more effective ways. Education concerning the integration of social, physiological, emotional, and mental aspects of forgiveness is recommended" (p. 21).

OBJECTIONS TO THE MINGLING OF THERAPEUTIC AND CHRISTIAN FORGIVENESS

We have articulated points that could, and we believe should, be made in a discussion of the concerns raised by our student when she said, "Somehow, leaving God out the discussion of forgiveness just really did not fit into my worldview at all." Yet, if we responded with the above arguments and left the matter there, we suspect her apprehensions would remain, and legitimately so.

The Methodist theologian L. Gregory Jones's (1995) theological study of forgiveness devotes a full chapter to a discussion of "therapeutic forgiveness," something of which he is highly critical (pp. 35–69). Jones introduces his critique by relating a story told by the psychiatrist Robert Coles of a devout Roman Catholic friend who, while hospitalized for a chronic life-threatening condition, had been visited by a priest. Coles arrived at his friend's bedside shortly after the priest had left, and found him in a state of anger. The hospitalized man said that the priest had asked,

> How the patient was managing to "cope" [and] proceeded in what Coles calls, "a relentless kind of psychological inquiry". How was the patient "feeling"? How was he "managing," in view of the "stress" he had to "confront"? The friend was enraged by such questions; he wanted to talk with the priest about God and God's ways, about Christ's life and death, about Luke's Gospel (a particular favorite), about Heaven and Hell—only to be approached repeatedly with words and phrases drawn from the vocabulary of popular psychology. As the friend characterized it to Coles: "He comes here with a Roman Collar, and offers me psychological banalities as God's word!" (Jones, 1995, p. 35)

Jones goes on to quote this comment from Coles:

> There are, of course, many kinds of burdens in this life. I wonder whether the deepest mire, the deepest waters, for many of America's clergy, not to mention us laymen, may be found in the dreary solipsistic world so many of us have learned to find so interesting: the mind's moods, the various "stages" or "phases" of "human development" or of "dying," all dwelt upon (God save us!) as if "Stations of the Cross." (p. 36)

A "PROZAC GOD"?

Part of what Coles and Jones are protesting is what Jones and others have described as our contemporary culture's "therapeutic mindset." This is a mindset that places the highest of priorities on individual fulfillment and that fosters the pursuit of personal serenity for its own sake. Acts of altruism, when identified as a value, are framed as a secondary achievement, the fruits of the prior attainment of a healthy sense of self and personal wholeness, rather than a means by which the self is discovered. In a culture with a therapeutic mindset, religion can easily be seen as a commodity which may be used to aid individuals in achieving fulfillment but which leaves them no less self-absorbed.

Dueck (2006) quotes T. S. Elliot (1940/1968): "It is a very dangerous inversion to advocate Christianity, not because it is true, but because it might be beneficial." Dueck goes on to say:

> In the application of religion/health research, a *utilitarian* view of religion emerges....If one engages in particular kinds of devotional behaviors such as regular church attendance, meditation, or prayer, the effort will be rewarded with increased health. Just as medication alters moods, so a "*Prozac* God" becomes the dispenser of health when we engage in personal acts of piety. It is one thing to affirm that persons with shared religious beliefs and practices live longer or spend less on healthcare, but it is quite another matter to argue that *for those reasons* one should be religious or spiritual. (p. 46)

Unfortunately for this instrumental view of religion, not all religious convictions and practices have positive effects. A violation of a deeply held belief may appropriately (if we may say so) occasion depression; a prophet may pay with his or her life for taking a specific stance. For some contemporary Christians, practicing radical faith in public—taking up the cross of Jesus—does not pay off with good mental health. Historic religions have been concerned less with teaching their adherents to live long and more with how to live *faithfully*. Shuman and Meador (2003) point out that the Christian can "live hopefully with the certainty that the ultimate meaning of history—including each individual's personal history of sickness and health—is determined not by scientific or religious cause and effect but by the cross and resurrection of Christ" (p. 2).

EMBODYING FORGIVENESS IN THE CHURCH

The point that an overemphasis on the individual self distorts the message of Christianity was made persuasively in a figural essay, "Saint Paul and the Introspective Conscience of the West," by New Testament scholar and former dean of the Harvard Divinity School, Krister Stendahl. Stendahl (1976) argued that Paul's message of righteousness by faith had been widely misunderstood and misinterpreted by Christians who see it as concerned with freeing individuals from the effects of a guilty conscience. But, Stendahl pointed out that Paul's overriding purpose in promulgating the doctrine of righteousness by faith was to remove the barrier of hostility that the law (as it was understood) created between Jews and Gentiles and prevented them from becoming one, harmonious community. It is especially noteworthy for our current purposes that Stendahl's essay, which is widely known in the field of New Testament studies, was presented for the first time in English at an annual meeting of the American Psychological Association. While aspects of Stendahl's overall argument merit criticism, his argument that Paul's purpose in emphasizing justification by faith was communal before it was individual is a needed corrective to an individualistic interpretation that is predominant today.

While he is critical of what he calls "therapeutic forgiveness," L. Gregory Jones (1995) points to deficits in the church as being at least partly responsible for the popularity of the therapeutic approaches. Christian psychologist Henry Cloud (Cloud & Townsend, 2001) makes a related point when he cites deficiencies in the way churches frequently conceptualize the healing process. Cloud refers to his own experience as an example when he writes about the disillusionment he experienced when he took his first job in a Christian psychiatric hospital, just a few months following his seminary education. He was enthusiastic about putting his learning in theology and counseling into practice, but his enthusiasm diminished as he came to the realization that many of the people with whom he worked—who suffered from addictions, marital problems, parenting difficulties, emotional trials, and work struggles—did not seem to respond to the ordinary spiritual answers they had been taught. Cloud writes:

> I saw people who had walked with God for years and many who knew more about God's truth than I did. These people, lay people and pastors alike, had been very diligent about prayer, Bible study, and other spiritual disciplines. Nevertheless, they were hurting and for one reason or another had been unable to walk through their valley. (Cloud & Townsend, 2001, p. 17)

Many of the Christians with whom Cloud had worked, both in a hospital setting and in church congregations, had repeatedly tried without success to change through what Cloud calls "…the common evangelical mode of operation [which is] a good picture of the law at work. Give the standard, offer forgiveness for falling short, and then ask for a deeper commitment to do better by trying harder (Cloud & Townsend, 2001, p. 69). What he found did help people heal or recover in most cases was becoming part of a small, caring group of fellow sufferers or grace-filled believers where it was safe to be honest about their struggles and where they were loved and brought into a relationship that provided ongoing support and mutual accountability.

A central theme of Cloud and Townsend's analysis of what the Bible teaches about personal growth is that the approaches typically taught as biblical in many contemporary evangelical churches fail to adequately represent the role the Bible gives to human beings in the healing process. They note that most believers would be quick to acknowledge that God works through people; but when it comes to personal growth, they live as though relying on people is God's back-up plan, when the Bible pictures it as God's "Plan A" (2001, p. 119). One of the things Cloud and Townsend (2001) call for is a better appreciation for the body of Christ as a healing agent. "We wanted pastors to know," they wrote, "how a small group ministry that addresses people's emotional problems is an important application of the doctrine of the church, not just a good idea from secular humanism" (p. 120).

L. Gregory Jones (1995) also looks to the body of Christ (the church) as the environment in which forgiveness is to be learned and practiced:

> Learning to embody forgiveness involves our commitment to the cultivation of specific habits and practices of the Church. This learning, typically at the hands of exemplars who are more skilled than we are, is similar to the ways in which a person learns to become an excellent physician or an accomplished pianist. Indeed, just as Aristotle emphasized the importance of learning a "craft" for learning how to live, so there is a craft of forgiveness that Christians are called to learn from one another, and particularly from exemplars, as we seek to become holy people. (p. xii)

Forgiveness is a habit that is fostered and reinforced when people are part of a church community that practices forgiveness. Forgiveness is initiated and empowered by God, who works through individuals and communities. It is not surprising that many of the people who have participated in psychologically based programs to promote forgiveness report that they made their journey to forgiveness a matter of prayer. Rice illustrates the power of faith in practicing forgiveness in a comment about the story of Christ's healing of the paralytic, as recorded in Mark 2 when Jesus tells the man his sins are forgiven and his opponent responds by saying, "Who can forgive sins, but God alone?" As Rice (2000) notes,

> If forgiveness is really something that God does, then to the extent that we forgive others, we are participating in God's act and extending the forgiveness that God offers....It seems to me that this is a relief for an individual to not have to develop within himself/herself all the resources of charity and forbearance that enable that person to be forgiving. Instead, the person becomes the vehicle by which God's own forgiveness is offered to others. (p. 14)

The biblical worldview sees history moving toward a time when violence, deception, and injustice will come under the judgment of God who will destroy evil and bring victory over death and pain. The meaning of individual acts of forgiveness is increased when they are part of this wider vision. It is this knowledge of how things will turn out in the end which empowers us to give up our right and need to exact vengeance.

CONCLUSION

The capacity to forgive is an essential ingredient for the building and maintenance of human relationships. Forgiveness is a central concern of all of the world's major religions, and the attention forgiveness has received from social scientists only serves to further highlight and reinforce its importance (Rice, 2000; Rye & Pargament, 2000). This paper has been specifically concerned with how the theoretical and methodological framework developed by social science fits together with the historic role of forgiveness in Christian faith and practice. We have, at particular points, narrowed our focus further to consider areas of theological emphasis within the Christian tradition that have been important in the experience of Seventh-day Adventists. These areas include the degree of value Adventists have placed on the study of science (e.g., in the areas of medicine and health) and to the belief that nature is God's second book and that its study is an important source of revelation about divine truth. A further point is the importance Adventists have placed on understanding God's character of love and on the conviction that His laws are not arbitrary but are designed for the betterment and happiness of humankind. While these perspectives are by no means unique to Seventh-day Adventists, they are not universally taught or emphasized by Christians.

There is much to appreciate about psychology's attention to forgiveness. Because forgiveness is a fundamental principle for achieving peace and maintaining good relationships, it will provide blessings apart from whether those who practice it know or consciously rely upon God. At the same time, therapeutic forgiveness lacks important aspects of the biblical understanding of forgiveness. While it may support the biblical understanding, it cannot be a replacement for it. The Christian concept of forgiveness cannot be removed from its religious foundations and framed in psychological language without being diminished. This fact has been recognized by psychologists working in the field of forgiveness, as well as by theologians (Jones, 1995; McCullough & Worthington, 1999; Meek & McMinn, 1997; McMinn et al., 2008). The Christian concept of forgiveness is intricately connected with other fundamental components of Christian theology, including the doctrines of sin, redemption, the church, the person and work of Christ, and the final triumph of good taught in biblical eschatology. The theological framework of forgiveness is also linked to the moral and ethical language of religion which emphasizes qualities like virtue, truth, charity, and character. The most important element of the biblical view of forgiveness, however, is not its connection to these other biblical themes we have mentioned. It is the certainty that in practicing forgiveness we are connected to God Himself, whose very nature is to forgive.

We began this paper by asking if the road to forgiveness mapped out by social science is parallel and complementary to the road of religious faith, or if it takes its travelers on a different road or even to a different destination. We believe that the insights of social science can help people of faith understand and practice forgiveness. This may be especially true for Christians in western cultures like the United States who have been heavily influenced by a therapeutic worldview and mindset. At the same time, those who have been most influenced by that mindset may most need to be reminded of its shortcomings and of the significant dimensions that a Christian understanding of forgiveness can provide. These can facilitate the goals of intentional spiritual growth and may clear the heart that is resistant to faith of bitterness so that it can be receptive to the love of God. But these ideas cannot be a substitute for faith. The power of forgiveness is diminished when it is exclusively identified with a modern trend to see self-fulfillment as the ultimate goal of life.

REFERENCES

Baskin, T. W., & Enright, R. D. (2004). Intervention studies on forgiveness: A meta-analysis. *Journal of Counseling & Development, 82,* 79–90.

Berry, J. W., & Worthington, E. L. (2001). Forgiveness, relationship quality, stress while imagining relationship events, and physical and mental health. *Journal of Counseling Psychology, 48,* 447–455.

Burman, B., & Margolin, G. (1992). Analysis of the association between marital relationships and health problems: An interactional perspective. *Psychological Bulletin, 112,* 39–63.

Cloud, H., & Townsend, J. (2001). *How people grow: What the Bible reveals about personal growth.* Grand Rapids, MI: Zondervan.

Cole, R. (1988). *Harvard diary.* New York: Crossroads.

Danker, F. (Ed.). (2001). *A Greek-English lexicon of the New Testament and other early Christian literature,* 3rd ed. Based on Walter Bauer's *Griechisch-deutsches Worterbuch zu den Schriften des Neuen Testaments und der fruhchristlichen Literatur,* 6th ed., Eds. Kurt Aland and Barbara Aland, with Viktor Reichmann and on previous English editions by W. F. Arndt, F. W. Gingrich, and F. W. Danker. Chicago: University of Chicago Press.

DiBlasio, F. A. (1998). The use of decision-based forgiveness interventions within intergenerational family therapy. *Journal of Family Therapy, 20,* 77–94.

DiBlasio, F. A. (2000). Decision-based forgiveness treatment in cases of marital infidelity. *Psychotherapy, 57,* 149–158.

DiBlasio, F. A., & Benda, B. B. (2002). The effect of forgiveness treatment on self-esteem of spouses: Initial experimental results. *Marriage and Family: A Christian Journal, 5,* 511–523.

Dueck, A. (2006). Thick patients, thin therapy and a Prozac god, *Theology News and Notes.* Retrieved on July 8, 2008, from: http://documents.fuller.edu/news/pubs/ tnn/2006_ Winter/TNN_Winter_06_Dueck.asp

Enright, R. D., & Coyle, C. T. (1998). Researching the process model of forgiveness within psychological interventions. In E. L. Worthington, Jr. (Ed.), *Dimensions of forgiveness: Psychological research and theological perspectives* (pp. 139–161). Philadelphia: Templeton Foundation Press.

Enright, R. D., Eastin, D. L., Golden, S., Sarinopoulos, I., & Freedman (1992). Interpersonal forgiveness within the helping professions: An attempt to resolve differences of opinion. *Counseling and Values, 36,* 84–103.

Enright, R. D., & Fitzgibbons, R. P. (2000). *Helping clients forgive: An empirical guide for resolving anger and restoring hope.* Washington, D.C.: American Psychological Association.

Enright, R. D., & The Human Development Study Group (1991). Five points on the construct of forgiveness within psychotherapy. *Psychotherapy, 28,* 493–496.

Enright, R. D., & The Human Development Study Group (1996). Counseling within the forgiveness triad. *Counseling and Values, 40,* 107–126.

Enright, R. D., & Zell, R. L. (1989). Problems encountered when we forgive one another. *Journal of Psychology and Christianity, 8,* 52–60.

Farrow, T. F. D., Zeng, Y., Wilkinson, I., D., Spence, S. A., Deakin, J. F. W., Tarrier, N., et al. (2001). Investigating the functional anatomy of empathy and forgiveness. *Neuroreport, 12,* 2433–2438.

Freedman, S. R., & Enright, R. D. (1996). Forgiveness as an intervention goal with incest survivors. *Journal of Consulting and Clinical Psychology, 64,* 983–992.

Gorsuch, R. L., & Hao, J. Y. (1993). Forgiveness: An exploratory factor analysis and its relationship to religious variables. *Review of Religious Research, 34,* 333–347.

Guthrie, D. (1981). *New Testament theology.* Downers Grove, IL: InterVarsity.

Harris, A. H. S., Luskin, F., Norman, S. B., Standard, S., Bruning, J., Evans, S., & Thoresen, C. E. (2006). Effects of a group forgiveness intervention on forgiveness, perceived stress, and trait-anger. *Journal of Clinical Psychology, 62,* 715–733.

Hernandez, B., Vonderfecht, H., Smith, S., Cress, P., Davis, R., & Bigger, D. (2011, submitted for publication). Evaluation of a faith-based psychoeducational approach to forgiveness. *Journal of Spirituality and Religion in Social Work.*

Jones, L. G. (1995). *Embodying forgiveness: A theological analysis.* Grand Rapids, MI: Eerdmans.

Kiecol-Glaser, J. K., Kennedy, S., Malkoff, S., Fisher, L., Speicher, C. E., & Glaser, R. (1988). Marital discord and immunity in males. *Psychosomatic Medicine, 50,* 213–229.

Koenig, H. G., McCullough, M. E., & Larson, D. B. (2001). *Handbook of religion and health.* New York: Oxford University Press.

Lamberton, H. H. (2004). The resurgence of interest in spirituality and health, in S. Sorajjakool & H. Lamberton (Eds.), *Spirituality health & wholess* (pp. 1–14). Binghamton, NY: Haworth.

Lawker-Row, K. A., Karremans, J. C., Scott, C., Edlis-Matityahou, M., & Edwards, L. (2008). Forgiveness, physiological reactivity and health: The role of anger. *International Journal of Psychophysiology, 68,* 51–58.

Lawler, K. A., Younger, J. W., Piferi, R. L., Billington, E., Jobe, R., Edmondson, K., & Jones, W. H. (2003). A change of heart: Cardiovascular correlates of forgiveness in response to interpersonal conflict. *Journal of Behavioral Medicine, 26,* 373–393.

Lawler, K. A., Younger, J. W., Piferi, R. L., Jobe, R. L., Edmondson, K. A., & Jones, W. H. (2005). The unique effects of forgiveness on health: An exploration of pathways. *Journal of Behavioral Medicine, 28,* 157–167.

Loma Linda University (2007). *Catalogue of Loma Linda University, 2007–2008, 97(1).* Loma Linda, CA: Loma Linda University.

Lundahl, B. W., Taylor, M. J., Stevenson, R., & Roberts, K. D. (2008). Process-based forgiveness interventions: A meta-analytic review. *Research on Social Work Practice, 18,* 465–478.

Luskin, F. A. (2002). *Forgive for good: A proven description for health and happiness.* San Francisco: Harper.

Maltby, J., Macaskill, A., & Day, L. (2001). Failure to forgive self and others: A replication and extension of the relationship between forgiveness, personality, social desirability and general health. *Personality and Individual Differences, 30,* 881–885.

Mauger, P. A., Perry, J. E., Freeman, T., & Grove, D. C. (1992). The measurement of forgiveness: Preliminary research. *Journal of Psychology and Christianity, 11,* 170–180.

McCullough, M. E., Fincham, F. D., & Tsang, J. A. (2003). Forgiveness, forbearance, and time: The temporal unfolding of transgression-related interpersonal motivations. *Journal of Personality and Social Psychology, 84,* 540–557.

McCullough, M. E., Pargament, K. I., & Thoresen, C. E. (2000). The psychology of forgiveness: History, conceptual issues, and overview. In

M. E. McCullough, K. I. Pargamet, & C. E. Thoresen (Eds.), *Forgiveness: Theory, research, and practice* (pp. 1–14). New York: Guilford Press.

McCullough, M. E., Rachal, K. C., Sandage, S. J., Worthington, E. L. Jr., Brown, S. W., & Hight, T. L. (1998). Interpersonal forgiving in close relationships: II. *Journal of Personality and Social Psychology, 75,* 1586–1603.

McCullough, M. E., & Worthington, E. L. Jr. (1995). Promoting forgiveness: A comparison of two brief psychoeducational group interventions with a waiting-list control. *Counseling and Values, 40,* 55–68.

McCullough, M. E., & Worthington, E. L. Jr. (1999). Religion and the forgiving personality. *Journal of Personality, 67,* 1141–1164.

McCullough, M. E., Worthington, E. L., Jr., & Rachal, K. C. (1997). Interpersonal forgiving in close relationships. *Journal of Personality and Social Psychology, 73,* 321–336.

McMinn, M. R., Fervida, H., Louwerse, K. A., Pop, J. L, Thompson, R. D., Trihub, B. L., et al. (2008). Forgiveness and prayer. *Journal of Psychology and Christianity, 27,* 101–109.

Meek, K. R., & McMinn, M. R. (1997). Forgiveness: More than a therapeutic technique. *Journal of Psychology and Christianity, 16,* 51–61.

Miller, M. C. (2008, March). Learning how to say, "I'm sorry." *Harvard Mental Health Letter, 24(9),* 4–5.

Miller, T. Q., Smith, T. W., Turner, C. W., Guijarro, M. L., & Hallett, A. J. (1996). Metanalytic review of research on hostility and physical health. *Psychological Bulletin, 119,* 322–348.

Morales-Gudmundsson, L. E. (2007). *I forgive you but… We know we should. Why is it so hard?* Nampa, ID: Pacific Press.

Neblett, W. R. (1974). Forgiveness and ideals. *Mind, 83*(330), 269–275.

Pargament, K. I., McCullough, M. E., & Thoresen, C. E. (2000). The frontier of forgiveness: Seven directions for psychological study and practice. In M. E. McCullough, K. I. Pargament, & C. E. Thoresen (Eds.), *Forgiveness: Theory, research, and practice* (pp. 299–319). New York: Guilford Press.

Recine, A. G., Werner, J. S., & Recine, L. (2007). Concept analysis of forgiveness with a multi-cultural emphasis. *Journal of Advanced Nursing, 59,* 308–316.

Rice, R, in an unpublished presentation at the [G. A.] Keough lectures at Columbia Union College, Takoma Park, MD, on March 17, 2000.

Rice, R. (2000, Spring). "Forgiving and forgiven: A conversation" moderated by James Londis with Linda Gilbert, Kent Hansen, Richard Rice, and Bev Sedlacek. *Spectrum, 28*(2), 7–14.

Rye, M. S., & Pargament, K. I. (2002). Forgiveness and romantic relationships in college: Can it heal the wounded heart? *Journal of Clinical Psychology, 58,* 419–441.

Rye, M. S., Pargament, K. I., Ali, M. A., Beck, G. L., Dorff, E. N., & Hallisey, C., et al. (2000). Religious perspectives on forgiveness. In M. E. Mc-Cullough, K. I. Pargament, & C. E. Thoresen (Eds.), *Forgiveness: Theory, research, and practice* (pp. 17–40). New York: Guilford Press.

Rye, M. S., Pargament, K. I., Pan, W., Yingling, D. W., Shogren, K. A., & Masako, I. (2005). Can group interventions facilitate forgiveness of an ex-spouse? *Journal of Consulting and Clinical Psychology, 5,* 880–892.

Schmaling, K. B., & Sher, T. G. (1997). Physical health and relationships. In W. K. Halford & H. J. Markman (Eds.), *Clinical handbook of marriage and couples interventions* (pp. 323–345). New York: Wiley.

Seybold, K. S., Hill, P. C., Neumann, J. K., & Chi, D. S. (2001). Physiological and psychological correlates of forgiveness. *Journal of Psychology and Christianity, 20,* 250–259.

Shuman, J. J., & Meador, K. (2003). *Heal thyself: Spirituality, medicine, and the distortion of Christianity.* New York: Oxford University Press.

Smedes, L. B. (1984). *Forgive and forget: Healing the hurts we don't deserve.* New York: Harper & Row.

Smedes, L. B. (1998). Stations on the journey from forgiveness to hope. In E. L. Worthington, Jr. (Ed.), *Dimensions of forgiveness* (pp. 341–354). Philadelphia: Templeton Foundation Press.

Stendahl, K. (1976). *Paul among Jews and Gentiles.* Augsburg: Fortress Press.

Subkoviak, M. J., Enright, R. D., Wu, C. R., & Gassin, E. A. (1995). Measuring interpersonal forgiveness in late adolescence and middle adulthood. *Journal of Adolescence, 18,* 641–655.

Tangney, J., Fee, R., Reinsmith, C., Boone, A. L., & Lee, N. (1999, August). Assessing individual differences in the propensity to forgive. Paper presented at the annual meeting of the American Psychological Association. Boston.

Thomas, G. (2000, January). The forgiveness factor. *Christianity Today, 4,* 38–45.

Thompson, L. Y., Snyder, C. R., Hoffman, L., Michael, S. T., Rasmussen, H. N., Billings, L. S., Heinze, L., Neufeld, J. E., Shorey, H. S., & Roberts, D. J. (2005). Dispositional forgiveness of self, others, and situations. *Journal of Personality, 73,* 313–359.

Thorensen, C. E., Alex, H. S., & Luskin, F. Forgiveness and health: An unanswered question. (2000). In M. E. McCullough, K. I. Pargament, & C. E. Thorensen (Eds.), *Forgiveness: Theory, research, and practice.* New York: Guilford Press.

Toussaint, L. L., Williams, D. R., Musick, M. A., & Everson, S. A. (2001). Forgiveness and health: Age differences in a U.S. probability sample. *Journal of Adult Development, 8,* 249–257.

Tutu, D. (1998). Without forgiveness there is no future. In R. D. Enright & J. North (Eds.), *Exploring forgiveness* (pp. xiii–xiv). Madison: The University of Wisconsin Press.

Wade, N. G., & Worthington, E. L. Jr. (2002). In search of a common core: A content analysis of interventions to promote forgiveness. *Psychotherapy: Theory, Research, Practice, Training, 42,* 160–177.

White, E. G. (1900, 1928). *Thoughts from the mount of blessing.* Mountain View, CA: Pacific Press.

Witvliet, C. V., Ludwig, T. E., & Van der Laan, K. L. (2001). Granting forgiveness or harboring grudges. *Psychological Science, 121,* 117–123.

Witvliet, C. V. O., Phipps, K. A., Feldman, M. E., & Beckham, J. C. (2004). Posttraumatic mental and physical health correlates of forgiveness and religious coping in military veterans. *Journal of Traumatic Stress, 17,* 269–273.

Worthington, E. L. Jr. (1998). An empathy-humility-commitment model of forgiveness applied within family dyads. *Journal of Family Therapy, 20,* 59–76.

Worthington, E. L. Jr., & Wade, N. G. (1999). The psychology of unforgiveness and forgiveness and implications for clinical practice. *Journal of Social & Clinical Psychology, 18,* 385–418.

Worthington, E. L., Berry, J. W., & Parrott, L. III (2001). Unforgiveness, forgiveness, religion, and health. In T. G. Plante & A. C. Sherman (Eds.), *Faith and health: Psychological perspectives* (pp. 107–138). New York: Guilford Press.

Worthington, E. L. Jr., Mazzeo, S. E., & Canter, D. E. (2005). Forgiveness-promoting approach: Helping people REACH forgiveness through using a longer model that teaches reconciliation. In L. Sperry, E. P. Shafranke (Eds.), *Spiritually oriented psychotherapy* (pp. 235–256). Washington, D.C.: American Psychological Association.

Worthington, E. L. Jr., Sandage, S. J., & Berry, J. W. (2000). Group interventions to promote forgiveness: What researchers and clinicians ought to know. In M. E. McCullough, K. I. Pargament, & C. E. Thoresen (Eds.), *Forgiveness: theory, research, and practice* (pp. 228–253). New York: Guilford Press.

Worthington, E. L. Jr., & Scherer, M. (2004). Forgiveness is an emotion-focused coping strategy that can reduce health risks and promote health resilience: Theory, review, and hypotheses. *Psychology and Health, 19,* 385–405.

Worthington, E. L. Jr. (2005). More questions about forgiveness: Research agenda for 2005–2015. In E. L. Worthington Jr. (Ed.), *Handbook of forgiveness* (pp. 557–574). New York: Brunner-Routledge.
Worthington, E. L. Jr. (2006). *Forgiveness and reconciliation: Theory and application.* New York: Routledge/Taylor & Francis Group.
Wuthnow, R. (2000). How religious groups promote forgiveness: A national study. *Journal for the Scientific Study of Religion, 39,* 125–139.

APPENDIX A

THE PROCESS OF FORGIVING ANOTHER

UNITS	COGNITIVE, BEHAVIORAL, AND AFFECTIVE PHASES
	UNCOVERING PHASE
1.	Examination of psychological defenses
2.	Confrontation of anger; the point is to release, not harbor, the anger
3.	Admittance of shame, when this is appropriate
4.	Awareness of cathexis
5.	Awareness of cognitive rehearsal of the offense
6.	Insight that the injured party may be comparing oneself with the injurer
7.	Realization that oneself may be permanently and adversely changed by the injury
8.	Insight into a possibly altered "just world" view
	DECISION PHASE
9.	A change of heart/conversion/new insight that old resolution strategies are not working
10.	Willingness to consider forgiveness as an option
11.	Commitment to forgive the offender

UNITS	COGNITIVE, BEHAVIORAL, AND AFFECTIVE PHASES
	WORK PHASE
12.	Reframing, through role taking, who the wrongdoer is by viewing him or her in context
13.	Empathy and compassion toward the offender
14.	Acceptance/absorption of the pain
15.	Giving a moral gift to the offender
	DEEPENING PHASE
16.	Finding meaning for oneself and others in the suffering and in the forgiveness process
17.	Realization that oneself has needed others' forgiveness in the past
18.	Insight that one is not alone (universality, support)
19.	Realization that oneself may have a new purpose in life because of the injury
20.	Awareness of decreased negative affect and, perhaps, increased positive affect, if this begins to emerge, toward the injurer; awareness of internal, emotional release

Taken from: Enright, R. D., & Fitzgibbons, R. P. (2000). *Helping clients forgive: An empirical guide for resolving anger and restoring hope.* Washington, D.C.: American Psychological Association.

APPENDIX B

13-STEP FORGIVENESS TREATMENT FOR MARRIED COUPLES:

1. Discussion of definitions of forgiveness
2. Establish focus on each person having the opportunity to seek forgiveness for his or her wrongful actions
3. Introduction to the forgiveness treatment and the decision whether to participate
4. Statement of offense
5. Offender provides explanation
6. Questions and answers about the offense
7. Offended person gives emotional reactions
8. Offender shows empathy and remorse for the hurt he/she caused the other
9. Offender develops a plan to stop/prevent behavior
10. Offended shows empathy for the offender's hurt
11. Emphasis on choice and commitment involved in letting go
12. Formal request for forgiveness
13. Ceremonial act

Taken from: DiBlasio, F. A., & Benda, B. B. (2002). The effect of forgiveness treatment on self-esteem of spouses: Initial experimental results. *Marriage and Family: A Christian Journal, 5,* 511–523.

APPENDIX C

NINE STEPS TO FORGIVENESS:

1. Know exactly how you feel about what happened and be able to articulate what about the situation is not okay. Then, tell a trusted couple of people about your experience.
2. Make a commitment to yourself to do what you have to do to feel better. Forgiveness is for you and not for anyone else. No one else even has to know about your decision.
3. Understand your goal. Forgiveness does not necessarily mean reconciling with the person who upset you or condoning his or her action. What you are after is peace. Forgiveness can be defined as the peace and understanding that come from blaming less that which has hurt you, taking the experience less personally, and changing your grievance story.
4. Get the right perspective on what is happening. Recognize that your primary distress is coming from the hurt feelings, thoughts, and physical upset you are suffering now, not what offended you or hurt you two minutes—or ten years—ago.
5. At the moment you feel upset, practice the Positive Emotion Refocusing Technique (PERT) to soothe your body's flight or fight response.
6. Give up expecting things from other people, or your life, that they do not choose to give you. Recognize the unenforceable rules you have for your health or how you or other people must behave. Remind yourself that you can hope for health, love, friendship, and prosperity and work hard to get them. However, you will suffer if you demand that these things occur when you do not have the power to make them happen.
7. Put your energy into looking for another way to get your positive goals met than through the experience that has hurt you. In other words, find your positive intention. Instead of mentally replaying your hurt, seek out new ways to get what you want.

8. Remember that a life well lived is your best revenge. Instead of focusing on your wounded feelings, and thereby giving the offender power over you, learn to look for the love, beauty, and kindness around you.
9. Amend your grievance story to remind you of the heroic choice to forgive.

Taken from: Luskin, F. A. (2001). *Forgive for good: A proven description for health and happiness.* San Francisco: Harper, pp. 211–212.

A Personal Integration of God in Psychiatric Treatment: Alcoholics Anonymous as a Paradigm

David Mee-Lee and Bruce Anderson

In mental health and addiction treatment there is intense focus on the brain, neural pathways, and neurotransmitters and the role they play in how we think, feel, and behave. At the same time, there is also an increasing interest in the role of religion and spirituality in behavioral health and medical care (CASA Study, 2001; Fosarelli, 2008; Milstein, 2008; Shafranske, 2000; Sloan, Bagiella, & Powell, 1999). In addiction treatment in particular, a recent study developed a comprehensive annotated public-domain bibliography of the literature on spirituality and addictions to facilitate future research and scholarship. A search of all citations listed in the major databases covering a period from 1941 to 2004 discovered a total of 1,353 papers that met the search parameters (Geppert, Bogenschultz, & Miller, 2007). Some are exploring the integration of these two trends in a new discipline, neurotheology, that argues that the structure and function of the human brain predispose us to believe in God (Joseph, 2001; Muller, 2008).

Long before this interest in neurotheology, some psychoanalysts posited that there are many patients and therapists who already have concepts and experience with God and religion. Ana-Maria Rizzuto, an analyst, in her book *The Birth of the Living God*, draws on clinical experiences with patients as she examined the history of their belief or lack of belief in God. Rizzuto argues that everyone has a God representation, "private God." She sees an individual's God representation as primarily an object representation of father or mother (Rizzuto, 1979, pp. 44–45, 14).

If Rizzuto is correct, it behooves clinicians to have some conceptual framework about where God fits into psychiatric and addiction treatment. To leave God out of our theory and practice may well be akin to leaving patients' parents out of our theory and practice. The introduction of God into psychiatric and addiction treatment, however, involves the same sensitivity as well as evaluative and timing skills that accompany the subject of parents in therapy. Just as therapists respect the complexity of feelings, attitudes, and individual meaning of parental representations, the same sensitivity is needed concerning God.

In this paper we provide a perspective on how God might be integrated into psychiatric care based on our clinical experience working in addiction treatment programs. Alcoholics Anonymous (AA) is a self-help/mutual help group that was founded in 1935 as a fellowship of people whose primary purpose is to stay sober and help others also suffering from alcoholism. AA grew and blossomed out of the Oxford Group, which was "a non-denominational, theologically conservative, evangelically styled attempt to recapture the impetus and spirit of what its members understood to be primitive Christianity" (Kurtz, 1979). The Oxford Group's popularity peaked in the late 1920s and early 1930s.

Many addiction treatment programs in the United States, and to a lesser extent internationally, embrace the Twelve Steps of AA as guiding principles in helping substance-dependent patients. At first glance, the principles and practices in AA would appear to be the farthest from any approaches in mental health or health care in general. The success of AA in the treatment of alcoholism has been examined from a systems theory viewpoint by Bateson (1972) and a psychoanalytic one by Mack (1981, pp. 128–162). Over the past decade, Galanter (2008, 2007, 2006) and others (Fiorentine & Hillhouse, 2000; Glickman et al., 2006; Magura, 2007; Piderman et al., 2007) have written extensively on the useful role AA has played as an adjunct to evidence-based addiction treatment. There is even evidence developing for a specific role that spirituality plays in AA's effectiveness (Galanter, 2008). We will examine how AA treatment principles may be understood from a theological point of view and attempt to show how these principles may be applied to psychiatric treatment in general.

As Mack says: "Our understanding of the religious aspect of AA may have importance for the mental health field beyond the treatment of alcoholism" (Mack, 1981, p. 145). We suggest that the Twelve Steps of AA provide a helpful framework for understanding how God and spiritual principles of the Seventh-day Adventist (SDA) church might assist patients in psychiatric and addiction treatment. Firstly, we will provide an historical context for the SDA church's worldview and health mission, especially as it relates to alcoholism and chemical dependence.

THE SDA CHURCH AND ITS HEALTH AND TEMPERANCE MISSION

Early nineteenth-century America was a time and place of great religious diversity. Reform movements flourished in this period, including those devoted to the abolition of slavery, the reform of prisons, the education of the blind and the deaf, the humane treatment of the mentally ill, and the right of free public education (Schwartz & Greenleaf, 2000, pp. 15–16). Among other reform movements of the day, health issues also came to the fore because in many ways care of the sick was primitive and prescientific. Medicine relied on methods such as purgation, blistering, and bloodletting, and physicians knew little of the causes of disease or the importance of diet and sanitation. Surgery was dangerous and was done without benefit of anesthesia or asepsis, and mortality rates were very high. The ineffectiveness of medical care along with its attendant risks stimulated increasing interest in health reform, including the improvement of health habits and the use of natural healing methods.

Today concerns about health and temperance are considered an essential part of Adventist belief and practice. Early Adventist preachers opposed the use of alcohol, but the greatest concern of the Millerite preachers of the 1830s and 1840s was not advocating health reform but was preaching the imminent return of Christ to this world. However, even then temperance, especially abstinence from liquor, was an accepted virtue and use of hard liquor was proscribed. A somewhat different attitude was evident regarding "domestic wine" used for medicinal or sacramental purposes. John Harvey Kellogg remembered that his Adventist parents kept a keg of ale in the basement to be used for a "weak stomach" (Schwartz & Greenleaf, 2000, p. 102).

An example of early Adventist attitudes towards the use of alcohol is the experience of Joseph Bates. In 1821, Bates, then a sea captain and later an Adventist preacher, began to worry that he looked forward to his single glass of liquor each evening with greater anticipation than he did to his food. That year he forsook the liquor which he believed had become too important to him, and a year later he also abandoned the use of wine. In 1827 he organized one of the first temperance societies in the nation (Schwartz & Greenleaf, 2000, p. 101).

Ellen Gould White was an extraordinarily productive and influential person who had a prophetic role in the founding and growth of the Seventh-day Adventist church. On June 5, 1863, during family worship at the Hilliard home in Otsego, Michigan, she experienced a forty-five-minute vision related to temperance. This "health reform vision" dealt not only with abstinence from liquor but also with moderation in work and eating. It also included the importance of water as a medicine superior to the drugs then in common use and the benefits of a meatless diet (Schwartz & Greenleaf, 2000, p. 104). She later advocated abstinence not only from liquor but also from what she described as "the milder intoxicants," such as wine, beer, or cider (White, 1905).

Three years later, in 1866, the church put the ideas stemming from the Otsego vision into practice with the founding of the Western Health Reform Institute in Battle Creek, Michigan. On October 1, 1876, John Harvey Kellogg, a twenty-four-year-old physician and protégé of James and Ellen White, reluctantly agreed to become medical director of the Battle Creek institution (Schwartz & Greenleaf, 2000, p. 112). Kellogg was a remarkably gifted and energetic young physician, surgeon, and entrepreneur. Many health initiatives of the Adventist church resulted from the indefatigable energies of Dr. Kellogg and his collaboration with James and Ellen White. In addition to founding a medical school, the American Medical Missionary College (1895), Kellogg authored dozens of books and publicized health reform by attracting many celebrities and political figures to Battle Creek. In 1878 he co-founded the American Health and Temperance Association. He also invented ready-to-eat breakfast foods, peanut butter, and a variety of exercise machines. This diminutive and charismatic doctor was an innovator in the treatment of alcoholism and discovered the tranquilizing benefits of wet sheet packs in patients with delirium tremens as well as the soporific effects of neutral baths (Schwartz, 1970, pp. 49–50).

The American Health and Temperance Association ended after fifteen years, a casualty of Kellogg's conflicts with the Adventist church over theological and financial issues. In 1932 the American Health and Temperance Association was reactivated as the American Temperance Society (ATS) and promoted its programs within the Adventist church on a modest scale. A reorganization of the ATS in 1947 was accompanied by the launch of the International Temperance Association headed by the dynamic W. A. Scharffenberg. He established a National Committee for the Prevention of Alcoholism and Drug Dependency (NCPADD) and later persuaded King Saud of Saudi Arabia to be honorary chair of the International Commission for the Prevention of Alcoholism. These efforts culminated in a World Congress of the International Commission which was held in Kabul, Afghanistan, in 1972 (Schwartz & Greenleaf, 2000, p. 490).

Scharffenberg also led in Adventist efforts to combat tobacco smoking. The 1954 film *One in 20,000* linked smoking and lung cancer, and was seen by as many as 75 million viewers, including members of the British Parliament. Five more anti-tobacco films were produced by the Adventist church. These efforts contributed to concerns about smoking which led to the publication of *Smoking and Health*, the first Surgeon General report on health hazards of smoking (Schwartz & Greenleaf, 2000, p. 492).

The Five-Day Plan to Stop Smoking was developed by physician J. Wayne McFarland and Pastor Elman J. Folkenberg. Adopted by the Adventist church in 1962, this program featured a pastor-physician team which contributed greatly to its effectiveness. Over five consecutive evenings, attendees were presented with medical information, reasons to quit smoking, dietary recommendations, and a group process which fostered the goal of abstinence from tobacco. The American Cancer Society was a frequent collaborator in the United States, and overseas the program was often supported officially by various governments. By 1974 sixty Five-Day Plans per week were occurring in various parts of the world (Schwartz & Greenleaf, 2000, p. 493).

Another Temperance Department program was the 4 DK Plan (Four Dimensional Key) developed by E. H. J. Steed and Laurence Senseman, M.D. A four-evening presentation was directed to alcoholic individuals and their families, exploring the physical, mental, social, and spiritual dimensions of the patient, followed by eight counseling sessions designed to assist those dependent on alcohol. Modeled on the Five-Day Plan to Stop Smoking, this program also featured a minister-physician leadership team (Schwartz & Greenleaf, 2000, p. 491).

Additional Adventist Twelve-Step programs include the Regeneration program developed by pastor Hal Gates, affiliated with the General Conference Health and Temperance Department, and currently coordinated by Ray Nelson. The Institute for Prevention of Addictions has had a prominent role on the campus of Andrews University. Its role is to generate research, educate, and produce policies pertaining to prevention and treatment of addictions. Other Adventist affiliated addiction programs include The Bridge developed by Paul and Carol Cannon and the Drug Alternative Program developed by Cliff and Freddie Harris.

In recent years, Adventist efforts to treat persons suffering from alcoholism and other chemical dependencies have been largely carried out in chemical dependency units of general or psychiatric hospitals. Alcoholics Anonymous and related recovery organizations have furnished a spiritual and philosophical underpinning for the creation of these units. Although AA Twelve-Step principles are designed to appeal to anyone suffering from addiction, AA's emphasis on unflinching honesty and its dependence on an undefined Higher

Power fit the metaphors of Christianity and readily harmonize with the Adventist philosophy of wholism.

Pioneered by physician-ethicist Jack Provonsha, founder of the Loma Linda University Center for Christian Bioethics, wholism stresses the unity of mind and body and the interdependence of physical and spiritual well-being. It minimizes any distinction between factors which promote physical health and those which promote spiritual growth. The cultivation of physical health becomes a moral imperative providing a religious motive and sanction for health care and a temperate lifestyle (Bull & Lockhart, 2007, p. 313). It provides a rationale for lifestyle change and recovery programs that deal with addictions and related disorders. The philosophy of wholeness takes in the whole array of Adventist medical and educational institutions and programs. This belief in restoring the divine in humans by means of healing people physically, mentally, and spiritually is the most convincing philosophical and moral justification for the massive Adventist investment in medical and educational institutions worldwide.

ALCOHOLICS ANONYMOUS AS A FRAMEWORK FOR GOD IN PSYCHIATRIC CARE

The higher one's level of abstract thinking and education, the more likely one is to reject religious doctrine, the church, and God. Personal experience and observation suggests this; research and surveys confirm this (Hanser, 1981; Muffler, Langrod, & Larson, 1992; Musseu, Conger, & Kagan, 1979; Shafranske, 2000), and theorists from Freud to Kohlberg rationalize this (Freud, 1927; Hanser, 1981; Musseu, Conger, & Kagan, 1979).

Since clinicians are well-educated and cognitively developed, many reject God. Psychiatrists and psychologists have significantly lower rates of belief in God compared to the general population: 73% (psychiatrists) and 72% (psychologists) believe in God in contrast to 96% of the general public. Only 37% of psychiatrists responded affirmatively to the question, "If it were scientifically demonstrated that the use of a spiritual intervention (e.g., prayer) improved patient progress, would you perform that intervention?" (Shafranske, 2000). In addition, spiritual aspects are not fully embraced as part of conventional medical "culture" (Milstein, 2008).

Against this attitudinal backdrop, it is especially confounding to witness the success of Alcoholics Anonymous (AA) and the Twelve Steps—success which cuts across educational, socioeconomic, and cognitive levels. Fifty percent of the twelve guiding principles refer to a relationship with God or a power outside ourselves, and most refer to morality, right and wrong, spirituality, and prayer and meditation. The Twelve Steps are described as a "group of principles, spiritual in their nature, which if practiced as a way of life, can expel the obsession to drink and enable the sufferer to become happily and usefully whole" (AA Twelve Steps and Twelve Traditions, 1952, p. 15).

CASE VIGNETTE

Robert W. is a fifty-five-year-old self-employed businessman who had progressively grown weaker from over fifteen years of chronic alcoholism. Jaundiced, edematous, and deteriorated in every aspect of his personal and social life, he had no perception of himself as sick. He had never before agreed to, nor received, primary alcoholism treatment. The only treatment he had received twice was for the secondary complications of his alcoholism. Mr. W's eight children had been prepared for an intervention session in four preparatory sessions. After only one fifty-minute intervention session, Mr. W. agreed to, and followed through with, primary inpatient alcoholism treatment which lasted over one month. The successful outcome of that session was particularly confounding considering that these same eight children had, without success, been variously urging, pleading, demanding, and cajoling their father to obtain treatment for years. His wife had given up, bitterly, years before.

What was done in the four preparatory sessions was to review with Mr. W's children specific descriptions of events which related to their father's drinking (e.g., "Last Sunday, you were so drunk that I had to pick you up off the floor and unbutton your coat. I feel so hurt and embarrassed that I can never safely bring home any of my friends when you drink."). When each person had compiled a list of specific events, the intervention session was rehearsed to help the children present the data with an attitude of concern and non-judgment. They were, however, to be specific, detailed and factual "to demonstrate the legitimacy of the concern being expressed" (Johnson, 1980, p. 56). For example, "Dad, I'm so worried when you go out drinking. In October last year, the car was weaving all over the road and I feared for my life and yours. After you were arrested for driving while intoxicated in January, I got so concerned that I vowed not to ride with you whenever you have been drinking."

"The goal of the intervention is to have the alcoholic see and accept enough reality so that, however grudgingly, the need for help can be accepted" (Johnson, 1980, p. 57). In essence, the goal of the intervention session was to bring Mr. W. to his first glimpse of Step One: "We admitted we were powerless over alcohol—that our lives had become unmanageable." Whenever Mr. W. began to waver about his need for treatment, both before and after he was admitted for inpatient treatment, I (DML) would remind him of that one powerful intervention session. In genuine surprise, he had said then: "I didn't know my drinking was hurting them like that." We would review in detail again the events and incidents specifically, bringing him back to Step One. Much of the initial focus in addictions treatment revolves around Step One work, without which Mr. W. would not have experienced and accepted the need for help.

As Mr. W. began to recuperate, emphasis in treatment shifted to helping him see his inability to control his drinking by his own willpower. He had past failed attempts to stop or decrease his drinking, but did achieve a year of sobriety in AA. Such work began the ground work for Step Two: "Came to believe that a Power greater than ourselves could restore us to sanity."

By meaningful daily attendance at scheduled treatment groups and AA, Mr. W. began work on Step Three: "Made a decision to turn our will and our lives over to the care of God as we understood Him." AA emphasizes that Step Three is not mystical or esoteric, but very practical. Every man and woman who has joined AA and intends to stick has, without realizing it, made a beginning on Step Three. "Each of them has decided to turn his or her life over to the care, protection, and guidance of AA. Already a willingness has been achieved to cast out one's own will and one's own ideas about the alcohol problem in favor of those suggested by AA.…Now if this is not turning one's will and life over a new-found Providence, then what is it?" (AA Twelve Steps and Twelve Traditions, 1952, pp. 36–37).

THE TWELVE STEPS: A THEOLOGICAL VIEW

Thus far, we have referred to the first three steps. At this point, we examine these steps, as illustrated by Mr. W's treatment, from the viewpoint of theology. We examine AA principles from an Adventist theological perspective with whose theology and heritage we are most familiar. However, the spiritual and theological principles likely cut across all faiths. While the terms may vary, the essence remains the same.

STEP ONE

Step One says: "We admitted we were powerless over alcohol—that our lives had become unmanageable." Theologically, we see this powerlessness and unmanageability described thus: "No one has ever really followed God's paths or even truly wanted to. Everyone has turned away; all have gone wrong. No one anywhere has kept on doing what is right; no one" (Rom. 3:11–12, LB). "When I want to do good, I don't and when I try not to do wrong, I do it anyway. Now if I am doing what I don't want to, it is plain where the trouble is: sin still has me in its evil grasp (Rom. 7:19–20, LB).

Step One, then, may be viewed as bringing patients to an awareness of sin and their powerlessness over it. Since the word "sin" can have negative connotations, further explanation is warranted. Karl Menninger, in his book, *Whatever Became of Sin?,* explains what he means by sin. "I mean any kind of wrong doing that we used to call sin. I have in mind behavior that violates the moral code or the individual conscience or both; behavior which pains or harms or destroys my neighbor—or me, myself. You know what wrong doing is and if a better word than sin is available, use it" (Menninger, 1973, p. 17). Menninger further defines sin: "Sin is transgression of the law of God; disobedience of the divine will; moral failure. Sin is failure to realize in conduct and character the moral ideal, at least as fully as possible under existing circumstances; failure to do as one ought towards one's fellow man (Webster)" (Menninger, 1973, pp. 18–19).

Viewing Step One as an awareness of sin does not add depression and gloom, but hope for change. "The assumption that there is sin in it somewhere implies both a possibility and an obligation for intervention. Presumably something is possible which can be reparative, corrective, meliorative, and that something involves me and mercy. Hence sin is the only hopeful view.... When no one is responsible, no one is guilty, no moral questions are asked, when there is, in short, just nothing to do, we sink to despairing helplessness. We wait from day to day for improvement, expectantly, but not hopefully" (Menninger, 1973, p. 188).

Mr. W's family had sunk into despairing helplessness, waiting day to day for improvement, but becoming more and more hopeless and frustrated. Hope returned when they saw that there might be a different way to help their father see what he was doing to himself and others. Such awareness provided the possibility and obligation for intervention and a reparative, corrective recovery program. Mr. W's surprised and painful awareness of how his drinking had inflicted such harm and pain on his family led him to the first step, and acceptance of hopeful treatment. As AA summarizes it: "the admission of powerlessness is the first step in liberation" (AA Twelve Steps and Twelve Traditions, 1952, p. 5).

STEP TWO

Step Two says: "Came to believe that a Power greater than ourselves could restore us to sanity." If Step One can be understood theologically as bringing people to an awareness of sin, then Step Two may be viewed theologically as the solution to sin—salvation. Alcoholics, Seventh-day Adventists, and the Jews Paul was addressing in the book of Romans have great difficulty with Step Two. Alcoholics may admit they have a problem, but then keep trying to control their drinking by their own willpower. They share "the widely internalized belief that it is a shameful and embarrassing failure to admit that this function (controlling their drinking) is no longer within the governing capabilities of the self" (Mack, 1981, p. 134).

Seventh-day Adventists may admit they are sinners; but like the Jews Paul was addressing, they have too often kept trying to save themselves by emphasizing all kinds of good works. Some Seventh-day Adventists have found it a shameful and an embarrassing failure to admit that salvation (solving the sin problem) is no longer within the governing capabilities of the self. "Now do you see it? No one can ever be made right in God's sight by doing what the law commands. For the more we know of God's laws the clearer it becomes that we aren't obeying them. Now God says he will accept and acquit us if we trust Jesus Christ to take away our sins" (Rom. 3:20, 22, LB).

Step Two emphasizes that through humility and an open mind, alcoholics can be led to faith. Every AA meeting is an assurance that God will restore them to sanity if they rightly relate themselves to Him (AA Twelve Steps and Twelve Traditions, 1952, p. 34). For Mr. W, the first step was to present him with the reality of his actions in the intervention session (his "sins"). Step Two was to help him see he could not stop drinking by himself (accept "salvation").

STEP THREE

Step Three says: "Made a decision to turn our will and our lives over to the care of God as we understood Him." Having established

Step One (the problem) and Step Two (the solution), AA then begins to address the practical day-to-day application of the solution. "Like all the remaining steps, Step Three calls for affirmative action, for it is only by action that we can cut away the self-will which has always blocked the entry of God—or, if you like, a Higher Power in our lives. Faith, to be sure, is necessary, but faith alone can avail nothing. We can have faith, yet keep God out of our lives" (AA Twelve Steps and Twelve Traditions, 1952, p. 35).

Theologically, being aware of sin and the powerlessness to save ourselves (Step One) led us to faith in God for salvation (Step Two). Then begins the practical day-to-day application of salvation. The parallel to AA is clear in this quote: "What's the use of saying that you have faith and are Christians if you aren't proving it by helping others? Will *that* kind of faith save anyone?...It isn't enough just to have faith. Faith that doesn't show itself by good works is no faith at all—it is dead and useless" (James 2:14–17, LB).

In the treatment of people with alcoholism, the progression from Step One through to Step Three is a difficult one. It presents the paradox of personal powerlessness versus personal responsibility. This is a struggle not only for alcohol-dependent people, but also for health professionals, Seventh-day Adventists, and the Jews Paul was addressing in Romans.

The alcoholic understandably questions: "If you tell me my life is unmanageable and I'm powerless to do anything about it, then what am I supposed to do? I've got plenty of willpower to stop drinking. I think I can kick the habit this time." Likewise, clinicians express concerns that if patients are told that their life is unmanageable and they are powerless to do anything about it, then this will only foster passivity and irresponsibility. Patients may blame their substance use on their disease and think they do not have to take personal responsibility. Some Seventh-day Adventists and the Jews in Romans question, "Well then, if we are saved by faith [powerless], does this mean that we no longer need obey God's laws?" (responsibility) (Rom. 3:31, LB).

Step Three and the remainder of the Twelve Steps shed light on the process by which this paradox is resolved. AA does not say that sustained and personal responsibility is not required to stay sober. It talks more of the misdirection of that effort. "Our whole trouble has been the misuse of will power. We had tried to bombard problems with it instead of attempting to bring it into agreement with God's intention for us" (AA Twelve Steps and Twelve Traditions, 1952, p. 42). Mr. W. had tried all kinds of efforts to stop drinking on his own—gardening, burying himself in work, and taking disulfiram (Antabuse). He found himself defeated and frustrated because he had not first integrated Step One and Step Two before the affirmative action of Step Three.

Seventh-day Adventists have correctly emphasized the need for personal exertion and responsibility. However, like alcoholics, they have often misdirected that obedience. Bombarding our shortcomings with a barrage of "works," we have failed to see the destructive, personally erosive effects of skipping Steps One and Two—the "faith" part. The productive sequence of faith and works is this: "Only when we trust Jesus [faith] can we truly obey Him [works]" (Rom. 3:31, LB). Or as AA says: "It is when we try to make our will conform with God's that we begin to use it [our will power] rightly" (AA Twelve Steps and Twelve Traditions, 1952, p. 42).

It may be clear by now that what we are proposing is that Steps One and Two of AA may be conceptualized as justification by faith and Steps Three through Twelve as sanctification. Even a cursory reading of the remaining steps will demonstrate this, but another quote under Step Six will illustrate further: "If we ask, God will certainly forgive our derelictions. But in no case does He render us white as snow and keep us that way without our cooperation. That is something we are supposed to be willing to work towards ourselves. He asks only that we try as best we know how to make progress in the building of character. So Step Six—"were entirely ready to have God remove all these defects of character"—is AA's way of stating the best possible attitude one can take in order to make a beginning on this lifetime job

(AA Twelve Steps and Twelve Traditions, 1952, p. 66). Clinically, it is a fascinating experience to observe the change in patients' personal and interpersonal lives as they progress in AA through the steps.

Table 1. Twelve Steps of AA as a Paradigm for God in Psychiatric Care

TWELVE STEPS OF ALCOHOLICS ANONYMOUS	SEVENTH-DAY ADVENTIST THEOLOGICAL VIEW	GOD IN PSYCHIATRIC CARE (EXPLICITLY OR IMPLICITLY)
1. We admitted we were powerless over alcohol—that our lives had become unmanageable	Justification by faith—sinner cannot save self by justification through works	Awareness of repetitive ineffective thought and behavior patterns leads to self acceptance, the possibility for intervention, and hope for change
2. Came to believe that a Power greater than ourselves could restore us to sanity	Justification by faith—salvation: saved and accepted just the way we are (just as if we had not sinned)	Recognition that current coping knowledge and skills are not effective; faith that therapy can bring recovery and improve life
3. Made a decision to turn our will and lives over to the care of God *as we understood Him*	Sanctification—choosing God, giving our heart to God	Acceptance of need for help and committing to treatment process
4. Made a searching and fearless moral inventory of ourselves	Sanctification—faith with works	Responsibility to open, honest exploration in treatment

TWELVE STEPS OF ALCOHOLICS ANONYMOUS	SEVENTH-DAY ADVENTIST THEOLOGICAL VIEW	GOD IN PSYCHIATRIC CARE (EXPLICITLY OR IMPLICITLY)
5. Admitted to God, to ourselves, and to another human being the exact nature of our wrongs	Sanctification—confession, honesty	Ongoing opening up and acceptance of ineffective patterns
6. Were entirely ready to have God remove all these defects of character	Sanctification—transformation	Therapeutic alliance and readiness to change
7. Humbly asked Him to remove our shortcomings	Sanctification—forgiveness	Ongoing process to change ineffective patterns
8. Made a list of all persons we had harmed, and became willing to make amends to them all	Sanctification—reconciliation	Responsibility to repair past and present relationships
9. Made direct amends to such people wherever possible, except when to do so would injure them or others	Sanctification—reconciliation	Responsibility to improve relationships, including acceptance and relationship with "self"
10. Continued to take a personal inventory and, when we were wrong, promptly admitted it	Sanctification—daily devotions	Maintain personal awareness and responsibility for integrity

TWELVE STEPS OF ALCOHOLICS ANONYMOUS	SEVENTH-DAY ADVENTIST THEOLOGICAL VIEW	GOD IN PSYCHIATRIC CARE (EXPLICITLY OR IMPLICITLY)
11. Sought through prayer and meditation to improve our conscious contact with God *as we understood Him,* praying only for knowledge of His will for us and the power to carry that out	Sanctification—daily devotions	Maintain recovery strengths, resources, and supports to grow mentally, socially, and spiritually
12. Having had a spiritual awakening as the result of these Steps, we tried to carry this message to alcoholics and to practice these principles in all our affairs	Sanctification—witnessing; message to all the world	Service to others, community, and "giving back"; self help and mutual help recovery groups

GOD IN PSYCHIATRIC TREATMENT

Arguably, controversies in the SDA church concerning righteousness by faith have some of their psychological roots in confusion over the role of personal responsibility. Many of the debates and theoretical battles on psychiatric treatment also focus around the issue of personal responsibility. Debate over nature or nurture, genetics or psychodynamics, neurotransmitters or maladaptive behavior patterns, and systems theory or intrapsychic theories all have implications for the role of personal responsibility.

It is in the relationship of the Twelve-Step principles to personal responsibility that AA has much to teach Seventh-day Adventists and mental health professionals. AA teaches us about where God fits into treatment in the way it resolves the paradox of personal powerlessness versus personal responsibility. We will now propose some concepts about how God might fit into psychiatric treatment, using AA as a paradigm. It is our hope that God in psychiatric treatment will take on a broader and more sophisticated significance than the simplistic, often destructive interpretation of attributing mental illness to the workings of the devil. God in psychiatric treatment means much more than simply handing a patient some religious material, or even simply praying with a patient.

Just as it seems AA would have little to offer mental health treatment in general, it would seem even less likely that there would be any comparison between psychoanalysis and AA. Yet, here is a personal clinical vignette. It is a case I (DML) know very well: David ML is a thirty-two-year-old married psychiatrist who would begin the psychoanalytic hour feeling that he clearly had no contribution or responsibility in the latest argument with his wife. He was convinced that it was all her problem and what needed to happen was for her to understand him better or change her neurotic ways. The patient would settle back on the analyst's couch, waiting to have his astute evaluation of the impasse vindicated by the psychoanalyst.

It was always surprising to find myself walking out of that analytic session fully aware of what *I* was doing to my wife and *my* part in the impasse. Despite this painful fresh awareness of my "addiction" (pathological patterns leading to personal and interpersonal negative effects), I was strangely accepting of that and realized I was powerless to change it by power of positive thinking or any other psychic manipulation. Feeling hopeful and optimistic that things could improve, I would often pick up the phone, make amends for my "neurotic" ways, and resolve to make it better between us.

In that fifty minutes, my analyst had brought me through Steps One to Three and probably up to Step Ten. With a tone of concern and non-judgment, he would intervene in my harangue of projected blame with specific, piercing interpretations of my behavior and ideas. Designed to help me see reality (or at least his perception of it), the interpretations served to bring me to an awareness that, in a way, my life had become unmanageable and that I was "doing it again." At that point, feeling embarrassed and remorseful for having been obstinate and self-righteous, I would remind myself that I am who I am and that my feelings and the past could not be instantaneously changed by legislating an immediate improvement in my attitudes or patterns; indeed, I was powerless over my past and who I am (Step One—"We admitted we were powerless over alcohol—that our lives had become unmanageable").

The natural next step was then to turn to my analyst, believing he could "restore me to sanity" (Step Two—"Came to believe that a Power greater than ourselves could restore us to sanity"). I would determine to continue analysis believing that things could improve. The affirmative action of Step Three or the "works" I needed to do consisted of lying on the analyst's couch and rambling about all manner of free associations. From one view, this is a ridiculous, expensive obsession. From another, this is a restorative healing investment. But no matter what your view, it certainly parallels the kind of commitment Step Three in AA demands: "Made a decision to turn our will and our lives over to the care of God as we understood Him."

Although my analyst rarely told me specifically what to do, his searching interpretations of my behavior left no doubt as to what needed to change (Step Four—"Made a searching and fearless moral inventory of ourselves"). Accepting his interpretations and insights led me to make amends and pick up the phone (Step Nine—"Made direct amends to such people wherever possible, except when to do so would injure them or others").

Here is a second clinical vignette:

Mary P. is a 31-year-old married factory worker who has been in psychiatric treatment of one kind or another on and off for ten years. She has been variously diagnosed as schizophrenic, histrionic personality, borderline personality, and with a variety of other affective and anxiety disorders. About two years ago, she joined a charismatic group of the Catholic Church and found great comfort and support there. Now that the Bible and God are meaningful to her, we talked very directly about Scripture and God. She has already firmly assented to Steps One through Three. Indeed she at times would accuse me of a lack of faith when I express skepticism about the healing services she witnessed. In our sessions together, we frequently dealt with her anger and rage for not getting the understanding and support from her husband she feels she deserved. Much of my work with her was to help her take some responsibility in changing her situation with her husband.

On the surface of it, the session sounds like a Bible study as I quoted Ephesians 4:26 for her: "If you are angry, don't sin by nursing your grudge. Don't let the sun go down with you still angry—get over it quickly" (LB). We talked about how being angry is not a sin, but nursing the grudge is and she began to look at what she might do to get over it quickly such as talking to her husband and expressing her anger. Other times, we would talk about how her husband may not be able to change or how he may be hurt. Pointing out that she may need to understand and accept him, we would discuss examples where Jesus accepted people for who they were, even though He was hurt when His disciples couldn't stay awake just before His crucifixion or when Peter denied Him.

MAKING SENSE OF THE CLINICAL VIGNETTES

What do these two clinical vignettes illustrate about how God may fit into psychiatric treatment? In the first example, there was no mention made of God; in the second vignette, God and the Bible are referred to extensively. We will first discuss how God fits into psychiatric treatment even *without* direct reference to Him, and then discuss how He fits into psychiatric treatment *with* direct reference to Him.

In the first example, the therapist made the patient aware of his harmful, hurtful behavior; his powerlessness to change it alone; and how to take hopeful affirmative action to improve things—all without invoking God by either the patient or the therapist. Indeed, if the insight had been achieved by referring to sins, evil, and the injunction to follow God's ways of acceptance and love with my wife, I might have experienced my analyst as unempathic to my pain and unaccepting of who I am. This may well have resulted in more resentment and alienation both with him and my wife.

The sequence of Steps One, Two, and Three and so on was followed in that analytic session. Or, viewed theologically, justification was followed by sanctification all without direct reference to God. Bringing patients through the progression from Step One to Step Three firmly asserts God's presence and principles in psychiatric treatment even if God is not directly referred to.

The generalized point is this: If a patient has negative connotations or associations about God, it is likely to be more destructive to invoke God's name and methods directly in psychiatric treatment. This does not prevent God's presence in treatment. If the therapist believes in the positive benefits of the concepts of sin, powerlessness, personal responsibility, justification, sanctification, and God, that framework and knowledge can guide treatment. Such principles can help evaluate psychiatric theories and methodologies by raising questions: How does the theory deal with the issue of personal responsibility and personal powerlessness? How does the methodology provide hope? How is the process and sequence of behavior and attitude change explained? What is the role of the therapist in the school of thought?

Besides helping evaluate various schools of thought, the guiding principles also help in specific treatment with patients whether in outpatient psychotherapy or inpatient acute care. In listening to patients, such questions arise: What are they doing to harm themselves and others? How can I help them see that reality and accept that their lives are unmanageable? How can I help them see that they are powerless and give up their old ways of repetitively and counterproductively dealing with the problem? How can I help them to look beyond their own efforts and establish hope? Yet, how can I help them accept responsibility to change what they can and accept the things they cannot change? If I am successful in all of this, I believe God and His methods have been at work, even if I have never mentioned His name.

In the second vignette, God was referred to extensively. All of the "God treatment principles" naturally apply here also, but this example illustrates how it may be far more efficient and effective to talk about God and Scripture directly. If the patient has positive concepts of and meaningful experience with God, not using the language and experience of that patient robs her or him of valuable treatment interventions and interpretations. When Mary P. would find herself harboring resentment, it was productive and reassuring to her to remember her own acceptance by God. Noting the Bible's attitude about anger, she realized her need to resolve differences quickly. This facilitated positive action more effectively than simply telling her about anger without appeal to a higher authority. Her ability to identify with Jesus' hurt and acceptance of others facilitated her empathy and acceptance of her husband more effectively than hours of couples therapy focused on establishing empathic contact.

In the treatment of psychiatric disorders, the paradox of personal powerlessness versus personal responsibility is always an issue. For example, if you believe the schizophrenic has a brain disorder and is therefore powerless, he is still personally responsible for accepting treatment and taking medication. Or if you believe the "neurotic" is shaped by past experiences and is therefore powerless over her past, she is still responsible for whether she continues her self-defeating ways.

In the matter of personal responsibility, the sequencing of the Twelve Steps of AA from unmanageability to making amends and helping others resolves the paradox of powerlessness versus personal responsibility; of faith versus works; of God versus human effort—in short, how God might fit into psychiatric treatment.

DISCUSSION AND CONCLUSION

While it may be interesting to see parallels between AA, psychoanalysis, justification, and sanctification, why bother framing things in terms of sin, God, and religion? Why not just use the treatment principles without involving God and religion either with patients or in the thinking of the therapist? Part of the answer draws on the observation that psychoanalysis, long-term psychotherapy, addictions treatment, and Christianity contain more coherent, complementary, and consistent principles than might be apparent at first glance. Apparently incompatible approaches to behavior change enhance each other to produce a synthesis far more rewarding and integrated for both the patient and therapist. To examine how God might fit into psychiatric treatment promises to enhance treatment, not regress it.

Or, if Rizzuto is correct, God in psychiatric treatment is not a technique or "icing on the cake," but a major part of treatment to be addressed with the same respect and skill that accompanies work on other primary objects. John Mack provides a part of the answer to the question of involving God. "Throughout the history of civilization, human beings have had great difficulty managing their childish desires, their self-oriented drives and grandiose wishes, their narcissism, without reference to a greater power in the universe, someone or something they call God. From a historical perspective, no reference to moral values... that is not perceived as deriving from a force in the universe greater than man himself has generally proved powerful enough to prevail in the face of man's egoistic desires" (Mack, 1981, p. 144).

A final part of the answer comes from Bean and Zinberg who suggest that involving "higher authority" in treatment has implications for meaning to life. They also point out that much of AA's success has to do with "higher authority" and reliance on a moral code. "The reliance on a moral code is far too little understood by most of the 'self-help' organizations that have attempted to copy one or another aspect of AA" (Bean & Zinberg, 1981, p. 31). Does God fit into psychiatric treatment? The answer is a frustrating yes and no. "Yes," we propose, always, if you are talking about how to understand people's problems and how to help them change. But "no" if you are talking about the automatic or superficial invocation of God's name and direct references to Him in treatment with all patients. This process demands a sophisticated understanding of how God historically insinuated Himself into people's lives; a sensitive ability to listen and evaluate a patient's private God and spiritual orientation; and a skillful sense of the timing of references to God.

REFERENCES

AA Twelve Steps and Twelve Traditions (1952). New York: Harper and Brothers.

Alcoholics Anonymous World Services (1952). *Twelve steps and twelve traditions.* New York: Hazelden Publishing & Educational Services.

Bateson, G. (1972). The cybernetics of "self": A theory of alcoholism. In *steps to an ecology of mind* (pp. 309–337). New York: Ballentine Books.

Bean, M., & Zinberg, N. (Eds.) (1981). *Dynamic approaches to the understanding and treatment of alcoholism.* New York: The Free Press.

Bull, M., & Lockhart, K. (2007). *Seeking a sanctuary.* Bloomington, IN: Indiana University Press.

CASA Study (2001). So Help Me God: Substance Abuse, Religion and Spirituality. New York: The National Center on Addiction and Substance Abuse at Columbia University.

Fiorentine, R., & Hillhouse, M. P. (2000). Exploring the additive effects of drug misuse treatment and Twelve-Step involvement: Does Twelve-Step ideology matter? *Substance Use and Misuse, 35*, 367–397.

Fosarelli, P. (2008). Medicine, spirituality, and patient care. *Journal of the American Medical Association, 300*, 836–838.

Freud, S. (1927). The future of an illusion. In C. L. Rothgeb (Ed.) (1973). *Abstracts of the standard edition of the complete psychological works of Sigmund Freud* (p. 238). New York: Jason Aronson.

Galanter, M. (2006). Spirituality and addiction: A research and clinical perspective. *American Journal on Addictions,15*, 286–292.

Galanter, M. (2007). Spirituality and recovery in 12-step programs: An empirical model. *Journal of Substance Abuse Treatment, 33*, 265–272.

Galanter, M. (2008). The concept of spirituality in relation to addiction recovery and general psychiatry. *Recent Developments in Alcoholism, 18,* 125–140.

Galanter, M. (2008). Spirituality, evidence-based medicine, and alcoholics anonymous. *American Journal of Psychiatry, 165,* 1514–1517.

Galanter, M., Dermatis, H., Bunt, G., Williams, C., Trujillo, M., & Steinke, P. (2007). Assessment of spirituality and its relevance to addiction treatment. *Journal of Substance Abuse Treatment, 33,* 257–264.

Geppert, C., Bogenschutz, M. P., & Miller, W. R. (2007). Development of a bibliography on religion, spirituality and addictions. *Drug and Alcohol Review, 26,* 389–395.

Glickman, L., Galanter, M., Dermatis, H., & Dingle, S. (2006). Recovery and spiritual transformation among peer leaders of a modified methadone anonymous group. *Journal of Psychoactive Drugs, 38,* 531–533.

Hanser, J. (1981). Adolescents and religion. *Adolescence, 16*(62), 309–320.

Johnson, V. (1980). *I'll quit tomorrow.* San Francisco: Harper & Row.

Joseph, R. (2001). The limbic system and the soul: Evolution and the neuroanatomy of religious experience. *Zygon, 36,* 105–136.

Kurtz, E. (1979). *Not-God: A history of Alcoholics Anonymous.* Center City, MN: Hazelden.

Mack, J. E. (1981). Alcoholism, A.A., and the governance of the self. In M. H. Bean & N. E. Zinberg (Eds.), *Dynamic approaches to the understanding and treatment of alcoholism* (239–251). New York: The Free Press.

Magura, S. (2007). The relationship between substance user treatment and 12-step fellowships: Current knowledge and research questions. *Substance Use and Misuse, 42,* 343–360.

Menninger, K. (1973). *Whatever became of sin?* New York: Hawthorn Books, Inc.

Milstein, J. M. (2008). Introducing spirituality in medical care: Transition from hopelessness to wholeness. *Journal of the American Medical Association, 299,* 2440–2441.

Muffler, J., Langrod, J. G., & Larson, D. (1992). "There is a balm in Gilead": Religion and substance abuse treatment. In J. H. Lowinson, P. Ruiz, R. B. Millman, & J. G. Langrod (Eds.), *Substance abuse: A comprehensive textbook* (2nd ed., pp. 584–595). Baltimore, MD: Williams & Wilkins.

Muller, R. J. (2008). Neurotheology: Are we hardwired for God? *Psychiatric Times, 25*(6), 24–25.

Musseu, P. H., Conger, J. J., & Kagan, J. (1979). *Child development and personality* (5th ed.). New York: Harper and Row.

The National Center in Addiction and Substance Abuse at Columbia University. *CASA Study - So help me God: Substance abuse, religion and spirituality*. Retrieved July 11, 2008, from www.casacolumbia.org.

Piderman, K. M., Schneekloth, T. D., Pankratz, V. S., Maloney, S. D., & Altchuler, S. I. (2007). Spirituality in alcoholics during treatment. *American Journal of Addiction, 16*, 232–237.

Rizzuto, A. M. (1979). *The birth of the living God: A psychoanalytic study*. Chicago: The University of Chicago Press.

Schwartz, R. (1970). *John Harvey Kellogg*. Nashville, TN: Southern Publishing Association.

Schwartz, R., & Greenleaf, F. (2000). *Light bearers*. Nampa, ID: Pacific Press.

Shafranske, E. (2000). Religious involvement and professional practices of psychiatrists and other mental health professionals. *Psychiatric Annals, 30*, 525–532.

Sloan, H. P., Bagiella, E., & Powell, T. (1999). Religion, spirituality and medicine. *Lancet, 353*, 664–667.

White, E. G. (1905). *The ministry of healing*. Mountain View, CA: Pacific Press.

"For as he thinketh in his heart, so is he": Seventh-day Adventists with Maladaptive Beliefs and Compensatory Strategies in Psychotherapy

Kendal C. Boyd

Religious beliefs and behavior are strikingly associated with increased mental health. Religiosity is linked with increased optimism, hope, self-esteem, sense of meaning, and internal locus of control; lower levels of depression, substance abuse, and suicide also accompany religiosity. In particular, religion is intrinsically motivated and integrated widely into a person's life who is associated with well-being during times of stress (Pargament, 2002). If this type of religion were a medication, it would probably be commonly prescribed. However, misapplied religious ideas can have detrimental side effects. Clinicians (Cloud & Townsend, 1995) have pointed out several beliefs and coping behaviors in Christian contexts which are associated with increased psychopathology. It is this less frequent, but still important, phenomenon that is the focus here.

Before exploring this further, it is first of all important to delineate the type of religion I am referring to: misapplied or misinterpreted Seventh-day Adventist (SDA) belief, and what is generalizable to it. It has been observed that SDA clients by and large are similar to clients from evangelical, fundamental, Pentecostal, and Latter-day Saint backgrounds (Richards & Bergin, 2000). Clinical issues may involve perfectionism, authority issues, sexual inhibitions, and guilt. In a survey of Protestant classification studies through 1985, the denominations classified most similarly to SDA were Nazarene, Assembly of God, Church of Christ, Church of God, Pentecostal, Southern Baptist, and Missouri Synod Lutheran (Smith, 1990). It is probable that the general religious beliefs described in this paper would apply to any religious believer, but the more specific beliefs, behaviors, and examples would most easily generalize to the mentioned denominations.

As noted previously, religiosity is significantly related to positive mental health. More specific to Adventism, belief in the Sabbath and positive eschatological expectations have been related to good mental health (Davis, 2006), allowing one to consider the added benefit of being an SDA over and above being generically religious. However, again illustrating that religion can cut both ways, fearful or confused SDA eschatological attitudes were related to poor mental health in the same study. In 1952 a psychoanalyst presented a paper at a conference entitled "An example of psychopathology of religion: The Seventh-day Adventist denomination" (Yarnell, 1957). Despite the title, the author concluded that SDAs didn't have any unique psychopathology that set them apart from other Protestants who fell victim to the neurosis of religion (Freud's conceptualization), although she expressed concern about SDA belief in the soon second coming of Christ and the resulting destruction of the world. Recently, a much more helpful overview of the manner in which SDA theology interacts with psychotherapy has been compiled (Fayard, Harding, Murdoch, & Brunt, 2007).

Second, the psychotherapeutic orientation I will be working from is cognitive behavior therapy (CBT), which has the reputation of being the most empirically supported psychotherapy in the field. Although any of the mainstream psychotherapeutic orientations are appropriate for Christians, it has been argued that the emphasis on evaluating thoughts with reference to an objective standard, such as doctrine or Scripture, might make cognitive therapy a particularly intuitive therapeutic choice (McMinn, 1991).

Third, it is important to note that this paper is written for the clinical professional who is engaged in psychotherapy with SDAs or similar clients whose religious beliefs are interacting with marked psychopathology. Failure to keep this in mind could lead the reader to think that SDA church members are inherently psychopathological, which is false. In addition, for a majority of SDA clients, religion is not implicated in their psychopathology, and for most it will be a positive resource. Also, not all clients have marked psychopathology, such as in a counseling setting. In sum, this is a paper which targets both a limited audience and scope.

COGNITIVE BEHAVIOR THERAPY

Cognitive Behavior Therapy (CBT) asserts that pathology-prone individuals learn negative global core beliefs about themselves in childhood, such as "I'm unlovable" (Alford & Beck, 1997; Beck, 1995). These become the lenses through which the person views the world. As such an individual tries to cope with these painful core beliefs, intermediate beliefs develop, such as, "If I am continually entertaining people, then they will love me," or behavioral compensatory strategies such as trying to be the class clown in school. These give rise to disturbing situation-specific automatic thoughts, such as "Of course they won't want me to be part of their activity," or "I'm boring to these people." The thoughts come and go so quickly, and the beliefs and strategies are so deeply ingrained, that the person only recalls that he was sad after talking to some acquaintances.

Many beliefs can be categorized within the cognitive triad of the self, the environment, and the future (Beck, 1976). When a person has a negative view of the self, perceives the environment as unsafe, and is pessimistic about the future, the natural reaction is distress. However, if even one leg of this negative triad can be weakened, it makes a significant difference. For instance, if a student views herself as a poor scholar, the faculty as hostile, and the situation as never getting better, she will probably become depressed. Conversely, making a change on any one of these will result in hope: "It's not that I'm horrible at math; I just need to study more effectively," or "The faculty are trying to ensure high-quality graduates," or "It will get easier once I get through this statistics course." I propose that when working with Christian clients, it is important to include Christian beliefs within the traditional cognitive triad and to also consider their concept of God.

CBT holds that the roots of psychopathology are core beliefs, which are general and global in nature. These are ideas about the self that are learned from one's parents or other important authority figures. Some common core beliefs are listed in the outline below. At this macro level the psychopathology is not specific to SDAs. There is not an Adventist way that clients believe they are worthless, for example, and the core beliefs about God generalize to most religious believers.

MALADAPTIVE CORE BELIEFS

- ◊ Cognitive Triad
    - Self
        - Self-Worth
            - "I'm unlovable"
            - "I'm defective"
            - "I'm incompetent"
        - Self-Efficacy: *"I'm helpless"*
    - Environment
        - Other People: *"They're untrustworthy"*
        - The World: *"It's dangerous"*
    - Future: *"It's hopeless"*
- ◊ Concept of God
    - "God is Wrathful"
    - "God is Weak"
    - "God is Uncaring"

My focus here is on the intermediate layer of beliefs and compensatory strategies, and ones that evangelical or fundamentalist Christians, including SDAs, might adopt as they struggle with painful core beliefs, resulting in their entering into psychotherapy. Intermediate beliefs can be assumptions, with an if-then form akin to the example above such as, "If people are laughing at my jokes, then they are loving me." They can also be rules, such as "I must always be the center of attention," and attitudes like, "It would be horrible to be ignored." Intermediate beliefs are not quite as global as core beliefs, nor are they as situation-specific as automatic thoughts (Beck, 1995). Compensatory strategies are behavioral patterns that develop in response to the painful core belief. Another plausible compensatory strategy in the example could be the person becoming passive-aggressive, "joking" with acquaintances that they must hate him because "you never invite me to come with you anymore."

With the increasing specificity of intermediate beliefs, psychotherapists might begin to detect content that is more idiosyncratic to Adventism. Some may be core beliefs operationalized in a particular context such as those listed in the outline below. Here, too, they are still general enough that they are common to most other evangelical or fundamental Christians struggling with negative core beliefs.

MALADAPTIVE INTERMEDIATE BELIEFS AND COMPENSATORY STRATEGIES COMMON TO SDA/CHRISTIAN CLIENTS

- ◊ Cognitive Triad
    - Self
        - Self-Worth
            - *Love worthy*: "It's unhealthy to have my needs met"
            - *Good enough:* "Guilt and shame are good for me"
            - *Achievement*: "I must be perfect"; "Shoulds are good"
        - Self-Efficacy: Pleading for direct intercession; Passive religious deferral
    - Environment
        - People: "If I rely on God, I don't need people"; Interpersonal religious discontent
        - World: "Popular culture will contaminate me"
    - Future: "Everything is falling apart"; "I'll be in great danger then"
- ◊ Concept of God
    - Wrathful: Punishing God appraisal
    - Weak: Reappraisal of God's powers
    - Uncaring: Spiritual discontent

CBT emphasizes the therapist establishing a warm, collaborative relationship with the client (Beck, 1995), and this has been shown to have an important influence on CBT treatment outcome (Butler, Chapman, Forman, & Beck, 2006). In the spirit of collaboration, the therapist explores the maladaptive ideas with the client in order to come to a mutual opinion regarding their validity and utility. The tools in the session are the client's and therapist's pooled logic, experience, and intuition.

Although I will be examining religious maladaptive beliefs and compensatory strategies, it is worth noting again that in the broader context religion is a tremendous psychological resource. For instance, a loving and supportive God concept has been associated with positive coping efforts (Pargament, Koenig, & Perez, 2000). The religiosity discussed in these examples of psychopathology clearly occurs in a minority of cases.

CBT therapists use various techniques for clients who have maladaptive intermediate beliefs and compensatory strategies. A handful of these will be described below as I outline possible therapeutic interventions for the examples generated.

SELF

In CBT terms, the schema of the self can be further divided into self-efficacy and self-worth, with the latter further subdivided into beliefs about being worthy of love, being good enough, and being capable of achieving life goals (Beck, 1995).

SELF-WORTH: LOVE WORTHY

The core belief associated with the love worthiness is "I'm unlovable" and a typical nonreligious example was given above. One could imagine that Christians who are struggling with this core belief could listen to stories of Christ's humble, sacrificial suffering and develop an attitude such as "It's unhealthy to have my needs met" (Cloud & Townsend, 1995; Rayburn, 2000).

Note that the unhealthy core belief about love worthiness came first in this example, likely from early interactions with parents and other influential adult figures. However, chronic low self-worth can lead to the construction of mental filters that might prompt the individual to ignore the positive elements of a biblical character and only notice aspects that support a "martyr" worldview.

This illustrates an important point: Seventh-day Adventism in particular, and Christianity in general, are probably not normally the direct causes of clients' maladaptive beliefs or compensatory strategies. The most appropriate initial hypothesis is that their psychopathology that includes religious content is an interaction between a person's cognitive triad and concept of God that developed in the context of the quality of that person's early environment and attachment to caregivers. However, once developed, these religious maladaptive beliefs and compensatory strategies can then cause their own problems. This is particularly true because deeply held beliefs often feel so true that a person assumes they are beyond question (Beck, 1995). They become basic assumptions, the lenses through which a person views the world. For devout Christians, an unfortunate extension may be to feel that God must ordain their pathological beliefs and compensatory strategies.

One technique that CBT therapists use with clients expressing maladaptive beliefs is Socratic questioning (Beck & Weishaar, 2005). Beck (1995) defines this as the therapist asking leading questions designed to guide the client to a more valid belief. The therapist does not impose the new belief, but works collaboratively and gradually with the client to reconstruct the old belief into a new, more functional, and less rigid belief.

In the example in which the client expresses, "It's unhealthy to have my needs met; look at Jesus' silent suffering," the therapist has one obvious foothold in that Christians believe that Jesus was God on a particular mission. The client, being human, has a different nature and a different mission. This therapist might start the process by asking, "I wonder what some of the differences are between you and Jesus." As the client acknowledges that the purpose of Jesus' silent suffering was theological and may not have the most direct application to the client's circumstances, the therapist may decide that the next beneficial step is to nudge the client toward exploring her personal experience. One of the sources of this client's problematic attitude is that during her youth she watched her mother dutifully suffer in silence. The therapist then explores with the client what her recollections are of her mother in this role, and elicits the client's assessment of how effective this strategy was for her mother. The therapist can continue this line of thought as he evaluates the client's current relationships in which she is not being assertive.

SELF-WORTH: GOOD ENOUGH

The assumption that there is something inherently faulty with the self supports the core belief that one is defective. There is a fine line between the doctrine of original sin (Rice, 1985) and this core belief. Ideally this theology does not damage a Christian's self-concept because of a similar belief in the doctrines of justification, or overcoming sin through Christ, and sanctification, or being transformed by the Holy Spirit (Rice, 1985). The core belief "I'm defective" differs from the doctrine of original sin in that it is learned by experiencing the way one's parents or other powerful authority figures related to him or her.

As previously mentioned, sexual inhibitions can distress some SDA clients. When these lead to expectations of the self that are contradicted by experience, a typical response is the negative core belief of being defective. A clinical example would be a young woman in her third month of marriage who experiences guilt, shame, and confusion related to her sexual feelings. She cites the years she maintained her virginity before marriage and was initially eager to finally be able to participate in sexual relations with her husband. However, she grew up in a home with parents who talked about sex being "dirty," referred to women who liked sex as "tramps," and stated that Ellen White referred to sex as "animal propensities" and "carnal lust" (White, 1952,

p. 127). She therefore feels guilty by any enjoyment of sex, and has the attitude, "Guilt and shame are good for me." Although her husband is understanding and supportive, her conflicted feelings have led her to become inorgasmic which also makes her think that there is something wrong with her. She begins therapy with symptoms of depression.

After first confirming that the client's inorgasmia is not related to a medical condition, the therapist uses both psychoeducation and historical reframing (Beck, 1995). The therapist first points out that it is not uncommon for women who have subdued sexual impulses for a period of time to have some small degree of conflict when they are finally able to turn their feelings into action. The therapist further discusses various comments by Ellen White (1952) which suggest that marital sexual activity is pleasing to God, placing her parents' remarks in the context of the times in which these words were written.

In addition, the therapist asks the client to read a modern translation and commentary of the *Song of Songs* that brings out the strong feminine sexuality of the book (Falk, 2004), and they later process this biblical view of sexuality. Later, the attitudes of the client's parents are explored with an emphasis on what forces likely shaped their views of sexual expression, appropriate sexual attitudes of women, and any experiences that may have influenced their ideas. Finally, the therapist processes what sexual activity means about her: that she is a normal woman who desires a physically and emotionally intimate relationship with a man, which God has ordained as a good thing in marriage. This leads to discussion about how she can take back her sexuality and increase her enjoyment during sexual relations.

SELF-WORTH: ACHIEVEMENT

The negative core belief, "I'm incompetent," has a negative impact on self-worth. This basic self belief leads to several unfortunate assumptions, rules, attitudes, and compensatory strategies. In some people it can lead to publicly deriding themselves so as to lower everyone else's expectations of them. This is most likely true for individuals who also have issues with the third leg of the cognitive triad: self-efficacy or helplessness, discussed below. For those who do not feel helpless, the opposite reaction can have religious overtones: perfectionism.

Perfectionism is an attempt to cope with the painful core belief, "I'm incompetent." It often takes the form of the dueling assumptions: "If I try, prepare, practice, or study perfectly, then I'll be competent. If I don't, then I'll be incompetent." Perfectionism can be distinguished from a healthy drive for excellence in how the person deals with not meeting the top standard. A perfectionist will feel it is a grave defeat, but someone striving for excellence will be able to gain some satisfaction from the process of his or her effort (Hamachek, 1978).

A person struggling with perfectionism might develop the rule, "I must be perfect," along with the attitude, "Shoulds are good for me." Both of these beliefs have been observed clinically as common pitfalls for Christian clients (Cloud & Townsend, 1995). Christians sometimes attempt to deal with a sense of helplessness by developing a set of rigid rules for themselves with the assumption that God expects perfection (Propst, 1996). A familiar imperative is, "Be ye therefore perfect, even as your Father which is in heaven is perfect" (Matt. 5:48, ASV). Although this is best interpreted as a standard that only Christ can meet (France, 2007), this verse is an example of how a religious or theological message can become destructive when caught in someone's unique psychopathology.

Further complicating the picture is that perfectionists can achieve a degree of success and be rewarded for their pathology. For instance, a hard-working perfectionist manager can increase production, pleasing the boss. This will be particularly true in the short-term. However, longer-term problems will emerge for perfectionists. Their fear will drive them to achieve at the expense of relationships and their own well-being.

An example of perfectionism manifesting itself in a SDA client might be someone who has attempted to cope with his fear of being incompetent by adopting a strict behavioral code around his diet, enforcing this on his family to the point of having difficulty functioning because of the family conflict this has generated. Many SDAs have a commitment to healthy living (Rice, 1985) and many follow a vegetarian diet. The Apostle Paul's assertion that the body is the temple of the Holy Spirit supports this (1 Cor. 6:19). The clinical difference is that the fear of being incompetent is the primary motivation for perfectionists.

A CBT treatment technique that has demonstrated some effectiveness with clinical perfectionism is the use of behavioral experiments in which intermediate beliefs and compensatory strategies are recast as hypotheses and tested (Farmer & Chapman, 2008). In this case, the client's attempt to cope with the painful core belief regarding self competency has generated the assumption, "If I can be a perfect Adventist, then I might not be incompetent," and its inverse, "If I am *not* a perfect Adventist, then I probably am incompetent." For this client, these assumptions have also generated this self talk: "If I can be perfect in my diet, then I might not be incompetent." Also in this case there is the client's rule: "A perfect Adventist father must make his family keep strict dietary standards," which is where the problem in our example superficially appears to be.

After a family session in which the father's assumption of diet determining competence comes to light, the therapist asks the father if he will participate in several individual sessions. Part of the client's homework is to have a family meeting, asking the members each what they would like to include in the family dietary practices if they could, such as keeping some things and changing others. Eating dessert, chips, candy, and dairy products appear on the list. In the next session, the therapist asks the client to arrange these on a dietary standards hierarchy, including a dimension of frequency such as eating dessert once a week and eating dessert three times a day. After constructing this lengthy hierarchy, the therapist asks the client to start testing the once-a-week items, such as allowing the family to eat a dessert of the childrens' choosing, and then writing about how this affected his perception of competency. After two weeks the client's assumption morphs into a less rigid assumption: "If I'm pretty good with my diet, then I'm still OK." The eventual goal is for the client to take the focus off diet as a basis for a sense of self-competence, discover where those early messages of incompetence came from, and develop more appropriate criteria for judging his competence.

SELF-EFFICACY

The core belief of people struggling with their self-efficacy is "I'm helpless." Coping behaviors of Christians dealing with helplessness often include religion. Pleading for direct intercession, where a person asks God for a miracle, has been associated with very poor psychological and spiritual outcomes. Likewise, although not associated with quite as much pathology, passive religious deferral is a poor compensatory strategy (Pargament, et al., 1998).

An example here could be a Christian who is having difficulty with his spouse. There is a range of adaptive active strategies such a husband can take. Unfortunately, this Christian husband was raised in an emotionally abusive environment where he could not escape or effectively manage these negative events. He consequently developed a basic fatalistic sense of helplessness and assumed that the main control for his happiness lay outside of himself. Being religious, he resorted to passive religious deferral thinking, "My marriage is in God's hands," and prayed for a miracle, asking God to "change my wife's heart."

The therapist asks what it means to the client that his marriage is in God's hands, and eventually his helpless attitude of "There is nothing I can do to improve my marriage" is uncovered. While the therapist admits that this might be true, she uses Socratic questioning, asking if she and the client can really establish that this is true without testing it multiple times. She encourages him to try some behavioral experiments. They then brainstorm for several good tests of this hypothesis and plan for the client to ask his wife if she would be willing to come to the couple's therapy. This will allow him to work on his communication skills, talk to his wife about his experience, and work on his listening skills while effectively hearing her experience.

ENVIRONMENT

The second leg of Beck's cognitive triad is that of the personal environment. This environment includes other people and all the milieus within which one operates, such as home, school, work, church, and shopping. The distressing core beliefs here involve themes of danger.

OTHER PEOPLE

When clients are concerned in therapy about other people, it is often accompanied by the core belief, "They're untrustworthy." Growing up in an unsafe environment can form this chronic mindset. Certainly there are dangerous environments filled with treacherous, powerful people, but in most circumstances it is maladaptive to constantly view the environment in this manner. While physical danger is more salient, emotional danger is probably more widespread. A person growing up under emotional attack or manipulation by their caregivers or other powerful adults will likely become suspicious of other individuals in authority, including clergy. Here, religion can interact with such a Christian's compensatory strategy in the form of suspicion toward religious leaders or their church community. Individuals who are confused or dissatisfied with clergy or other church members experience what Pargament terms "interpersonal religious discontent," which is associated with a poor outcome (Pargament, et al., 1998).

An example is a Christian who was previously active but is now depressed and is reluctant to go to church because of perceived slights by the ministers or church members. The therapist in this case rightly sees church attendance as a potentially rich resource for this client because, as formerly mentioned, religious practices, including church attendance, are associated with lower depression. As the therapist and client explore this, they uncover an attitude—"They [church members] are spiteful and manipulative"—and an assumption: "If anyone is hypocritical, then this church is awful."

The therapist decides to use the cognitive continuum technique in which the client is encouraged to conceptualize people and situations more accurately on a range of good to bad, rather than in two polar opposite categories of excellent and awful (James & Barton, 2004). He asks the client to imagine the most spiteful, manipulative person she can imagine. The middle-aged client concludes this would be Leona Helmsley, dubbed the "Queen of Mean" by the media during the 1980s for screaming profanities at her New York hotel workers while firing them over insignificant offenses. The therapist tells the client, "OK, let Leona be a 100 on the spiteful and manipulative scale. Now, who would be a 0, or have the most profound absence of spite you can possibly imagine?" The client suggests a public television children's show character from her formative years, Mister Rogers, a famously warm and friendly man. The therapist continues: "So now, on this scale anchored by Mister Rogers at a 0 and the Queen of Mean at 100, where would these people at church fall?" After some deliberation, the client replies, "Well, I guess about a 70." This then allows the client to admit that since they aren't all bad that they probably have some good; she may later be more open to trying the church again.

Another possibility for Christian clients who have a core belief that others are untrustworthy is the development of the assumption "If I rely on God, I don't need people" (Cloud & Townsend, 1995). As with most assumptions, this one lends itself to a behavioral experiment. The client is asked to test whether it is more effective to deal with her loneliness by solitary religious study or by interacting with groups of people, including church activities. The odds are that increased social interaction will prove to be more rewarding than the isolation.

THE WORLD

As previously mentioned, one's environment can be dangerous but often is not. However, Christians have developed a suspicion of the world, although they are called to preach the gospel to it. This has developed into what is often called the social doctrine of being in, but not of, the world (Fitz-Gibbon, 2000).

The development of the core belief that the world is dangerous is probably rooted in the experiences of both the client and her parents, and the avoidance of the aspects of the world then served a functional purpose in some way. In conservative Christian environments, this is often expressed in the attitude that "Popular culture will contaminate me." The Christian then seeks to maintain a lifestyle that is consistent with her concept of what God's ideal is. This dynamic is unlikely to cause clinical symptoms until it occurs in the context of a relationship with someone who does not share this belief system.

An example is the relationship between a conservative SDA mother and her strong-willed teenage daughter, who is oppositional and defiant. The specific issues concern music the young woman wants to listen to and the clothes and make-up she wants to wear, all of which are in the mainstream of current popular culture. As with the prior example of the perfectionistic father, the cognitive continuum technique is useful here, particularly the use of Socratic questioning. First, the therapist asks the mother if she thinks that all popular culture is contaminating, encouraging her to consider previously believed problem issues such as makeup foundation, pantsuits, and John Denver. When he then asks the daughter to offer some aspects of current popular culture that she grants are problematic for teens, she names the singer Pink, fishnet stockings, and nipple piercings. This allows the therapist to define a new attitude in which the mother and daughter can have some common ground: "Some popular culture is OK, some is contaminating." Now the stage is set for a cognitive continuum homework assignment where mother and daughter review current fashion, music, and makeup, with each constructing a continuum using *safe* and *dangerous* as the poles. They bring their continua to the next session, which is spent on negotiating compromises in the effort to construct a common continuum. As the daughter sees that her mother is trying to understand her and compromise, she becomes more willing to accept her mother's wisdom and larger frame of reference.

FUTURE

The last aspect of the cognitive triad is the person's schema regarding the future. The negative core belief here is, "It's hopeless." One of the important beliefs that leads to depression is the one that there is no hope—the negative situation will never change. As with the previous problematic core beliefs, this too likely has its roots in childhood. Hopelessness is related to dispositional pessimism (O'Connor & Cassidy, 2007). Pessimism about the future could be learned though personal experience or by observing the attitude and experience of the parents.

Although Christians also are subject to depression and hopelessness, the literature has not noted anything idiosyncratic about the manner in which Christians despair of their future. It is possible, however, that religious groups, such as Seventh-day Adventists who have an eschatology involving personal stress and fearful world-wide events (Rice, 1985), might have members who become fixated on this theology as an aspect of their depression or anxiety (Yarnell, 1957). Some initial findings in the *Adventist Health Study–2* suggested that respondents who feared God's return had poorer mental health and decreased life satisfaction (Walters & Lee, 2008).

Such an SDA client might espouse the attitude, "I'll be in great danger at that time," which could contribute to an already existing anxiety problem. In this case the client professes to have rational knowledge that he is safe theologically, claiming to know about the biblical promises that the Holy Spirit will be with those who are persecuted in God's name, but he has excessive fear about the Time of Trouble. The therapist uses the biblical example of Peter, who initially was fearful in the face of persecution but later became courageous as the Holy Spirit worked through him. This draws on the CBT technique of *Acting "As If,"* where the client imagines what a person who had a more adaptive belief would act like and then tries to imitate it (Beck, 1995). The client then tells himself, "The Holy Spirit will be with me" and imagines himself as Peter confidently speaking to the Sanhedrin.

Another possible attitude could be "The world is falling apart—why bother?" and the client decides not to pursue a meaningful career. For the therapist who is knowledgeable about Adventist history and the Great Disappointment of 1844, some Socratic questioning will probably help this client admit that it is poor judgment to cut occupational corners because of presuming that the second coming is very near.

CONCEPT OF GOD

People's beliefs about themselves, their environment, and the future are critical. For a Christian, however, this set of psychological beliefs and compensatory strategies would be incomplete without addressing a person's concept of God which includes the characteristics a person ascribes to God. Negative concepts of God correlate with an insecure attachment style and psychological distress. Early psychotherapists such as Freud, Jung, and Adler all gave marked consideration to their clients' God concept (Hall, 1971; Palmer, 1997). Since then, empirical psychologists have set about defining this concept's dimensions (Gorsuch, 1968; Wong-McDonald & Gorsuch, 2004).

Gorsuch developed an empirically derived set of dimensions regarding people's beliefs about the character of God (1968). Although he called them factors, let us make a clinical extension of the factor structure. There were two main positive core beliefs about God: "God is a companion" and "God is benevolent." Two core beliefs were neutral: "God is all" and "God is potently passive." The negative core belief was "God is wrathful."

To this latter core belief, one can add a couple of more after an examination of the religious coping strategies outlined by Pargament: "God is uncaring" and "God is weak." These three negative conceptualizations of God were all associated with poor physical health, poor mental health, and current distress.

WRATHFUL GOD

A wrathful concept of God appears to be at the root of Pargament's religious coping strategy of a punishing God appraisal, which is seeing a stressor as God's punishment for sins (Pargament, et al., 2000). This compensatory strategy of fear has been linked with a negative outcome, both psychologically and spiritually. A Christian client—who has experienced marked suffering, believes in an all-powerful God, and struggles with some of the previously mentioned painful self-worth core beliefs—could have a sense that it is God's will that she be punished. One example would be a Christian woman who was sexually abused as a girl and then married an abusive husband. Early on she developed the core beliefs "I'm unlovable" and "I'm helpless." These beliefs are then reinforced through the treatment she receives from her spouse. When a tragedy befalls her child, her beliefs about herself make it easy for her to assume that this is a punishment from God because of her sins.

As she and her therapist work together, the assumption "If bad things happen to me, then I deserved it" comes to light, as well as the rule "I should not try to escape from my abusive husband" and the attitude "I will always be punished." One CBT technique the therapist uses is to have the client imagine what her life would be like if she was not in the abusive relationship and not being punished (Beck, 1995). Another is what McMinn (1991) calls the "Contemplative Worship technique." The therapist may use guided imagery (Singer, 2006) to lead the client to view God as more benevolent and companionable. In this case, the imagery deals with God physically embracing the client, expressing understanding and support, and encouraging her to listen to God's Holy Spirit in guiding her actions and decisions.

WEAK GOD

An image of God as being unable to bring about any meaningful change for believers is unsatisfying to many. For clients who have believed in a powerful God but whose recent experiences lead them to question this and downgrade God's omnipotence, this view is particularly distressing. The religious compensatory strategy of reappraising God's powers is rooted in the core belief of a weak God. This hopeless reappraisal is associated with poor outcomes, both physical and emotional.

A clinical example is a woman who comes to therapy because her husband is having an affair. She is dealing with both the loss of her dream of a happy, permanent relationship and the decision regarding whether to try to save the relationship. In the course of this situation she prays regularly that God will change her husband's heart so that he will love her again. Instead of the outcome she is looking for, however, he continues his affair, and she becomes convinced that God is powerless to help her when she really needs it.

As the therapist processes her loss, he also encourages her to express her beliefs about God's ability to work in the world and bring about events that otherwise would not have occurred. He introduces the concept of God being self-constrained to being able to only actualize one of the potentials in an entity's prior state (Murphy, 1997), in this case her husband being the entity who, through his choices and developmental vulnerabilities, has probably not left God with any option of restoring the marriage relationship to health. However, the therapist encourages her to have faith that God can actualize her positive potential to survive her loss and reconstruct a fulfilling life.

UNCARING GOD

Spiritual discontent, or a compensatory strategy of viewing God with confusion or dissatisfaction, has also been associated with poor psychological and spiritual outcomes (Pargament, et al., 1990). An example is a person who developed with a relatively positive view of himself and of God, but later in life underwent a series of difficult interpersonal challenges. This became difficult for him to reconcile with his view of God as loving, and he reappraises his core belief about God to the more angry "God is uncaring."

After spending a couple of sessions listening and empathizing with the client, the therapist gives the client the homework of reading about Christ's passion in the Gospel of Mark, paying particular attention to the suffering of Christ in Mark 14:36 and 15:34. In *The Message* translation (Peterson, 2002) the former text reads, "Papa, Father, you can—can't you?—get me out of this. Take this cup away from me. But please, not what I want—what do you want?" In 15:34 Jesus says, "My God, my God, why have you abandoned me?" In the next session she uses a form of role play (Beck, 1995) where she asks the client to play the role of God while she plays the role of the client. One reason for this arrangement initially is so that the client does not cast her in a judgmental role; another is so she can further demonstrate her understanding of his situation, and a third is to encourage the client to begin to take a wider perspective. For the first half of the session she alternately uses her acting skill to vividly represent him in his misery for a few moments, and then she debriefs with him. During the second half of the session they switch roles, the therapist emphasizing God's empathy with his suffering and drawing the parallel of how God suffered along with Christ, who also felt abandoned by God in that awful circumstance. After this they debrief, with the therapist and the client discussing how God feels and identifies with the client's pain and disappointment.

CONCLUSION

Christianity in general and Seventh-day Adventism in particular are good for the soul. However, beliefs and strategies that have to do with Christianity and Adventism can interact with a client's personal issues and form a psychopathology that can present special challenges to psychotherapists. One reason for this is that the clients assume their belief or strategy is particularly valid because it has the apparent markings of religion. It is important for psychotherapists to keep a temporal sense of etiology when treating these psychopathologies. When these are driven by core beliefs of being unlovable, incompetent, and helpless, the most probable causes are negative messages the clients received as children from influential caregivers. Whether these caregivers were responding to invalid messages they received from their religion is certainly relevant.

Cases in which the psychopathology appears to be more related to the clients' concept of God may also be somewhat related to their parents. Early parental figures have been identified as important in the formation of a person's concept of God (Dickie, Ajega, Kobylak, & Nixon, 2006). In spite of this, it may be more directly helpful for therapists to start treatment by exploring a client's view of God.

A limitation to my interactional conceptualization of core beliefs and religion is that there are also occurrences of religious beliefs directly causing psychopathology. This is particularly true when the people who presented that religion to the client have their own marked psychopathology.

Much of what Christians do involves their core beliefs about themselves, the world, the future, and God. From these spring up many of the attitudes, rules, assumptions, and compensatory behavioral strategies that psychotherapists treat. As SDA clients and psychotherapists grapple with these issues, they can be assured that the God of healing will assist in the process.

REFERENCES

Alford, B. A., & Beck, A. T. (1997). *The integrative power of cognitive therapy.* New York: Guilford Press.

Beck, A. T. (1976). *Cognitive therapy and the emotional disorders.* New York: New American Library.

Beck, A. T., & Weishaar, M. (2005). Cognitive therapy. In R. J. Corsini & D. Wedding (Eds.), *Current psychotherapies* (pp. 238–268). Belmont, CA: Thomson Brooks/Cole Publishing Co.

Beck, J. S. (1995). *Cognitive therapy: Basics and beyond.* New York: Guilford Press.

Butler, A. C., Chapman, J. E., Forman, E. M., & Beck, A. T. (2006). The empirical status of cognitive-behavioral therapy: A review of meta-analyses. *Clinical Psychology Review, 26*, 17–31.

Cloud, H., & Townsend, J. S. (1995). *12 "Christian" beliefs that can drive you crazy: Relief from false assumptions.* Grand Rapids, MI: Zondervan.

Davis, L. E. (2006). Religious belief, coping, and mental health in Seventh-day Adventists. *Dissertation Abstracts International: Section B: The Sciences and Engineering, 67,* 2276.

Dickie, J. R., Ajega, L. V., Kobylak, J. R., & Nixon, K. M. (2006). Mother, father, and self: Sources of young adults' God concepts. *Journal for the Scientific Study of Religion, 45,* 57–71.

Eurelings-Bontekoe, E. H. M., Van Steeg, J. H., & Verschuur, M. J. (2005). The association between personality, attachment, psychological distress, church denomination and the God concept among a non-clinical sample. *Mental Health, Religion & Culture, 8,* 141–154.

Falk, M. (2004). *The Song of Songs: Love lyrics from the Bible.* Lebanon, NH: Brandeis.

Farmer, R. F., & Chapman, A. L. (2008). *Behavioral interventions in cognitive behavior therapy: Practical guidance for putting theory into action* (1st ed.). Washington, D.C.: American Psychological Association.

Fayard, C., Harding, G. I. V., Murdoch, W., & Brunt, J. (2007). Clinical implications for psychotherapy from the Seventh-day Adventist tradition. *Journal of Psychology and Christianity, 26,* 207–217.

Fitz-Gibbon, A. L. (2000). *In the world, but not of the world: Christian social thinking at the end of the twentieth century.* Lanham, MD: Lexington Books.

France, R. T. (2007). *The Gospel of Matthew* (The new international commentary on the New Testament). Grand Rapids, MI: William B. Eerdmans.

Gorsuch, R. L. (1968). The conceptualization of God as seen in adjective ratings. *Journal for the Scientific Study of Religion, 7,* 56–64.

Hall, R. W. (1971). Alfred Adler's concept of God. *Journal of Individual Psychology, 27,* 10–18.

Hamachek, D. E. (1978). Psychodynamics of normal and neurotic perfectionism. *Psychology: A Journal of Human Behavior, 15,* 27–33.

James, I. A., & Barton, S. (2004). Changing core beliefs with the continuum technique. *Behavioural and Cognitive Psychotherapy, 32,* 431–442.

Keijsers, G. P. J., Schaap, C. P. D. R., & Hoogduin, C. A. L. (2000). The impact of interpersonal patient and therapist behavior on outcome in cognitive-behavioral therapy: A review of empirical studies. *Behavior Modification, 24,* 264–297.

McMinn, M. R. (1991). *Cognitive therapy techniques in Christian counseling* (Resources for Christian counseling; v. 27). Dallas, TX: Word.

Moreira-Almeida, A., Neto, F. L., & Koenig, H. G. (2006). Religiousness and mental health: A review. *Revista Brasileira Psiquiatria, 28*, 242–250.

Murphy, N. (1997). Divine action in the natural order: Buridan's ass and Schrodinger's cat. In R. J. Russell, N. Murphy, & A. R. Peacock (Eds.), *Chaos and complexity: Scientific perspectives on divine action* (2nd ed.). Berkley, CA: Center for Theology and the Natural Sciences.

O'Connor, R. C., & Cassidy, C. (2007). Predicting hopelessness: The interaction between optimism/pessimism and specific future expectancies. *Cognition & Emotion, 21*, 596–613.

Palmer, M. F. (1997). *Freud and Jung on religion.* New York: Routledge.

Pargament, K. I. (2002). The bitter and the sweet: An evaluation of the costs and benefits of religiousness. *Psychological Inquiry, 13*, 168–181.

Pargament, K. I., Ensing, D. S., Falgout, K., Olsen, H., & et al. (1990). God help me: I. Religious coping efforts as predictors of the outcomes to significant negative life events. *American Journal of Community Psychology, 18*, 793–824.

Pargament, K. I., Koenig, H. G., & Perez, L. M. (2000). The many methods of religious coping: Development and initial validation of the RCOPE. *Journal of Clinical Psychology, 56*, 519–543.

Pargament, K. I., Zinnbauer, B. J., Scott, A. B., Butter, E. M., Zerowin, J., & Stanik, P. (1998). Red flags and religious coping: Identifying some religious warning signs among people in crisis. *Journal of Clinical Psychology, 54*, 77–89.

Peterson, E. H. (2002). *The Message: The Bible in Contemporary Language.* Colorado Springs, CO: NavPress.

Propst, L. R. (1996). Cognitive-behavioral therapy and the religious person. In E. P. Shafranske (Ed.), *Religion and the clinical practice of psychology* (pp. 391–407). Washington, D.C.: American Psychological Association.

Rayburn, C. A. (2000). Psychotherapy with Seventh-day Adventists. In P. S. Richards & A. E. Bergin (Eds.), *Handbook of psychotherapy and religious diversity* (pp. 211–234). Washington, D.C.: American Psychological Association.

Rice, R. (1985). *The reign of God: An introduction to Christian theology from a Seventh-day Adventist perspective.* Berrien Springs, MI: Andrews University Press.

Richards, P. S., & Bergin, A. E. (2000). Religious diversity and psychotherapy: Conclusions, recommendations, and future directions. In P. S. Richards & A. E. Bergin (Eds.), *Handbook of psychotherapy and religious diversity* (pp. 469–489). Washington, D.C.: American Psychological Association.

Riley, C., Lee, M., Cooper, Z., Fairburn, C. G., & Shafran, R. (2007). A randomised controlled trial of cognitive-behaviour therapy for clinical perfectionism: A preliminary study. *Behaviour Research and Therapy, 45*, 2221–2231.

Singer, J. L. (2006). Imagery applications in cognitive-behavioral therapies. In *Imagery in Psychotherapy* (pp. 105–128). Washington, D.C.: American Psychological Association.

Smith, T. W. (1990). Classifying Protestant denominations. *Review of Religious Research, 31*, 225.

Walters, J., & Lee, J. (2008). *Image of God, positive/negative eschatology, and health outcomes.* Paper presented at the Loma Linda University Adventist Health Studies Seminars, Loma Linda, CA.

White, E. G. (1952). *The Adventist Home.* Hagerstown, MD: Review and Herald.

Wong-McDonald, A., & Gorsuch, R. L. (2004). A multivariate theory of God concept, religious motivation, locus of control, coping, and spiritual well-being. *Journal of Psychology & Theology, 32*, 318–334.

Yarnell, H. (1957). An example of the psychopathology of religion: The Seventh-day Adventist denomination. *Journal of Nervous and Mental Disease, 125*, 202–212.

Comprehensive Oncology Patient Services and the Organizational Mission "To Make Man Whole": Implications and Challenges for the Adventist Health System

Deane L. Wolcott and Carlos Fayard

This paper presents a current comprehensive model for the provision of oncology supportive care services within the hospital cancer care delivery system for patients and their families. This model is based on current national clinical care delivery standards for the range of services included within the term "oncology supportive care services" (OSCS). This paper will use the terms "cancer" and "oncology" interchangeably.

The development of these national OSCS standards cumulatively reflects a major national shift in definition of the key objectives of, and models for, delivery of high-quality oncology patient care. This model shift can be briefly summarized as away from an earlier model focused almost exclusively on the role of individual providers in the diagnosis and treatment of cancer to the current model focused on the comprehensive, longitudinally coordinated, multidisciplinary team care of the cancer patient and provision of support to his or her family throughout all illness phases.

The development of these OSCS standards are highly consistent with the services delivery organization implications of Loma Linda University Adventist Health Sciences Center/Loma Linda University Medical Center/Adventist Health System (LLUAHSC/LLUMC/AHS) mission and vision statements as applied to oncology patient care.

This paper discusses the implications of the model for the following:

1. The provision of cancer patient/family supportive care services within LLUMC and other AHS hospitals in the context of LLUAHSC/AHS mission, and as a general template for the provision of these services to other medically ill populations within LLUMC/AHS hospitals.

2. The implications of this model for provision of psychiatric and mental health services to medical patients within LLUMC/AHS hospitals.
3. The education by LLUAHSC/other AHS-affiliated educational institutions of health care professionals who provide patient/family supportive care services in the medical setting and specifically those who provide oncology patient/family supportive care services.
4. How the principles behind this model may help LLUAHSC/AHS hospital leaders make future care delivery organization decisions as the health care system continues to evolve in response to quality and cost concerns.

LLUAHSC AND SELECTED MISSION STATEMENTS

LLUAHSC and the AHS are deeply rooted within the Seventh-day Adventist church by history, ongoing cultural commitment, and continuing organizational and leadership structure. This history and commitment are very clearly expressed in the mission/vision/value statements of AHS organizations. Selected statements from three organizations are presented as examples.

Adventist Health System: West (Mission, Vision, and Values, n.d.):

- ◊ Our Mission: "To share God's love by providing physical, mental, and spiritual healing"
- ◊ Our Vision: "Adventist Health will be a recognized leader in mission focus, quality care and fiscal strength"
- ◊ Our Values (Selected): "The compassionate, healing ministry of Jesus"; "Excellence in clinical and service quality"; "The health care heritage of the Seventh-day Adventist Church"

Adventist Health System: South East (Mission and Values, n.d.):

- ◊ Our Mission: "Extending the healing ministry of Christ"

◊ Our Values: "AHS employees draw motivation and direction from 6 strongly held principles [selected]...Christian Mission—We exist to serve the needs of our communities in harmony with Christ's healing ministry and incorporate Christian values at every level of service...Quality and Service Excellence... Compassion"

Loma Linda University Adventist Health Science Center (Loma Linda University, n.d.):

◊ Our Mission: "Loma Linda University, a Seventh-day Adventist Christian health sciences institution, seeks to further the healing and teaching ministry of Jesus Christ 'to make man whole' by:
- Educating ethical and proficient Christian health professionals and scholars...
- Expanding knowledge through research...and applying this knowledge to health and disease
- Providing comprehensive, competent, and compassionate health care for the whole person through faculty, students, and alumni."

BRIEF OVERVIEW OF THE RELATION OF RELIGION AND SPIRITUALITY TO ADJUSTMENT AND QUALITY OF LIFE IN CANCER POPULATIONS

A comprehensive review of the growing literature on religion/spirituality and cancer is beyond the scope of this article. Research has caught up with Adventists' long-held views on whole-person care, although perhaps it is, sad to say, Adventists who have not been as active in conducting the research or designing comprehensive treatment protocols, thus facilitating the implementation of AHS mission and values. Robust results have been obtained when measures of spirituality and religion have been related to measures of quality of life (McCullough, Hoyt, & Larson, 2000), pain management, social adjustment, emotional distress, and coping with end-of-life issues (Thune-Boyle, Stygall, Keshtgar, & Newman, 2006).

Although the literature is less than uniform on the positive role played by religion in the life of individuals with cancer and their families (see Thune-Boyle et al., 2006; Stefanek, McDonald, & Hess, 2004), strong religious beliefs, hope, optimism, freedom from regret, a sense of life satisfaction, a sense of meaning and peace, and positive religious coping (e.g., "God is interested in my well-being") have been associated with improved emotional adjustment and quality of life in the presence of high levels of pain and fatigue, posttraumatic growth, and perceived life threat (Jim & Jacobsen, 2008; Laubmeier, Zakowski, & Bair, 2004; Krupski, Kwan, Afifi et al., 2006; McCoubrie & Davies, 2006; O'Mahony, Goulet, Kornblith et al., 2005; Salsman, Brown, Brechting, & Carlson, 2005; Tarakeshwar, Vanderwerker, & Paulk et al., 2006; Thune-Boyle et al., 2006).

It could be argued that even the studies that found that higher levels of religiosity or spirituality were associated with higher levels of distress (see Thune-Boyle et al., 2006) may not necessarily argue against a spiritually sensitive approach to care. In fact, these individuals may be the ones who could benefit from specialized pastoral or psychological care as some of their discomfort is associated with failed spiritual expectations ("God is not answering my prayers") or negative religious coping ("God is angry with me—I am being punished by God").

The Institute of Medicine of the National Academy of Sciences recently released a report entitled *Cancer Care for the Whole Person: Meeting Psychosocial Health Needs* (Holland & Weiss, 2008) outlining evidence-based standards for clinical practice, which explicitly require the assessment of emotional, social, and spiritual needs as part of the routine care for cancer patients. The systematic use of psychological and spiritual aid in the treatment of cancer has a long and controversial history. Nevertheless, patients and their families tend to seek psychological and spiritual support on their own with mixed results (Kaplar, Wacholtz, & O'Brien, 2004).

A variety of non-medical intervention approaches delivered by a multidisciplinary team and integrated into cancer treatment are showing promise. For instance, structured multidisciplinary group interventions that incorporate psychological and spiritual considerations as part of cancer treatment have been shown to increase quality of life over time (Rummans et al., 2006). Training oncology physicians to provide a spiritual intervention has shown to be well received by patients—increasing their sense of personal care by their physician and reducing depressive symptoms (Kristeller, Rhodes, Cripe, & Sheets, 2005). Perhaps more controversial are the results of a randomized clinical trial that followed participants in such a psychological intervention over eleven years, showing that participants had significantly reduced risk for recurrence and survival rates when compared to control subjects who received treatment as usual (Andersen et al., 2008).

Given the overwhelming empirical evidence for the importance of whole-person cancer care, how would an Adventist Health System entity implement this mandate? Would it replicate what is being done in secular contexts, or would it attempt to dream ways of articulating the notion that "healing is ministry"? Would it rely on Eastern-based conceptualizations of spirituality that teach mindfulness meditation as a tool for coping, or would it seek to start with "where the patient is at," not unlike the Good Samaritan, and, like him, assist the patient in finding the care needed by *planting seeds* that may *incline* the heart of the patient to the Great Physician (White, 1905, p. 391)? Would it be organized around discipline boundaries, deferring spiritual care to the chaplain, or would it attempt to see that each team member is a participant in the "ministry of Jesus"? What does it mean today to participate in the healing ministry of Jesus?

CLINICAL SERVICE DELIVERY AS MINISTRY

Although a comprehensive answer to the question of what it means to participate in the healing ministry of Jesus is beyond the scope of this article, the following observations might be helpful to consider as most AHS-affiliated organizations no longer employ spiritually homogeneous, faith-oriented clinical providers. If AHS mission is to be successful, the training and recruitment of human resources committed to its fulfillment is crucial. We submit that the intentional development of the notion of clinical service as "ministry" can provide the organization focus to accomplish its mission in this environment.

This idea was brought home as one of us (CF) was sitting through a presentation of the strategic plan for a large AHS-affiliated institution. The word *ministry* was used to name the entire operation, but was never referred to again. It could have been used to articulate the reasons for the set of values selected, the emphases on why improving customer services was important, or the development of clinical services that could have advanced whole-person care. The rationale provided for the organization's core values was no different from that of other corporations. Customer service improvement was needed to improve competitiveness and market position, and additional clinical services to expand the organization's need to feed patients at the main hospital. Nothing is wrong with that; however, the notion of ministry as the prime motivator for the entire enterprise was lost. It is our suggestion that any organization needs to have a clear identity, and that articulating the idea of what it means to participate in the healing ministry of Jesus can be helpful. Here are some brief examples.

One of us (CF) has had an opportunity to work in different secular and church-related settings, each with its own distinct identity. As a psychologist working for the state of California, everyone knew who we were: bureaucrats. Service delivery was competent, in many cases compassionate, but clearly focused on discharging a duty. No sense of mission. When working in the mission field, everyone knew who we were: missionaries. Service delivery was not always competent as the strictures of the environment prevented state-of-the-art capacity; in most cases, compassion and dedication made up for whatever else was lacking. Uppermost in the minds of those providing services was the opportunity to witness directly, or to serve in a supportive capacity for the purposes of witnessing for Christ. The entire operation was built around this notion, with the development of comprehensive clinical services taking a second seat.

Very succinctly, how would a ministry look? Competent, compassionate, and clear about its motivation for being in business. In the Seventh-day Adventist church, it would be wise to follow Ellen White's counsel in her book *Ministry of Healing* (1905). The primary dedication would be to healing, with a clear dedication to planting seeds in the hearts of the patients that may incline them to God. It would be concerned every step of the way about the spiritual and emotional needs of the patient, just as much as about any medical concern. It would be personalized, respectful, and attentive to the patient's situation and need as the point at which whole-person care begins. To be effective, we suggest that every member of the treatment and support team would know what it means to be a "minister."

Let us now turn to the reality of the challenge and opportunity for providing comprehensive cancer care.

OVERVIEW OF CANCER IN THE UNITED STATES

CANCER EPIDEMIOLOGY AND COSTS

This paper uses the terms *oncology* and *cancer* to cover the entire range of malignant solid tumor and hematological diseases. Cancer is one of the most commonly diagnosed life-threatening conditions (about 1.3 million new cases per year, not including skin cancer) and is one of the leading causes of death in the United States (American Cancer Society, 2007; National Cancer Institute, n.d). Due to cumulatively dramatic improvements in cancer screening and diagnostic services resulting commonly in the diagnosis of cancer in earlier/curable stages; major advances in scientific understanding of the cellular and molecular biology of cancer; and major advances in cancer surgery, radiotherapy treatment, and medication treatment regimens; the average five-year patient survival rate for cancer in the United States has increased in the last thirty years from about 50% to about 67%. For certain conditions, the increased five-year survival rate has been even much more dramatic.

The result of the combination of increased cancer incidence due to the aging of the country's population and increased prevalence due to longer average patient survival has resulted in a rapidly increasing population of cancer survivors in the United States, currently estimated to be about twelve million (using the definition of cancer survivor as someone diagnosed with cancer until his or her death). Thus cancer is now increasingly being recognized as a chronic disease which needs to be cared for using chronic disease management models, not acute disease models.

The direct and indirect costs of cancer are very substantial. The NIH estimated that the total cost of cancer in 2006 was $206.3 billion, including $78.2 billion in direct medical costs and $128.1 billion in indirect costs (morbidity costs and mortality costs; Shih & Halpern, 2008). Per-case cancer care active treatment costs are rising very rapidly in the United States due to a combination of the costs of newer imaging and other diagnostic technology applied to cancer diagnosis and treatment, technology-based advances in cancer surgery (minimally invasive surgery and robot-assisted surgery), advanced radiotherapy treatment capabilities (brachytherapy, IMRT, IGRT, stereotactic radiosurgery, proton therapy), newer more complex and expensive chemotherapy/targeted therapies regimens, the costs of palliative care for patients with advanced cancer, and the costs of end-of-life care.

There are very great national concerns about the rapidly rising costs of cancer treatment, with special concerns about the costs of medication-based regimens, as individual "targeted agents" can now cost $50,000 to $100,000 per patient per year (Shih & Halpern, 2008).

OVERVIEW OF THE UNITED STATES CANCER-CARE DELIVERY SYSTEM

The United States cancer-care delivery system is very complex and fragmented. The most prominent cancer-care providers in the country are large dedicated cancer hospitals and academic medical centers with major research and educational missions (e.g., Memorial Sloan-Kettering Cancer Center, the University of Texas MD Anderson Cancer Center, and other NCI-designated Comprehensive Cancer Centers). While many excellent teaching hospitals and community hospitals provide a significant range of cancer services, about 80% of all chemotherapy and about 50% of all radiotherapy treatment in the United States are provided in the free-standing, office-based, or community cancer center environment. In general, these office/community-based cancer care providers offer a limited range of active treatment services, have limited off-hours urgent/emergent care provision capabilities, and are limited in their abilities to directly provide comprehensive, patient-centered supportive care services.

ONCOLOGY PATIENT CARE STANDARDS

Many explicitly articulated national standards exist for defining cancer patient care and cancer treatment excellence. These can be categorized as follows:

1. National hospital cancer program standards (American College of Surgeons Commission on Cancer, 2006; Association of Community Cancer Centers, 2008)
2. Clinical practice guidelines related to the care of the individual patient. These include cancer risk reduction, screening, and diagnosis care; active treatment of diagnosed cancer patients (e.g., by NCCN, ASCO, ACR, ASTRO, CAP, and others) (National Comprehensive Care Network, n.d.; American Society of Clinical Oncology, n.d.; American College of Radiology, n.d.); supportive care services (NCCN, n.d.; NCCN, Adult, n.d.); cancer survivorship services (Hewitt, Greenfield, & Stovall, 2006); and palliative and end-of-life care services (NCCN, Palliative; n.d.; National Quality Forum, n.d.; National Quality Forum, 2006)
3. General oncology services, excellence standards, and disease-

specific centers' excellence standards with associated clinical quality dashboards (Oncology Roundtable, 2004; Oncology Roundtable, 2005; Oncology Roundtable, 2007)

4. Specific oncology provider quality performance measurement standards and programs (e.g., ASCO QOPI and CMS PQRI) (National Quality Forum, n.d.; ASCO, 2008; Centers for Medicare and Medicaid, 2008; AMA, n.d.)

Figure 1 presents an overview of these categories of oncology care quality standards.

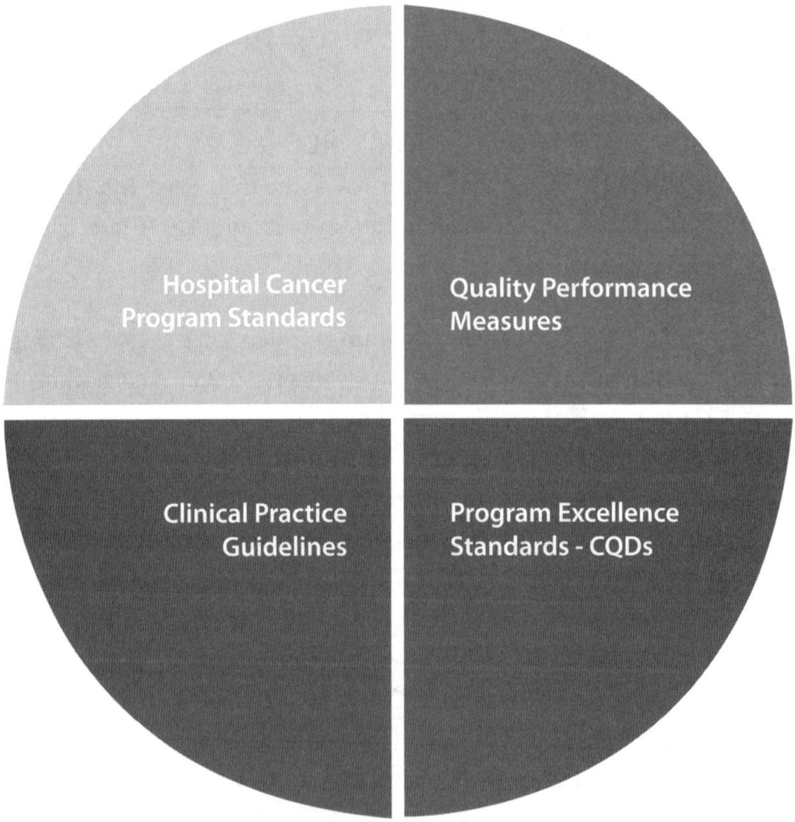

Figure 1. Oncology Care Quality Standards and Measures: Major Categories

The comprehensiveness of cancer care provided (e.g., multispecialty oncologist physicians, oncology nursing expertise and services, diagnostic/imaging services, ancillary clinical services, full range of active treatment services, and range of patient/family supportive care services) is an additional contributor to hospital ambulatory cancer center (HACC) provider cancer care excellence.

Several additional characteristics of HACC cancer clinical care excellence are widely accepted. These include the provision of truly integrated multidisciplinary team care, the provision of comprehensive disease-specific services/centers (e.g., breast centers, prostate centers), the provision of patient- and family-centered care (e.g., patient education; patient's active role in treatment decision-making, family education, and support), excellent provider information sharing and care coordination both internally and with all external care providers, and provision of longitudinal care coordination through all disease phases.

Certainly the clinical quality of care is one very important component of cancer care excellence. The patient experience of care (provider service quality and associated patient satisfaction levels with care) is another very important component. A third key component of care quality is the quality of the provider(s) relationships with the patient and with his or her family members as manifested by the quality of communication and the patient's experience of receiving compassionate, caring, respectful care.

ONCOLOGY SUPPORTIVE CARE SERVICES FOR PATIENTS AND FAMILIES

The role of oncology patient/family supportive care services (OSCS) has received much recent emphasis as a key component of cancer care excellence. In general, these services are directed at caring for the patient and family in order to contribute to the best possible active treatment of the cancer and the best possible patient quality of life (Institute of Medicine, 2007). The development of standards for the provision of OSCS is one of the most important indicators of the fundamental model change in oncology care to be further discussed later.

The older term for "oncology supportive care services" was historically psychosocial oncology services. While psycho-oncology and psychosocial oncology services are very important components of oncology supportive care services, more inclusive services delivery models include psycho-oncology services, oncology social worker services, oncology dietitian services, cancer pain/symptom management services, spiritual counseling services, integrative oncology/complementary therapies services, cancer survivorship services, and palliative care/end-of-life care/hospice services (see Figure 2).

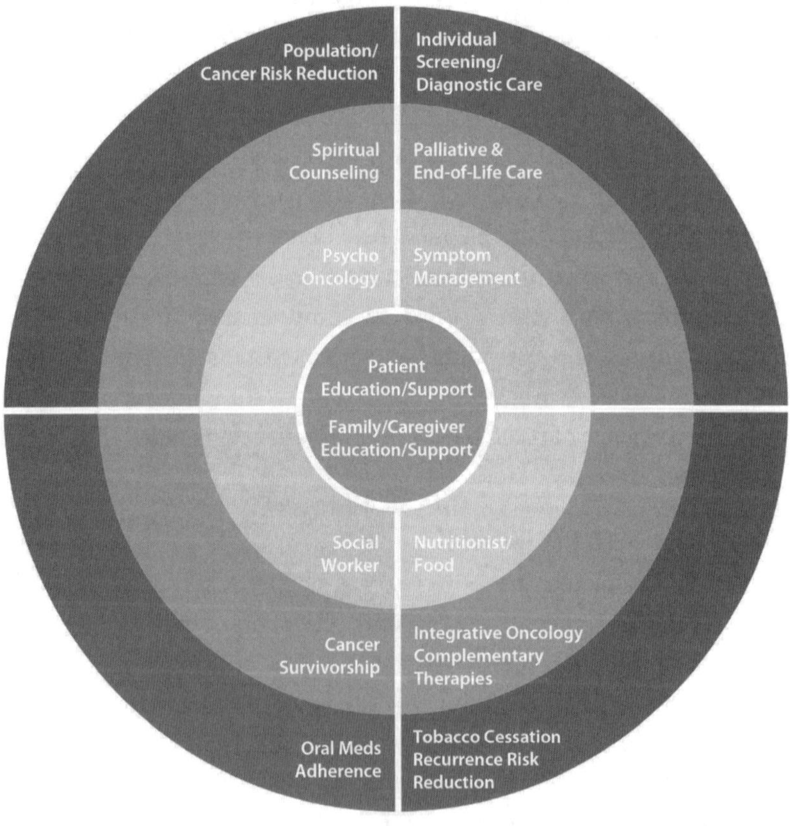

Figure 2. Comprehensive Oncology Supportive Care Services Model

Important factors in the provision of optimal OSCS cancer center services are:

- ◊ The development of the full range of these services provided by an internal, highly integrated multidisciplinary team which is itself physically based in the hospital ambulatory cancer center
- ◊ Full integration of these services within the hospital's larger cancer patient care delivery system (see Figure 3)
- ◊ The effectiveness of these services in contributing to optimal coordination of all cancer center services with all other internal and external care providers' services throughout all patient illness phases (see Figure 4)
- ◊ The effectiveness of these services in contributing to excellent palliative and end-of-life care (see Figure 5)

While many prestigious cancer hospitals in the United States provide the highest levels of professional and technical expertise in the diagnosis and treatment of cancer based on world-class research and educational capabilities, and while many of these also provide many oncology supportive care services, many of these do not provide optimally integrated/coordinated patient care services or the full range of oncology supportive care services. Thus hospital academic prestige and standing does not necessarily translate to the highest quality cancer patient care. Many community hospital cancer programs and community-based cancer care providers provide no or very limited OSCS.

Given the many criteria for cancer-care excellence outlined above, the specific care delivery-role limitations of hospital inpatient cancer services (focus on acute episodes of surgical care and other emergent cancer care situations), and the commonly limited range of office-based and community cancer care services, the authors' judgment is that truly outstanding cancer patient care needs to ideally be based in a hospital's outpatient oncology department/ambulatory cancer center. This assertion is based on the potential capability of the hospital ambulatory cancer

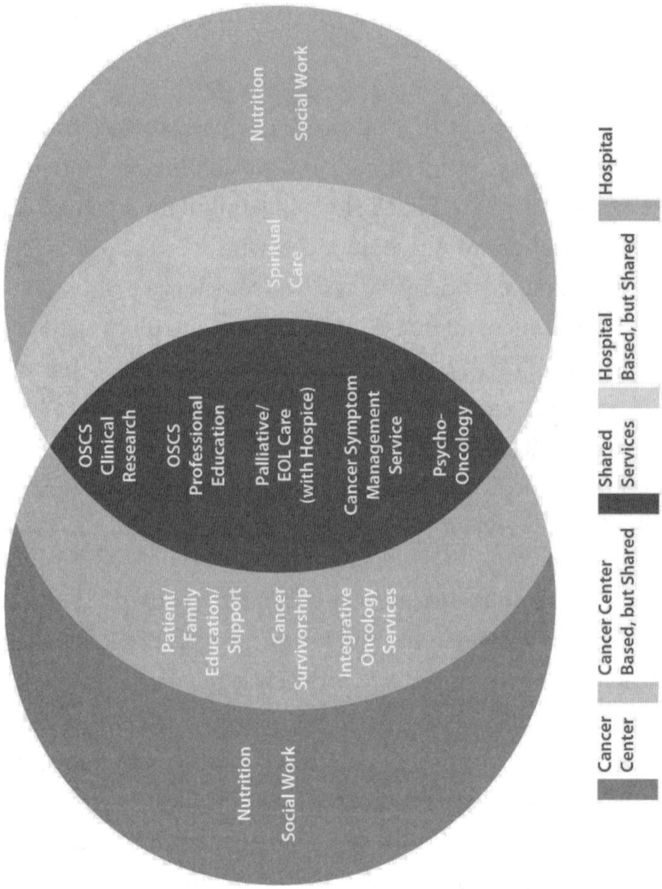

Figure 3. Cancer Center/Hospital OSCS Integration Model

center to provide a full range of integrated screening, diagnostic, professional, active treatment, ancillary clinical, and patient supportive care services; to provide the comprehensive, multidisciplinary, and longitudinally coordinated care delivery required to manage cancer as a chronic disease rather than as a time-limited acute episode of care; and the capability to longitudinally coordinate patient care delivery with

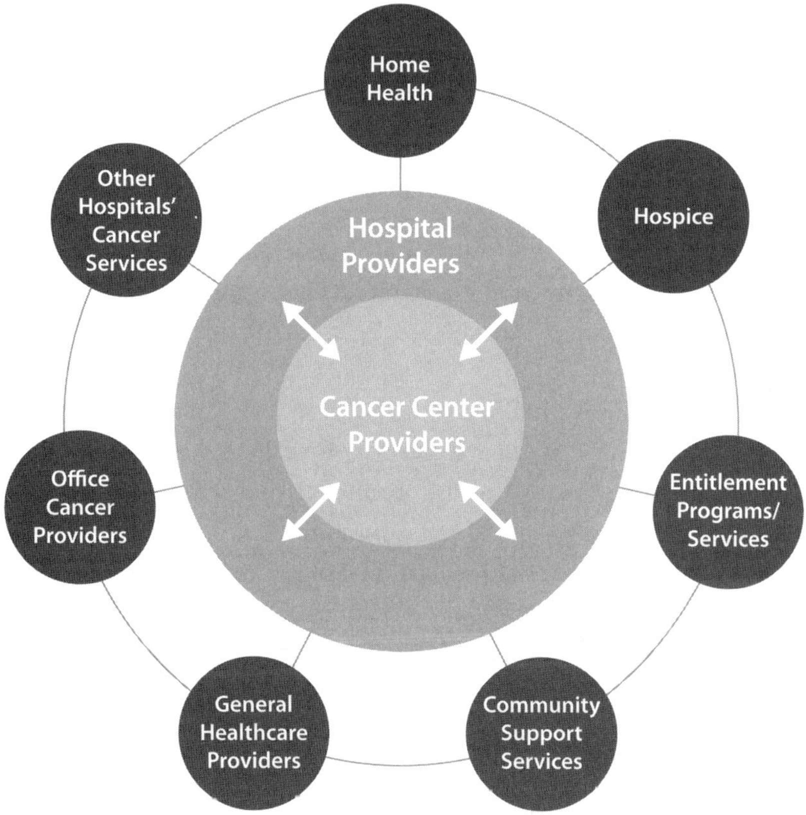

Figure 4. Cancer Center Oncology Supportive Care Services—Common Care Coordination Functions

a wide variety of hospital inpatient, community-based, and hospice services providers.

ONCOLOGY SERVICES AND ONCOLOGY PATIENT SUPPORTIVE CARE SERVICES: QUALITY STANDARDS

The health care system in the United States has entered the era of provider accountability for the quality of care delivered. This new era has been driven by multiple national stakeholders concerned about the high and rapidly rising costs of health care delivery, evidence of significant health care provider system deficiencies in meeting well-accepted quality of care standards, and evidence that many population health outcomes do not compare particularly well with population health outcomes in other first-world countries.

This general emphasis on health care provider quality accountability is rapidly spreading to cancer care services. The concern with cancer care provision is focused mostly on clinical quality and costs, with cancer patient outcomes in the United States comparing favorably with the patient outcomes achieved by most other first-world health care systems.

As described above, national oncology care quality standards are now applicable to almost all cancer care activities, including OSCS. These OSCS quality standards are also embedded in hospital cancer program services standards (Association of Community Cancer Centers, 2008), national clinical practice guidelines (National Comprehensive Cancer Network; n.d.; American Society of Clinical Oncology, n.d.; National Comprehensive Cancer Network, Adult, n.d.; National Comprehensive Cancer Network, Palliative, n.d; Carr, Goudas, & Lawrence, et al., 2002; ASCO, 2006; Elliott, Molseed, & McCallum, 2006; NCCN, Distress, n.d.), program excellence standards in services/Centers with associated clinical quality dashboards (Oncology Roundtable, 2004; Oncology Roundtable, 2005; Oncology Roundtable, 2007), and within oncology quality performance measures (National Quality Forum, n.d.; ASCO, 2008; Centers for Medicare and Medicaid, 2008; AMA, n.d.). Many of these standards relate to the full range of OSCS (see Table 1), while some relate to specific patient illness phases (e.g., cancer survivorship and palliative care/end-of-life care) (Hewitt, Greenfield, & Stovall, 2006; NCCN, Palliative, n.d; National Quality Forum, n.d.; National Quality Forum, 2006).

Thus the provision of comprehensive oncology patient/family supportive care services has moved in the last twenty years from being rarely considered within oncology care delivery models or standards of care to being firmly embedded in current standards of care (see Table 1).

Table 1. Oncology Patient Care Standards—Existing Services Standards

SERVICES	NATIONAL STANDARDS ORGANIZATIONS
Psychiatry/Psychology, Social Worker/Dietitian	American College of Surgeons Commission on Cancer Association of Community Cancer Centers Institute of Medicine National Comprehensive Cancer Network National Quality Forum Oncology Roundtable Professional Organizations
Symptom Management/ Oral Medication Adherence	Agency for Healthcare, Research, and Quality American Pain Society Association of Community Cancer Centers Joint Commission on Accreditation of Healthcare Organizations National Comprehensive Cancer Network National Quality Forum Oncology Roundtable
Spiritual Assessment/ Counseling	Association of Community Cancer Centers Joint Commission on Accreditation of Healthcare Organizations National Comprehensive Cancer Network
Integrative Oncology	Association of Community Cancer Centers Society for Integrative Oncology
Cancer Survivorship	Association of Community Cancer Centers Institute of Medicine

SERVICES	NATIONAL STANDARDS ORGANIZATIONS
Palliative/End-of-Life Care	Association of Community Cancer Centers National Comprehensive Cancer Network National Consensus Project for Quality Palliative Care National Quality Forum

Reasons for the current common limitations in provision of hospital ambulatory cancer center OSCS include the commonly low priority assigned to these services by hospital cancer program leaders, the relatively low direct reimbursement for provision of these services, major limitations in the size of the national pool of professionals with the appropriate expertise to provide high-quality services, the recent emergence of standards for some services such as cancer survivorship services, and the complexity of the provision of some services such as palliative care/end-of-life care (EOLC) services (National Quality Forum, n.d.; National Quality Forum, 2006; see Figure 5).

Cancer pain/symptom management, palliative care, and end-of-life care services require optimal coordination of services delivery among hospital ambulatory cancer center, hospital inpatient, home health agency, and hospice services providers (see Figure 5).

CHALLENGES TO ONCOLOGY CARE PROVIDERS

The health care system in the United States is in the early stages of a fundamental transition related to provider quality accountability and transparency and provider reimbursement models. The first stage of this major transition can be summarized under the general term, *Pay for Performance* (P4P). P4P programs have been developed by governmental and health care plan payers intended to both improve provider quality of care and to decrease the costs of care. The essential tools of P4P are to require provider documentation that services meet

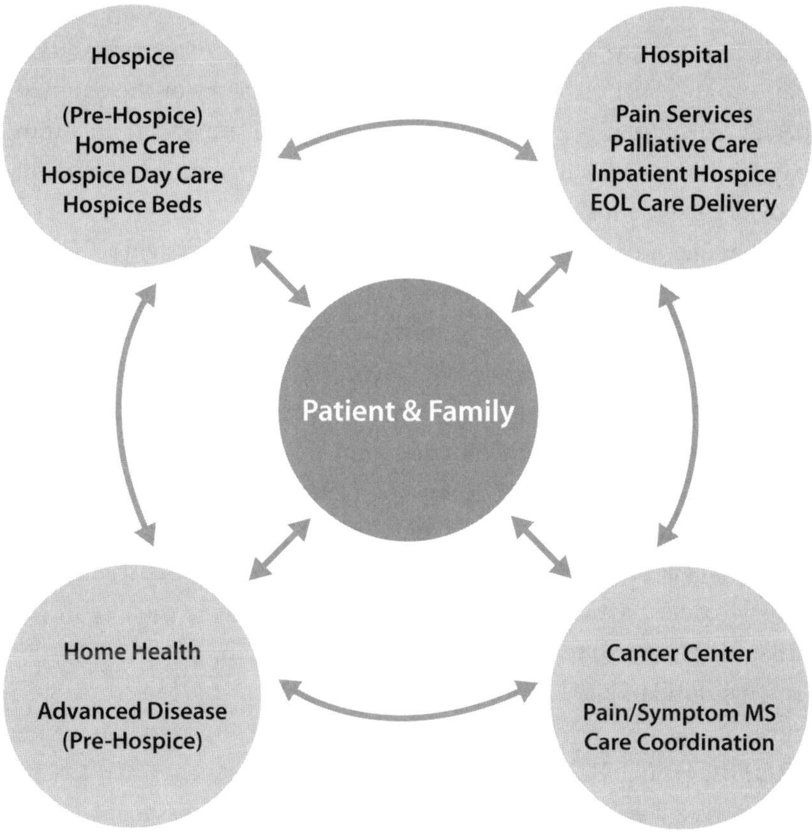

Figure 5. Comprehensive Model for Palliative and End-of-Life Care

specified quality standards, to measure and publicly report provider performance on these quality measures, and to offer economic incentives to providers based on their level of reporting and/or actual quality performance.

While P4P is seen as only a first step in provider system reform, and as only a modestly powerful tool, P4P has strong support from the Centers for Medicare & Medicaid Services (CMS) (US Department of Health and Human Services, 2007) and the major health care plans. P4P programs are very rapidly accelerating in number and scope, and are now beginning to be nationally standardized.

This movement from a "pure" provider services/activities volume-based payment system to one based at least partially on provider quality performance is a very significant event in the history of the country's health care system. However, probably the most important upcoming payer initiative which will impact the provider system is fundamental provider payment system reform.

The general goals of fundamental provider payment system reform are to move the payment system away from payment for individual patient care services or even brief acute episodes of care to "evidence-informed, extended episode of care, bundled payment (most/all providers), case rates" (as stated on many billing forms). This movement is also driven by the goals of overall care cost containment/care quality improvement, but additionally by the goals of decreasing overall administrative overhead costs for providers and payers, decreasing the frequency of non-aligned and perverse provider incentives which abound in the current health care provider payment system, and extending provider quality of care accountability to much longer time intervals/episodes of care.

This fundamental payment system reform approach has been most practically developed to this point by an organization named PROMETHEUS Payment® (Prometheus Payment, Inc., n.d.). CMS clearly has a policy goal of achieving fundamental payment system reform along the lines outlined above. This fundamental payment system reform could very early on be applied to oncology providers, because much oncology active treatment care (radiotherapy and medication-based regimens) consists of well-defined treatment regimens which are provided over relatively long periods of times (weeks to months) and could be quite easily "bundled."

The provider care delivery changes which will be required for hospital cancer care providers to survive and thrive under the reformed provider payment system will require that many oncology supportive care services be highly developed and effectively integrated within the provider's overall cancer care delivery system. Oncology care providers who thrive under this system will have the following characteristics:

1. High levels of internal coordination of all patient services delivery activities, so that patient visit flow and patient services provider productivity are optimal
2. Very effective patient and family education and support services so patients are (as much as possible) actively informed about their illness and treatment options, are active participants in personal treatment decisions, and are highly adherent to their treatment regimen
3. Effective early detection of patients at high risk for future medical systems/problems which can be prevented but which are potentially very expensive to treat (e.g., screening/care related to decreased oral intake and significant weight loss—e.g., oral mucositis)
4. Effective processes for rapidly moving patients between provider systems and coordinating patient care among all internal and external providers
5. Excellent and effective symptom management services which minimize the need for avoidable ER visits and hospitalizations, and which ensure that inpatient stay length is as efficiently short as possible (Strouse, Flanagan, Kerrihard, Williams, & Wolcott, 2006)
6. Outstanding medical supportive care services (e.g., prevention and early detection of and treatment for cancer-related infections)
7. Highly integrated and effective palliative and end-of-life care

Thus, the provision by hospital cancer care providers of excellent care which meets current quality of care standards, which supports provider success in the current oncology P4P environment, and which will be necessary to thrive under coming fundamental payment system reform is partially but significantly dependent on the hospital provider's development of comprehensive and well-integrated oncology supportive care services.

OPERATIONAL AND BUSINESS RATIONALE FOR PROVIDING OSCS

While a significant amount of time, effort, and resource is required to develop comprehensive and excellent Cancer Center/Hospital Cancer Program OSCS, the authors' experience in developing these services over many years at a wide variety of hospital ambulatory cancer centers (HACC) is that actual services and operating costs are a very small percentage of overall Cancer Center revenues. These services generate a modest to significant amount of direct revenues, with higher direct revenues associated with a successful cancer pain/symptom management service.

Well-developed and comprehensive MDT (multidisciplinary team) OSCS based which are well-integrated components of the hospital CC cancer care delivery system provide many clinical operational benefits to a Cancer Center. These benefits include helping ensure optimally efficient patient visit flow and treatment services productivity, supporting optimal CC physician and nursing staff productivity as complex and time-consuming patients with complex non-medical problems are cared for by OSCS staff members, improving coordination and efficiency of care environment transitions (e.g., CC to hospital, HHA referrals), and providing positive contributions to patient treatment adherence.

The well-developed and integrated hospital ambulatory cancer center (HACC) and hospital cancer program (HCP) OSCS can help achieve high levels of cancer services business success, decrease costs related to utilization of hospital ER and inpatient care resources for the care of patients with pain/symptom crises (Strouse, Flanagan, Kerrihard, Williams, & Wolcott, 2006), greatly contribute to the reputation of the hospital's overall cancer program, provide an excellent base for the clinical trials success of the hospital cancer program, and greatly contribute to a hospital's overall reputation and financial success in its community.

Additionally OSCS can greatly contribute to positive patient satisfaction with a wide variety of CC Services (Wolcott, Wolosin,

Macdonald, & Strouse, 2008). They can also positively contribute to the quality of provider relationships with patients and their family members. Commitment to providing OSCS does require the understanding that benefit and value cannot always be reduced to identifiable service-specific revenues.

MENTAL HEALTH IN ONCOLOGY SUPPORTIVE CARE SERVICES

The development of the OSCS model has profound implications for the role of formal mental health care services within oncology service delivery. Whereas twenty years ago psycho-oncology and psychosocial oncology services were in very early stages of development, and when present were mostly individual patient-focused consultation services provided by individual practitioners, they are now recognized as an integral component of a much broader group of OSCS provided by an ideally fully integrated multidisciplinary team of providers. In older parlance this transition has been from a consulting model (provision of an individual patient care service) to a "liaison" model (integrated team member with wide-ranging informal and formal relationships with other care delivery team members in support of overall patient care delivery effectiveness).

This OSCS model requires significant levels of individual discipline-specific oncology expertise, staff members who can work effectively in a MDT model, staff members who obviously really care about their patients and their family members, and staff members who can work effectively in support of the primary cancer care provided by oncologist physicians, nurses, and other professionals.

In models with the best practices, psycho-oncology and psychosocial oncology services are also fully involved in the provision of advanced cancer pain and symptom management services (Carr, Goudas, & Lawrence et al., 2002), as well as palliative care and end-of-life care services (National Quality Forum, n.d.; National Quality Forum, 2006; Strouse, Flanagan, Kerrihard, Williams, & Wolcott, 2006). The ideal psychiatrist or psychologist involved with OSCS is now one with advanced psycho-oncology expertise and advanced cancer pain/symptom management expertise.

The authors contend that the general principles of the OSCS model provide an excellent general model for the role of patient supportive care services within hospital inpatient and outpatient care delivery environments for a wide variety of (especially) chronic health care conditions. The management of chronic diseases (e.g., diabetes, hypertension, cardiovascular disease) is one of the most important and costly components of the health care delivery system in the United States.

IMPACT OF OSCS ON PROVIDERS, PATIENTS, AND FAMILIES

Well-functioning OSCS make many highly valued contributions to the clinical practice experience of Cancer Center physicians and nurses. These values include the OSCS team managing many complex, demanding, and time-intensive patient care situations that would otherwise require physician or nurse effort; rapid provider access to informal and formal consultation with OSCS team members regarding patients who may not be formally cared for by the OSCS team; OSCS team-member provision of informal and formal education to other providers concerning these human aspects of care; OSCS team-member informal and formal provision of support to CC physicians and nurses concerning the often very significant stresses associated with providing cancer care; and the professional rewards of knowing that CC patients are receiving truly outstanding, comprehensive care.

These services are also very highly valued by patients and their family members. Patients really want to receive comprehensive, caring treatment. The OSCS is another tangible manifestation to patients that the hospital cancer program is committed to providing "whole person" care. Family members also greatly benefit from and appreciate the access to a wide range of services the OSCS provides or helps ensure are provided.

ONCOLOGY CARE AND THE MISSION OF AHS

With respect to oncology care and the mission of AHS, the authors assert the following:

1. The current models of oncology supportive care services, and standards concerning their role in hospital ambulatory cancer center services, represent a major positive shift towards comprehensive, patient/family-centered, multidisciplinary team, longitudinally coordinated care.
2. The development of comprehensive oncology supportive care services is now the national standard of quality care for hospital cancer programs/ambulatory cancer centers. Implementation of fully developed OSCS can bring many clinical, operational, and business benefits to LLUAHSC/AHS hospitals which have cancer programs.
3. This comprehensive, multidisciplinary team OSCS model supports the appropriate role and specialized expertise of psycho-oncology and psychosocial oncology services providers, but fundamentally puts the patient, rather than the individual provider, at the core of the much expanded patient care delivery system.
4. The newer models of hospital ambulatory cancer center services, and of the role of OSCS within hospital cancer programs, represent a highly developed practical expression of the general mission statements and organizational vision of AHS institutions, including LLUMC/LLUAHSC, as applied to cancer care.
5. The more general development of comprehensive patient supportive care services is an equally powerful and applicable model for LLUAHSC/LLUMC/AHS in providing medical care in the inpatient setting and in the provision of chronic disease management care in the hospital ambulatory care setting.

OSCS MODELS: EDUCATIONAL AND RESEARCH OPPORTUNITIES

There exist specific educational opportunities for LLUAHSC/ LLUMC and other AHS institutions which provide advanced health care professional education to the range of disciplines which commonly comprise OSCS. These clinicians include psychiatrists, psychologists, oncology social workers, oncology dietitians, chaplains, cancer pain physicians, cancer pain/symptom management/palliative care service nurses, pharmacists, and potentially professional providers of integrative medicine and complementary therapy services.

The goals of these clinician education programs now go beyond developing individual professional knowledge and expertise to developing individual professional capabilities to work effectively in OSCS multidisciplinary teams and to developing the expertise to work most effectively with oncologist physicians, nurses, and other primary cancer care clinicians in the HACC and hospital inpatient environment.

The OSCS model also has implications for clinical research and clinical research training. While discipline-specific research questions can still be addressed, clinical research and research training can now expand to interdisciplinary approaches to research and health services delivery research related to the effectiveness of OSCS. The OSCS model also encourages and facilitates clinical and services research collaborations between OSCS team members and oncologist physicians/nurses who engage in "traditional" oncology clinical trials.

LLUAHCS/LLUMC/AHS LEADERSHIP OPPORTUNITIES

Given the religious heritage, culture, and mission statements of the above organizations, these institutions can be national leaders in developing innovative patient-centered supportive care services which fully realize organizational mission at the practical level of patient care delivery. This is an ongoing leadership challenge from the standpoints of vision, priority, creativity, and effectiveness in overcoming practical obstacles to implementation.

LLUMC and AHS hospital cancer program leadership should carefully review the structure of their cancer services, and particularly the development and function of their oncology supportive care services in the light of related national quality standards, oncology P4P programs, and coming fundamental provider payment system reform initiatives outlined above.

The provision of comprehensive, multidisciplinary OSCS is not only fundamentally consistent with LLUMC/AHS mission statements, but it is a key to the provision of the highest quality cancer patient care and the most successful hospital cancer services business models. This is an example where doing right from the clinical care delivery standpoint and doing well from a business standpoint are mutually compatible.

Using the principles of the OSCS model, LLUMC/AHS leaders should carefully review the status of the development and integration of patient supportive care services within their full spectrum of inpatient and ambulatory care services.

CAN THERE BE AN IMPROVED AHS VERSION OF OSCS?

From the authors' limited experiential perspective, in general AHS institutions have consistently had leadership which is strongly committed to the Adventist heritage of the institution and to realizing their institution's mission. Obviously depending on the size of the institution and the nature of its employee mix, preserving that strong cultural sense of mission throughout the entire organization is an ongoing leadership challenge. The authors' experience, based on the LLUAHSC/AHS organizations with which there is some extended (if limited in intensity) relationship, is that AHS institutions have in general succeeded admirably in preserving this institutional commitment to mission.

The question has appropriately been raised whether the uniquely Adventist Christian philosophy of healing can further inform and elevate the care of cancer patients in AHS institutions beyond the principles and practice of the OSCS delivery model described in this paper. Certainly having the OSCS team composed of members who are individually and collectively committed to providing comprehensive services which reflect the healing ministry of Christ is very important. This individual professional and OSCS MDT commitment can and should be evident to all those touched by the team.

Having this committed OSCS team providing care as part of a larger CC/hospital cancer patient care delivery system, where all primary cancer care providers (physicians, nurses, other clinicians, ancillary clinical care providers, and other professional staff members) are also highly committed to this comprehensive care and healing model adds additional benefit to patients and providers.

The cumulative impact of this commitment of all cancer care providers within AHS institutions should be that patients (and their family members) always sense that they are being cared for as integrated "bio-psycho-social-spiritual" beings, not simply as recipients of specific treatments directed towards their disease. While such a patient experience of comprehensive patient-centered care is not unique to AHS institutions, it should be powerfully pervasive within such institutions.

Probably the most important impact of the Adventist Christian philosophy of healing on cancer care delivery provided in AHS institutions should be the unwavering leadership commitment to creating and preserving this comprehensive patient/family-centered model of care in all organizational, operational, political, and financial circumstances. This sustained level of organizational leadership commitment would be a powerful testament that AHS leadership is absolutely determined to provide this model of care based on organizational mission, vision, and values. To do so successfully over time requires successful adaptation to changing organizational circumstances and needs while preserving the essence of the model.

AHS institutions can develop, implement, and sustain this model of care in widely varying hospital size and location circumstances.

However, this model is clearly more difficult to develop and maintain within smaller hospitals in more rural locations. In these circumstances, increased leadership commitment and creativity, appropriate use of community-based professional services and resources, and judicious use of telemedicine models for service delivery may all be required.

CONCLUSION

This paper has reviewed current models for delivery of comprehensive oncology supportive care services, and for the OSCS role in the hospital ambulatory cancer center and overall hospital cancer program services. These service models reflect a major shift in the model of cancer care excellence away from a narrow focus on the diagnosis and treatment of cancer to a broad focus on the comprehensive care of the patient.

The current OSCS model is fundamentally consistent with the mission and values of LLUAHSC/LLUMC and AHS. These organizations face both challenges and opportunities in implementing this OSCS model as part of their cancer programs and implementing the general supportive care services MDT model in other hospital inpatient and ambulatory care settings for other medical patient populations.

LLUAHSC/LLUMC/AHS institutions which offer health care professional education to the disciplines providing oncology or general patient supportive care services in the hospital setting can further strengthen their educational offerings by emphasizing the OSCS multidisciplinary model of care in the didactic and clinical training experiences they provide. The OSCS model also expands opportunities for clinical research models and research collaborations, which can and should be part of the education of the "OSCS disciplines."

This expanded educational focus will help prepare health care professional students for the far-reaching changes in the nation's health care system which focus on the provision of comprehensive, multidisciplinary, truly patient-centered care which is longitudinally coordinated. The OSCS model provides one opportunity in one domain of patient care and professional education to help LLUAHSC/LLUMC/AHS achieve their mission statements "To make man whole" and "To share God's love by providing physical, mental, and spiritual healing."

REFERENCES

Adventist Health: Mission, Vision and Values (n.d.). Retrieved July 1, 2008 from www.adventisthealth.com/aboutus/goDocDocument.asp?CN=77&DID=79.

Adventist Health System: Mission and Values (n.d.). Retrieved July 1, 2008 from www.ahss.org/AboutAHS/MissionValues/tabid/144/Default.aspx.

American Cancer Society (2007). *Cancer Facts and Figures 2007.* Atlanta, GA: American Cancer Society.

American College of Radiology (ACR) (n.d.). Retrieved July 23, 2008 from: www.acr.org/SecondaryMainMenuCategories/quality_safety/ro_section.aspx.

American College of Surgeons Commission on Cancer (2006). *Cancer Program Standards 2004, Revised Edition.* Chicago, IL: American College of Surgeons.

American Medical Association (AMA) (n.d.). Physician Consortium for Practice Improvement Performance Measure Status Report. Retrieved April 18, 2008 from www.ama-assn.org/ama1/pub/upload/mm/370/measures 110507.pdf.

American Society of Clinical Oncology (ASCO) (n.d.). Retrieved July 23, 2008 from www.asco.org/ASCO/Quality+Care+%26+Guidelines/Practice+Guidelines.

American Society of Clinical Oncology (ASCO) (2006). ASCO-ESMO Consensus Statement on Quality Cancer Care. *Journal of Clinical Oncology, 24,* 3498–3499.

American Society of Clinical Oncology (ASCO) (Spring 2008). Summary of QOPI™ Measures. Retrieved April 15, 2008 from www.asco.org/ASCO/Quality+Care+%26+Guidelines/Quality+Measurement+%26+Improvement/Quality+Oncology+Practice+Initiative.

Andersen, B., Yang, H., Farrar, W., Golden-Kreutz, D., Emery, C., Thornton, L., Young, D., & Carson, W. (2008). Psychological intervention improves survival for breast cancer patients: A randomized clinical trial. *Cancer, 113,* 3450–3458.

Association of Community Cancer Centers (2008). *Cancer Program Guidelines 2008, Chapter 4: Clinical Management and Supportive Care Services,* pp. 10–24. Retrieved April 16, 2008 from http://accc-cancer.org/publications/publications_cpguidelines.asp.

Carr, D., Goudas, L., Lawrence, D., Pirl, W., Lau, J., DeVine, D., Litt, M., Kupelnick, B., & Miller, K. (2002). Management of cancer symptoms: Pain, depression, and fatigue. *Agency for Healthcare Research and Quality Publication NO 02-E032.* Retrieved April 14, 2008 from //www.ahrq.gov/downloads/pub/evidence/pdf/cansymp/cansymp.pdf.

Centers for Medicare and Medicaid Services: Physician Quality Reporting Initiative: Overview (2008), PQRI. Retrieved April 17, 2008 from www.cms.hhs.gov/pqri/.

Elliott, L., Molseed, L.L., & McCallum, P.D. (Eds). (2006). *The clinical guide to oncology nutrition,* 2nd ed. Chicago, IL: American Dietetic Association.

Hewitt, M., Greenfield, S., & Stovall, E. (Eds.). (2006). *From cancer patient to cancer survivor: Lost in transition.* Washington, D.C.: The National Academies Press.

Holland, J., & Weiss, T. (2008). The new standard of quality cancer care: Integrating the psychosocial aspects in routine cancer from diagnosis through survivorship. *The Cancer Journal, 14,* 425–428.

Institute of Medicine (2007). *Cancer care for the whole patient: Meeting psychosocial health needs.* Washington, D.C.: National Academies Press.

Jim, H., & Jacobsen, P. (2008). Posttraumatic stress and posttraumatic growth in cancer survivorship: A review. *The Cancer Journal, 14,* 414–419.

Kaplar, M., Wachholtz, A., & O'Brien, W. (2004). The effect of religious and spiritual interventions on the biological, psychological, and spiritual outcomes of oncology patients: A meta-analytic review. *Journal of Psychosocial Oncology, 22,* 39–49.

Kristeller, J., Rhodes, M., Cripe, L., & Sheets, V. (2005). Oncologist assisted spiritual intervention study (OASIS): Patient acceptability and initial evidence of effects. *The International Journal of Psychiatry in Medicine, 35,* 329–347.

Krupski, T. L., Kwan, L., Afifi, A. A., & Litwin, M. S. (2005). Geographic and socioeconomic variation in the treatment of prostate cancer. *Journal of Clinical Oncology, 23,* 7881–7888

Laubmeier, K., Zakowski, S., & Bair, J. (2004). The role of spirituality in the psychological adjustment to cancer: A test of the transactional model of stress and coping. *International Journal of Behavioral Medicine, 11,* 48–55.

Loma Linda University Adventist Health Science Center: Loma Linda University Mission Statement (n.d.). Retrieved July 1, 2008 from www.llu.edu/mission/llumission.html.

McCoubri, R. C., & Davis, A. N. (2006). Is there a correlation between spirituality and anxiety and depression in patients with advanced cancer?

Support Care Cancer, 14, 379–385.

McCullough, M., Hoyt, W., & Larson, D. (2000). Religious involvement and mortality: A meta-analytic review. *Health Psychology, 19,* 211–222.

National Cancer Institute (n.d.). Surveillance Epidemiology and End Results (SEER); Cancer Stat Fact Sheets/Cancer of All Sites. Retrieved April 18, 2008 from http://seer.cancer.gov/statfacts/html/all.html.

National Comprehensive Cancer Network (NCCN) (n.d.). Retrieved July 23, 2008 from www.nccn.org/professionals/physician_gls/f_guidelines.asp.

National Comprehensive Cancer Network (NCCN) (n.d.). NCCN Clinical Practice Guidelines in Oncology™: Adult Cancer Pain V.1.2007. Retrieved April 16, 2008 from www.nccn.org/professionals/physician_gls/PDF/pain.pdf.

National Comprehensive Cancer Network (NCCN) (n.d.). NCCN Clinical Practice Guidelines in Oncology™: Distress Management V.1.2008. Retrieved April 16, 2008 from www.nccn.org/professionals/physician_gls/PDF/distress.pdf.

National Comprehensive Cancer Network (NCCN) (n.d.). NCCN Clinical Practice Guidelines in Oncology™: Palliative Care V.1.2008. Retrieved July 22, 2008 from www.nccn.org/professionals/physician_gls/PDF/palliativecare.pdf.

National Quality Forum (n.d.). List/Tables of Current National Voluntary Consensus Standards as of February 28, 2008 and of Candidate Consensus Standards as of March 24, 2008. Retrieved April 15, 2008 from http://www.qualityforum.org/.

National Quality Forum (2006). *A national framework and preferred practices for palliative and hospice care quality: A consensus report.* Washington, D.C.: National Quality Forum.

O'Mahony, S., Goulet, J., Kornblith, A., Abbatiello, G., Clarke, B., Kless-Siegel, S., Breitbart, W., & Payne, R. (2005). Desire for hastened death, cancer pain and depression: Report of a longitudinal observational study. *Journal of Pain Symptoms Management, 29,* 446–457.

Oncology Roundtable (2004). *Benchmarking clinical quality: Best practices for elevating the standard of cancer care.* Washington, D.C.: The Advisory Board Company.

Oncology Roundtable (2005). *Clinical quality strategy: 25 imperatives for instituting a world-class quality program.* Washington, D.C.: The Advisory Board Company.

Oncology Roundtable (2007). Inside the Mind of the Cancer Patient. *National*

Membership Meeting 2007, Investing for Excellence: Securing Strategic Advantage Through Principled Patient Service and Operational Reform, 95–103. Washington, D.C.: The Advisory Board Company.

Prometheus Payment, Inc.: Igniting Payment Reform (n.d.). Retrieved July 17, 2008 from www.prometheuspayment.org.

Rummans, T., Clark, M., Sloan, J., Frost, M., Bostwick, J., Atherton, P., Johnson, M., Gamble, G., Richardson, J., Brown, P., Mortensen, J., Miller, J., Piderman, K., Huschka, M., Girardi, J., & Hanson, J. (2006). Impacting quality of life for patients with advanced cancer with a structured multidisciplinary intervention: A randomized controlled trial. *Journal of Clinical Oncology, 24,* 635–642.

Salsman, J., Brown, T., Brechting, E., & Carlson, C. (2005). The link between religion and spirituality and psychological adjustment: The mediating role of optimism and social support. *Personality and Social Psychology Bulletin, 31,* 522–535.

Shih, Y. C. T., & Halpern, M. T. (2008). Economic evaluations of medical care interventions for cancer patients: How, why, and what does it mean? *CA: Cancer Journal for Clinicians, 58,* 231–244.

Stefanek, M., McDonald, P., & Hess, S. (2004). Religion, spirituality and cancer: Current status and methodological challenges. *Psycho-Oncology, 14,* 450–463.

Strouse, T. B., Flanagan, F., Kerrihard, T., Williams, C., & Wolcott, D. L. (2006). Managing cancer pain in a 24-hour outpatient cancer center. *Journal of Supportive Oncology, 4,* 351–354.

Tarakeshwar, N., Vanderwerker, L., Paulk, E., Pearce, M., Kasl, S., & Prigerson, H. (2006). Religious coping is associated with the quality of life of patients with advanced cancer. *Journal of Palliative Medicine,* 8, 646–657.

Thune-Boyle, I., Stygall, J., Keshtgar, M., & Newman, S. (2006). Do religious/spiritual coping strategies affect illness adjustment in patients with cancer? A systematic review of the literature. *Social Science & Medicine, 63,* 151–164.

US Department of Health and Human Services (November 21, 2007). *Report to congress: Plan to implement a medicare hospital value-based purchasing program.* Washington, D.C.: Centers for Medicare and Medicaid Services.

White, E. G. (1905). *Ministry of Healing.* Washington, D.C.: Review and Herald.

Wolcott, D. L., Wolosin, R. J., Macdonald, J. S., & Strouse, T. B. (2008). Cancer patients' use of supportive care services and cancer center services satisfaction. *Journal of Clinical Oncology, 26,* 20641.

Section 5

Education and Training

Supervision of Spiritual Issues in Psychotherapy Training: Contributions from an Adventist Worldview

Barbara Couden Hernandez

Supervision is a privileged mentoring relationship between a therapist in training and a clinician with a wider vision of therapy due to advanced education, experience, or skill. Literature abounds regarding the ethics, techniques, and processes of supervision. However, a Seventh-day Adventist (SDA) perspective on supervision, particularly as it pertains to therapy with spiritual and religious issues, has not been elucidated. Seventh-day Adventism is mentioned in the behavioral health literature as a feature of relational experience (Ali & Naidoo, 1999; Lee, 2007; Patzer & Helm, 2007) or as it pertains to health practices (Parmer & Rogers, 1997). In their foundational work, Fayard, Harding, Murdoch, and Brunt (2007) set forth dimensions of psychotherapy which are significantly influenced by SDA beliefs. This paper is an attempt to articulate what an SDA worldview contributes to supervision practices and attitudes. The remainder of this chapter will expand on the guiding principles of Aten and Hernandez (2004) regarding an SDA worldview for supervision of clinicians who work with spiritually oriented clients.

SUPERVISION AS DISCIPLESHIP

As I begin supervision with new therapist trainees, I often ask them to conceptualize their work with patients or clients in terms of a metaphor. This yields interesting images such as teacher, guide, walking companion, or partner. One family therapist's word picture vividly portrayed her perspective on this delicate helping role: "I join with the family to learn their dance; then I begin to lead." Surely, joining and maintaining a trusting relationship are central themes in mentoring relationships whether between therapist and client(s) or supervisor and supervisee.

Christians are given a wonderful ideal for supervision in the example of the kind and tender mentoring that Jesus provided to His disciples. These twelve men attached themselves to Him at His invitation. In studying the life of Christ, one can see that the disciples were mentored in several different ways. First, they learned by observation: "When he saw the crowds, he had compassion on them, because they were harassed and helpless, like sheep without a shepherd" (Matt. 9:36, NIV). They witnessed His gracious interactions and saw how He managed issues of power and privilege by manifesting kind regard for people without social stature: women, children, lepers, and Samaritans. Christ's parables of everyday agrarian life, His willingness to mingle with people of ill repute such as tax collectors and prostitutes, as well as His fearless contact with Pharisees, the spiritual stuffed shirts of the day, demonstrated the value of meeting people where they are. As the disciples were loved by Jesus, they in turn began the process of learning that divine love heals bodies and souls.

Second, Jesus taught the disciples by didactic means and by entertaining their questions. He helped them understand, as much as they could comprehend, issues related to His mission and the purposes of God. They were able to ask Him questions about the meaning of the parables as well as issues about the coming Kingdom. They brought to Him issues of justice, forgiveness, and existential concerns: "Who sinned, this man or his parents?" (John 9:2, NIV). Even though they were unable to understand many seemingly enigmatic things that He told them and were fearful of asking for clarification, Christ was constant in instructing them directly and through His conversations with others.

Third, Jesus paced instruction and spiritual activities according to what the disciples could assimilate. For example, after sending them out two by two into the surrounding communities, Jesus took them to a secluded place to help them process and consolidate their experiences. He withdrew from them when the crowds were about to forcefully put Him forward as a civic leader. He was mindful of their development when He stated, "You do not realize now what I am doing, but later you will understand" (John 13:7, NIV). By providing a learning base of activities, instruction, and example, Christ built a foundation upon which they would be able to carry forward His work after He was no longer with them.

Fourth, Jesus prayed for His disciples. Perhaps one of the most loving prayers is recorded in John 17. "I pray for them…for they are yours….Protect them by the power of your name" (John 17:9, 11, NIV). After Jesus did all that He could to prepare them for lives of service, He commended them to God's care knowing that the seeds sown during times of their spiritual infancy would yield a bountiful return as they matured.

The first three forms of Christ's mentorship—demonstration of skills (Zarski, Sand-Pringle, Greenbank, & Cibik, 1991) and apprentice learning (Schulman, 2005; White & Russell, 1997), didactic education (Anderson, Schlossberg, & Rigazio-DeGilio, 2000; Aten, Boyer, & Tucker, 2007), and attention to the developmental needs of supervisees (Bischoff, Barton, Thober, & Hawley, 2002; Protinsky & Coward, 2001)—are common themes in supervision literature. Considerably less is written regarding prayer or other Christian features of supervision.

In keeping with Christ's spiritual concern for His disciples, Butman and Kruse (2007) suggest that Christian supervisors need to take a holistic approach to the spiritual development of their supervisees. They recommend helping supervisees to become "uncommonly decent" human beings by learning how to be gracious, respectful, and to act with integrity in all things (p. 308). This may mean that Christian supervisees learn to speak the truth in love even though their input may not be what the clients wish to hear. In addition, the authors recommend that supervisors discuss the supervisees' spiritual growth and take a mentoring approach to them that goes beyond the mere teaching of therapy skills. Sorenson (2004) describes the importance of the supervisors' transparency regarding their own spiritual experiences and their bearing upon therapy as a means to experiential learning of supervisees. Jones (2007) recommends that supervisors utilize spiritual assessments such as a spiritual genogram with supervisees in preparation for their work with clients. However, it is important to carefully consider how to balance the ethical standards of one's profession with these recommendations in order to avoid performing therapy with supervisees, imposing the supervisor's values, or unethically using one's position of power as a supervisor. Pointing out areas that impact the supervisee's effectiveness may suffice, along with the encouragement to address personal issues with the therapist.

Two other elements central to Christianity frame supervision from an SDA worldview. The first is the power of relationship and the second is the power of prayer. Hubble, Duncan, and Miller's (1999) work on the common factors in therapy highlight the role of relationship, or the therapeutic alliance, in promoting change. This research validates the example of Jesus' warmth and goodness as He interacted with the disciples and those whom He sought to help. This element is described more fully later in the paper.

Prayer keeps alive our belief in a Creator who is able to do "exceedingly abundantly above all that we ask or think" (Eph. 3:20, KJV), whether that is in the lives of our clients or within our own personal lives. There is value in helping supervisees understand that knowledge and skills have their limitations but that God is able to work beyond the therapy room to move clients toward wholeness in ways that we as human therapists often fall short of doing. This also underscores the fact that therapists are not God, but rather His instruments.

I was recently approached by an intern who was very worried about his client's safety due to severe partner abuse. The intern had previously consulted with me on several occasions about how to proceed in this complex case. However, neither my recommendations nor those of other consulting clinicians had brought about any positive change for the victim. When interventions based on legal advice were ineffective and the client dropped out of therapy, the intern was scarcely able to conceal his dismay. After processing the difficulty he was having as he watched the client make poor choices and resist his efforts to help, we prayed together. Noting that we had no power to influence the outcome further, we put the client in God's hands and asked Him to continue to move her toward healing and wholeness. Including prayer in our supervision time served to remind the intern that the ministry of the Holy Spirit and involvement of other people in the client's life could help to mobilize her to make the necessary changes. An interesting discussion ensued regarding free will, self determination, and the job of therapy which sometimes is intended merely to "sow the seeds" that will benefit the client at a later date. This comforted the intern considerably by encouraging him to focus on his own countertransference issues and by recognizing the limitations that accompany his mandate to make reasonable and informed efforts to promote change in his clients. As I recognized his struggle and dedication to his personal and professional growth, I prayed for him several times over the next few days.

We have a great Exemplar who has shown us what infinite patience is when working with our supervisees. The pacing of learning opportunities according to the supervisees' level of development, the ability for learning both by observing therapy and practicing their skills on their own, and assistance understanding the process of therapy are all elements of Christ's method of mentorship.

We look now at some of the ways that spirituality and religion can be addressed in therapy and how supervisors can encourage interns and trainees to work with clients from various faith traditions. The following model was created by Aten and Hernandez (2004) as a way to incorporate issues of spirituality in supervision. The following is an expansion of this article in order to apply the model more specifically to SDA supervision issues.

A MODEL FOR RELIGIOUS INTEGRATION IN THERAPY

Using the eight domains from Stoltenberg and Delworth's (1987) integrative developmental model (IDM), Aten and Hernandez (2004) identified specific supervisor functions for the integration of religion in supervision. Regardless of the format of supervision—either live supervision through a one-way mirror, by case discussion, or via co-therapy—these domains are helpful to address with supervisees in order to appropriately assess and include client beliefs in therapy. A clear understanding of the client's worldview or of the diversity within a family in terms of ideology and spiritual practice is necessary in order to promote change sensitively.

INTERVENTIONS

The span of attitudes within the SDA church toward psychological interventions ranges from the belief that therapy is "of the devil" to its polar opposite belief that the Gospel is merely a collection of positive self-help aids. Devout SDA therapists in training sometimes consider therapy a platform for proselytizing. They may think that being a Christian and a therapist must by definition include use of Scripture references and prayer in their work by "Giving the trumpet a certain sound." This phrase, used by Ellen White (1904), was intended to spur the young SDA church to make ready the world for the second coming of Christ. When erroneously applied to therapy, this amounts to trying to set clients straight in regards to perceived moral lapses, spiritual views, or variance from the therapist's values. This attitude aligns with angry feedback I was given once by a pastor that unless baptisms resulted from therapy, my work was worthless. Aside from the obvious ethical implications of imposing one's beliefs and the devaluation of therapy as a healing art used to relieve suffering, the therapeutic impasses that result from this short-sighted approach require swift and tactful supervisory intervention.

Eck (2002) provides an excellent list of spiritual interventions that explicitly reference religious beliefs. Doherty's (1999) model of addressing religious concerns through the domain of moral values, spirituality, or clinical insight is most helpful in working with individuals whose beliefs differ from those of the therapist. A number of excellent texts also exist that provide guidance for therapists who wish to utilize spiritual resources in therapy (Aten & Leach, 2008; Helmeke & Sori, 2006; Onedera, 2007; Walsh, 2003).

Some therapists in training have seen little modeling in their social lives of spiritual interactions which do not coerce, manipulate, or shame clients for beliefs or moral behaviors that vary from their own. It is incumbent on the SDA supervisor to point supervisees to the example of Jesus Christ. While on this earth, much of His time was spent with people who were social and moral outcasts of the day and whose behaviors, even existence, were problematic in Jewish society: tax collectors, lepers, prostitutes, uncouth and unlearned individuals. "As He relieved their suffering, the truths He taught were associated with His acts of mercy, and were thus riveted in the memory" (White, 1940, p. 87). This is the God-With-Us (Matt. 1:23) approach to therapeutic interaction: a practice in which the therapeutic relationship embodies an experiential corrective emotional or spiritual experience. This is not necessarily in the absence of addressing clients' moral choices or, as Doherty (1995) suggests, serving as a moral compass in therapy. It is, however, a way of interacting that is Christ-like and that includes warmth, expression of concern for the individual, gentleness, and acceptance. This may be balanced with kind but firm confrontation, emphasis on personal accountability, and careful but gracious questioning. It may or may not include explicit reference to God, religion, or spirituality. In the book *Ministry of Healing*, Ellen White (1909) addressed physicians in the chapter "Mind Cure": "When the love and sympathy that Christ manifested for the sick is combined with the physician's knowledge, his very presence will be a blessing" (p. 245). The SDA supervisor thus not only focuses on the body of knowledge that guides her discipline to make therapeutic decisions, but also on promoting a healing relationship between supervisees and their clients through use of self.

ASSESSMENT

Not everyone is religious or desires spiritual issues to be addressed in therapy. This is an important issue to discuss with supervisees: Do they feel comfortable assessing clients' religious beliefs? Do they think that therapy is not the place to discuss religious concerns? Do they know how to recognize when clients use religion to skirt other pressing therapeutic issues? Inexperienced clinicians indeed often have difficulty differentiating between religious beliefs and psychopathology. For example, as an intern my therapeutic work was continually detoured by a client's explanations of her New Age beliefs of "third eye" communication until I realized she was exhibiting magical thinking consistent with schizotypal personality disorder.

There are at least five reasons for completing a religious assessment as part of the intake process (Richards & Bergin, 2005): (1) to enhance empathic attunement based on a clear understanding of the client's views, (2) to determine whether the client's religious views have a deleterious or salutary effect on the presenting problem, (3) to identify beliefs and religious community resources, (4) to match appropriate religiously oriented interventions, and (5) to identify unresolved religious issues as potential therapeutic foci. Religious beliefs and spiritual practices may indeed contribute to clients' presenting problems in such instances as the dissolution of mixed orientation marriages (Hernandez & Wilson, 2007) or variations of perceptions regarding domestic abuse due to the blending of ethnicity and religion (Poling, 2006). It is prudent to encourage supervisees to explore the range of spiritual and religious assessments to select one or two that they can easily use as part of the intake process.

Hodge (2005) offers five formalized qualitative assessment tools that provide a format for therapeutic exploration. These include a list of standardized questions, as well as the spiritual history, spiritual lifemap, spiritual genogram, and spiritual ecogram. Other qualitative tools include the spiritual life review with the elderly (Helmeke, 2006); spiritual journey mapping with gay, lesbian, or bisexual clients (MacDonald, 2006); and informal questions such as, "How do your personal religious beliefs influence your current concerns?"

In order to frame questions that assist the therapist to understand the role of religion in clients' lives, Richards and Bergin (2005) recommend query that elucidates the following: (1) beliefs about the role of God in a their experience, (2) religious affiliation, (3) the degree of adherence to beliefs and practices, (4) religious coping style (see Pargament, Murray-Swank, & Tarakeshwar, 2005), (5) spiritual identity and spiritual self-worth, (6) perceptions of how God views them personally, (7) congruence between beliefs and lifestyle or behaviors, (8) understanding of major doctrinal issues, and (9) spiritual maturity and religious development.

Formal assessment instruments include *Index of Core Spiritual Experiences* (Kass, Friedman, & Lesserman, 1991), the *Religious Commitment Inventory* (Worthington et al., 2003), *Inventory on Religiousness* (Rayburn, 2004), and *Religious-Spiritual Assessment* (Richards & Bergin, 1997). Readers are referred to *Measures of Religiosity* (Hill & Hood, 1999) for a compilation of over 120 assessments that address religious experience.

INDIVIDUAL AND CULTURAL DIFFERENCES

Understanding one's religious affiliation does not necessarily predict clarity about a client's practices, orthodoxy, or attitudes about God. For example, one evening I joined a Jewish colleague for dinner who ordered a pork chop and washed it down with a shrimp cocktail. Similarly, new clinicians are often exposed to variations of behaviors that are viewed as acceptable and consistent with clients' religious views but which are morally or spiritually repugnant to the therapist. This is evident in the judgments frequently made about SDAs whose attitudes and behaviors seem to be correlated to geographic regional norms. However, within each region is found a plethora of contextual factors that influence religious attitudes such as ethnicity, socioeconomic status, and education. As plurality and globalization increase, openness and sensitivity to the views of others are imperative.

There are two potential pitfalls expressed by therapists in training about this domain. It is often assumed that there must be wholesale acceptance of others' views without questioning congruence between belief and behavior, or without examining how clients' views serve them. The opposite extreme is to question clients in a leading manner, or to challenge the correctness of their beliefs or behaviors on the basis of the therapist's belief system. However, it is important that as SDAs we remember Christ's words, "Other sheep have I which are not of this fold" (John 10:16, ERV). In *Ministry of Healing*, Ellen White told physicians that when working with the very ill, "no word of creed or controversy should be spoken" (p. 120). Coach supervisees to first assist clients to deal with crisis issues, and then assist in making changes that improve their wellness and quality of life. Helping clients to think through religious beliefs that are related to their presenting problems may or may not occur. As stated earlier, Doherty (1999) points out that most issues have moral, clinical, and spiritual components. When a client views a behavior only through a spiritual lens without realizing the moral or clinical implications of this perspective, sensitive questioning by the therapist challenges the client to expand his or her lens to incorporate other important domains. Likewise, Doherty (1995) offers several steps of increasing intensity by which to address moral issues that impact clients in therapy.

Supervisees can obtain a clearer understanding of within-group differences and variations from group to group by becoming informed of the religious and cultural bases for their clients' beliefs and practices. It is helpful for clinicians to examine their own experiences with religion, spirituality, and various cultural groups by creating spiritual (Frame, 2000) and cultural (Hardy & Laszloffy, 1995) genograms. This is particularly useful when working with former SDAs whose early interactions with the church have been a polarizing experience. Identifying the sources of countertransference assists supervisees to consolidate their own beliefs and stay differentiated from their clients.

After constructing his own five-generation spiritual genogram, one supervisee was surprised to notice his tendency to be dismissive of religious beliefs expressed by male clients. His genogram examination highlighted the ways in which religious education and personal spirituality were systematically encouraged and embodied in the matriarchs of the family, while his male relatives tended to be irreligious, unreliable parental figures. These findings led the supervisee to seek therapy to deal with unresolved issues surrounding religion and his experience with parenting. His newfound awareness enabled him to follow his natural curiosity with more freedom and spontaneity as he addressed religious issues of other male clients.

INTERPERSONAL ASSESSMENT AND DIFFERENTIATION

Supervision involves professional socialization through instruction, modeling, and skill building. Another facet of supervision is professional mentoring. Collins (1993) describes a four-stage model of mentoring within social work education. *Interaction* involves instructional actions of a supervisor meant to model professional behaviors or skills. The development of a warm and respectful relationship between supervisor and supervisee marks the *investment* stage. *Facilitation* occurs as the supervisee begins to internalize the skills and values taught by the supervisor. Finally, *adaptation* occurs as the two begin to relate as peers. Serving as a mentor in addition to having a history of being mentored predicts the highest levels of professional satisfaction (Collins, 1994).

These findings are intuitive to Christians for whom mentorship is somewhat similar to the process that the disciples followed during their time with Jesus. Following the example of Christ, while the supervisor is intent on enhancing growth of the supervisee, her goal is not to obliterate the supervisee's unique characteristics, views, or practices in therapy. The supervisor assists the supervisee in developing a unique therapeutic style which may or may not be similar to her own, but which is based on sound practice principles. This process is progressive in nature and depends on the supervisor's encouragement for professional differentiation to take place.

Assessing interpersonal and spiritual differentiation may be initiated by a discussion of the Gestalt concept of confluence (O'Leary, 1997). This contact interruption may be mistaken for empathy or admiring emulation of the supervisor. Explicitly encouraging the supervisee to consider his or her unique ideas in supervision provides two useful functions. In addition to promoting the emergence of the supervisee's developing professional identity, the supervisee learns by example how to perform this same intervention with clients who may struggle with approval issues. Through parallel process (Kaiser, 1997), interactive dynamics between supervisor and supervisee are eventually transmitted to the supervisee-client relationship.

Basic to a strong working relationship is the formation and maintenance of appropriate boundaries. The relationship with therapists in training often mirrors other formative relationships in the supervisee's experience. Accompanying projections and introjects often require explicit acknowledgement and referral for personal therapy. A warm, trusting relationship often develops over time to become a mutually enjoyable experience. Supervisees often muse aloud about their religious and existential concerns, asking the supervisor for input as they refine their ideas. It is helpful to bear in mind that there may be a temptation to weigh in on the supervisee's issues more than may be helpful or requested. Remembering that supervision is to support the best professional interests of a therapist in training helps supervisors monitor comments they may make about their personal or religious experiences or views. Periodically reviewing the ethical guidelines of one's professional discipline in supervision sessions can clarify expectations as well as prompt the supervisee to consider how he maintains boundaries with his clients.

THEORETICAL ORIENTATION

Historically, psychology has labeled religion and its adherents as neurotic, psychosexually repressed, and as a sort of useful but unhealthy mental aid (Bankhart, 1997; Blazer, 1998; Brown & Srebalus, 1996). Commenting upon the current psychological therapy of her day, Ellen White (1862) clumped together phrenology, psychology, and mesmerism as being tools in the hands of Satan. Over two decades later she wrote, "The sciences which treat of the human mind are very much exalted. They are good in their place; but they are seized upon by Satan as his powerful agents to deceive and destroy souls" (White, 1884). This warning appears to discourage individuals from participating in therapy, particularly in conjunction with statements found in *Ministry of Healing* such as, "If you do not feel lighthearted and joyous, do not talk of your feelings. Cast no shadow upon the lives of others" (p. 488) and "It is not wise to look to ourselves and study our emotions. If we do this, the enemy will present difficulties and temptations that weaken faith and destroy courage" (p. 249). These statements would appear to support cognitive-behavioral methods and strength-based approaches while discouraging experiential models. SDA therapists in training often question whether there is one theoretical framework that is spiritually preferable to others. A full response to this issue is outside the scope of this chapter (see Burt, Mee-Lee, & Anderson chapters for a more complete discussion of this topic). However, it is interesting to note that although Ellen White warned against quackery and unsafe practices of her day, her own sons underwent a phrenological examination from a Dr. Jackson in Dansville, New York. She wrote, "Dr. Jackson gave an accurate account of the disposition and organization of our children. He pronounces Willie's head to be one of the best that has ever come under his observation. He gave a good description of Edson's character and peculiarities. He enjoined upon him outdoor exercise and not much study. I think this examination will be worth everything to Edson." (See Ellen G. White's *Manuscript Releases* [1990], vol. 6, p. 347). Ellen White appeared to be open to scientific advances of her day and although animal magnetism and clairvoyance had metaphysical components, phrenology did not (*Phrenology: Fad and Science—A Nineteenth Century American Crusade).*

There are numerous biblical principles that support the use of psychological, relational, and spiritual interventions in therapy. Discussion with SDA supervisees about the strengths and limitations of various therapeutic modalities allows therapists in training to determine what is most consistent with their beliefs, values, and therapeutic style.

A number of authors have discussed the religious integration efforts in psychoanalysis (Aron, 2004), Rational Emotive therapy (Ellis, 2000), postmodern therapies (Jankowski, 2003), Adler's approach (Weiss-Rosmarin, 1990), cognitive-behavioral therapy (D'Souza & Rodrigo, 2004), and family systems therapies (Cloud, Townsend, Carder, & Brawand, 1995; Friedman, 1985). Discussion of Ellen White's comments with attention to the guiding principles laid out in her work can prevent rigid literalist interpretation of her writings and promote the construction of helpful therapeutic practices that address the complexity of today's individuals, couples, and families.

PROBLEM CONCEPTUALIZATION

A major function of spiritually oriented supervisors is to model integration through case conceptualizations (Aten, Boyer, & Tucker, 2007). Routinely inquiring about religious affiliation and practices of clients helps therapists in training to be cognizant of how religion may influence their clients' presenting issues. Socratic questioning or a hermeneutic discussion about client beliefs may provide the supervisee with multiple entry points for intervention. For example, one intern reported that a bullied twelve-year-old client had an imaginary friend who was not visible to anyone but herself. This "friend" claimed to be the spirit of her beloved dead grandmother. Holding traditional SDA beliefs about the state of the dead, this intern construed her client's reports as evidence of demonic harassment and was alarmed about her spiritual welfare. As we explored the meaning of the imaginary friend and the communications reported, it became clear that this girl had never dealt with her grandmother's death and had unresolved loss issues. She also had no friends at school, quite possibly because her social skills and chaotic family life prevented social integration. It was helpful to clarify the principle of identifying the least pathologic explanation for client symptoms as a starting place for therapy. My supervisee's goals changed from delivering a sermonette on soul sleep to helping her client establish friendships while alternately grieving the loss of her grandmother. I explained that if our conceptualization from the least degree of pathology proved correct, positive change would occur and the "spirit" communications would cease, which, in fact, did stop within a short time. SDAs hold a number of unique beliefs that can augment our views of holistic client care. Ellen White's writings regarding self-care such as health maintaining behaviors, the role of a positive attitude, and contributing to the welfare of those less fortunate (White, 1973) may prove to provide a more well-rounded approach to treatment. The potential for incorporating elements of the health message in therapy by encouraging clients to adopt an exercise regimen can be helpful therapeutic adjuncts. This is true particularly when working with individuals with persistent mental illness who are reported to experience worse physical health and die twenty-five years earlier on average than other clients due to inactivity, smoking, obesity, and medication side effects (Elias, 2007).

Gingrich and Worthington (2007) point out that case conceptualization will differ according to the professional development of the supervisee. For example, new therapists in training are typically concerned with their skills and ability to manage the therapy hour while containing their anxiety. More advanced therapists are able to enter the worldview of their clients through empathic attunement, while licensed therapists are more likely to be able to simultaneously focus on the client's experience, their own experience, and movement in therapy. Jones (2007) suggests that Christian supervisors remain mindful of the spiritual development of their supervisees as this determines one's ability both to relate to God and to integrate spirituality in therapy. Through appropriate transparency about their own beliefs and relationship with God, supervisors encourage therapists in training to examine their religious ideas that will then influence their work. Support for this active mentoring process is an integral part of the SDA mission. "If we have been following Jesus step by step, we shall have something right to the point to tell concerning the way in which He has led us" (White, 1940, p. 340).

TREATMENT PLANNING

A treatment plan drawn up after conducting an intake can be considerably different than the treatment plan designed if a spiritual assessment is performed as part of the intake. This is also true of instances in which therapists are not afraid to probe moral and spiritual issues that are mentioned, or to serve as a moral consultant in therapy (Doherty, 1999). Clearly warning about typical fallout from inadvisable behaviors such as abandoning children, engaging in an affair, or failing to adhere to psychotropic medication regimens may require a change in goal setting and subsequent treatment planning.

For example, a devout Christian woman presented to therapy stated that she felt there was something in her past that prevented her from taking God at His word. Intake assessment revealed that she had previously been diagnosed with chronic major depression but had discarded her antidepressants after hearing a sermon which gave the impression that reliance on anything or anyone other than God was unacceptable. Over the last two weeks she had become increasingly tearful and incapable of caring for her four small children, three of whom were under the age of four. Supervision with the therapist involved role playing how to explain the moral aspects of her obligation to her children in the face of her increasingly disorganized and depressed state. The supervisor also recommended that her pastor be invited to attend a session the next day with the client. The ensuing session was pivotal for therapist, client, and pastor. The client was alarmed but motivated to reconsider psychotropic support after the therapist briefly summarized research findings regarding young children of depressed primary caregivers. The pastor had not realized that his words would be construed as condemnatory of parishioners with mental health concerns and he expressed support for the client to adhere to her antidepressant therapy. This was the therapist's first experience conducting a conjoint session with a clergy member and was delighted with the outcome. The treatment plan that would have resulted from the client's initial request for help was significantly different from the plan that included spiritual consultation with her pastor. It helped her explore her spiritual ideas regarding medication usage and assist her in making a moral choice regarding her ability to parent her children.

Therapists in training need encouragement to seek out spiritual resources in order to help them create treatment goals that are consistent with their clients' beliefs and practices. The vast majority of religious groups hold at least some values in common with SDAs which can be used to support change and growth in clients of different religions. Discussing goals with clients in view of their spiritual or religious experience strengthens congruence between beliefs and resulting behaviors.

PROFESSIONAL ETHICS

It would seem to be a fairly straightforward process to review legal and ethical issues in supervision. However, a number of ethics standards may confuse therapists. For example, the ethical requirement to avoid misrepresentation of the counselor's work is typically not considered when potential clients inquire as to whether one practices "Christian Counseling." Discussion concerning the difference between being a "Christian Counselor" and being a counselor who is a practicing Christian should clarify that the former connotes advanced training, certification, study, or affiliation with an organization that either grants certification or sets professional standards for Christian counseling. Being a therapist who happens to be a devout Christian but who has not engaged in study, affiliation, or training that forwards Christian counseling should not claim this specialization (ACA, 2005, Section C; APA, 2002, 5.01; AAMFT, 2001, 3.7; NASW, 2006, 1.04). Careful discussion and application of ethical standards in practice ensures that clients seeking both religiously oriented and nonreligious counseling may be ethically treated.

Religious clients are often concerned that the therapy process will in some way encourage them to violate their beliefs (McMinn, Chaddock, & Edwards, 1998). Interestingly, a number of SDA therapists fear that clients will request assistance in attaining a goal that violates the therapist's own values and beliefs. For example, individuals who request assistance in obtaining an abortion, leaving a spouse to continue an affair, or desiring to improve sexual function in a same-sex relationship lead many supervisees to either treat the client while ignoring their sense of internal conflict or immediately refer the clients to other therapists. It is helpful to encourage supervisees to discuss their ethical dilemmas in supervision or in an unscheduled phone consultation if warranted. Actual presenting issues often do not reflect the client's articulation or understanding of them. Therapist assumptions and premature referral should be avoided when possible.

For example, as an intern I once received a request to work with a transgendered person on his "personal issues." This caused me considerable dread before I met with him, as I was not knowledgeable about transgendered people or the gender-change process. As I internally catastrophized about the ethical dilemmas I was fearful of facing in regards to the client's sexual issues, my supervisor pointed out that until I knew what the real presenting problem was, I could not presume that my role was to help him decide which gender to assume, how to have a sexual relationship with another individual of either gender, or to help him do something that was against my own moral values. My supervisor's calming remarks prepared me to compassionately work with this client who had been living with the results of failed surgical procedures and an abusive partner. There were plenty of issues to address that improved my client's quality of life and his spiritual well-being without violating any of my beliefs. The complexity of the human condition that exists in a world created by a God who loves purity is part of endless debates by theologians, philosophers, and politicians. As mental health practitioners, we seek to heal and uplift the lot of our clients in every way possible.

> Every association of life calls for the exercise of self-control, forbearance, and sympathy. We differ so widely in disposition, habits, education, that our ways of looking at things vary. We judge differently. Our understanding of truth, our ideas in regard to the conduct of

> life, are not in all respects the same. There are no two whose experience is alike in every particular. The trials of one are not the trials of another. The duties that one finds light are to another most difficult and perplexing. (White, 1909, p. 483)

Some therapists will choose not to work with individuals or families who are dealing with issues that to the therapist are morally distasteful or unacceptable due to their religious views. While it is sometimes unwise to insist that supervisees do or do not work with various cases, it is critical that their concerns are voiced and explored in order to avoid unresolved issues which create therapist preoccupation, a therapeutic impasse, imposition of supervisee beliefs, or the exercise of undue influence.

Therapist disclosure statements, which are required in a number of states, include information such as educational background, office hours and emergency information, theoretical or practice approaches, and work with special populations. It is recommended that supervisors coach supervisees to clarify and articulate important aspects of therapy pertaining to spiritual integration as they create their own disclosure statement.

Chapelle (2000) outlines additional legal and ethical issues to be considered for those who include spiritual interventions in therapy. First, therapists must not hold themselves out as religious leaders and should clarify their role as therapists, as well as their purpose for utilizing spiritual interventions. Supervisees who are both therapists and clergy should function as the client's mental health providers and should take care that their remarks do not minimize the role of the client's own clergy. Additionally, it is important when working in prisons, schools, or other public venues to check with the agency administration to be certain that use of spiritual interventions will not jeopardize federal funding for the agency. Informed consent for use of spiritual interventions should be obtained at the outset of therapy. Subsequent religious discussions or interventions should be germane to the treatment issues.

Increasing research on empirically based spiritual interventions allows practitioners to utilize techniques that are consistent with several theoretical approaches to treat a variety of problems. Use of such interventions as well as how these contribute to the overall treatment goals must be documented, particularly for third-party reimbursement purposes. Any intervention, plan, or interaction must be weighed against the ethical mandate to provide assistance that is in the client's best interest and that promotes well-being.

CONCLUSION

Supervision by Seventh-day Adventist practitioners and educators requires spiritual discernment, knowledge of ethical and legal mandates, interest in the spiritual development of supervisees, and ability to model and integrate religion appropriately in the supervisory relationship. As Aten and Hernandez (2004) suggest, many religious clients appreciate the opportunity to speak candidly about their beliefs in therapy. Given that many mental health practitioners do not feel that their education provides this expertise (Shafranske, 1996; Shafranske & Malony, 1990), it is crucial that attention be given to this emerging emphasis in mental health care delivery. It is anticipated that this work provides a starting point for further discussion, development of practice guidelines and policy, and improved contributions to the lives of those clients and supervisees whom we serve.

REFERENCES

AAMFT (2001). *Code of Ethics.* Washington, D.C.: American Association of Marriage and Family Therapy.

ACA (2005). *ACA Code of Ethics.* American Counseling Association, www.counseling.org.

APA (2002). *Ethical principles of psychologists and code of conduct.* Washington, D.C.: American Psychological Association.

Ali, H. K., & Naidoo, A. (1999). Sex education sources and attitudes about premarital sex of Seventh-day Adventist youth. *Psychological Reports, 84*(1), 312.

Anderson, S. A., Schlossberg, M., & Rigazio-DeGilio, S. (2000). Family therapy trainees' evaluation of their best and worst supervision experiences. *Journal of Marital and Family Therapy, 26*(1), 79–91.

Aron, L. (2004). God's influence on my psychoanalytic vision and values. *Psychoanalytic Psychology, 21*(3), 442–451.

Aten, J. D., Boyer, M. C., & Tucker, B. T. (2007). Christian integration in clinical supervision: A conceptual framework. *Journal of Psychology and Christianity, 26*(4), 313–320.

Aten, J. D. & Hernandez, B. C. (2004). Addressing religion in clinical supervision: A model. *Psychotherapy: Theory, research, practice and training, 41*(2), 152–160.

Aten, J. D., & Leach, M. M. (Eds.) (2008). *Spirituality and the therapeutic process: A comprehensive resource from intake to termination.* Washington, D.C.: American Psychological Association.

Bankart, C. T. (1997). *Talking cures: A history of Eastern and Western psychotherapies.* Pacific Grove, CA: Brooks/Cole.

Bischoff, R. J., Barton, M., Thober, J., & Hawley, R. (2002). Events and experiences impacting the development of clinical self-confidence: A study of the first year of client contact. *Journal of Marital and Family Therapy, 28*(3), 371–382.

Blazer, D. (1998). *Freud vs. God: How psychiatry lost its soul and Christianity lost its mind.* Downers Grove, IL: InterVarsity Press.

Brown, D., & Srebalus, D. (1996). *Introduction to the counseling profession.* Needham Heights, MA: Allyn & Bacon.

Butman, R. E., & Kruse, S. J. (2007). On creating a healthy supervisory environment: A Christian relational and developmental perspective. *Journal of Psychology and Christianity, 26*(4), 307–312.

Chapelle, W. (2000). A series of progressive legal and ethical decision-making steps for using Christian spiritual interventions in therapy. *Journal of Psychology and Theology, 28*(1), 43–53.

Chen, C. T. (2007). Model of contact interruption, unfinished business, and psychological wellbeing. *Bulletin of Educational Psychology, 39*(1), 45–68.

Cloud, H., Townsend, J., Carder, D., & Brawand, A. (1995). *Secrets of your family tree: Healing for adult children of dysfunctional families.* Chicago: Moody Bible Institute.

Collins, P. (1993). The interpersonal vicissitudes of mentorship: An exploratory study of the field supervisor-student relationship. *The Clinical Supervisor, 11*, 121–135.

Collins, P. (1994). Does mentorship among social workers make a difference? An empirical investigation of career outcomes. *Journal of the National Association of Social Workers, 39,* 413–419.

D'Souza, R. F., & Rodrigo, A. (2004). Spiritually augmented cognitive behavioural therapy. *Australasian Psychiatry, 12*(2), 148–152.

Doherty, W. J. (1995). *Soul searching: Why psychotherapy must promote moral responsibility*. New York: Basic Books.

Doherty, W. J. (1999). Morality and spirituality in therapy. In F. Walsh (ed.), *Spiritual Resources in Family Therapy,* pp. 179–192. New York: Guilford Press.

Eck, B. E. (2002). An exploration of the therapeutic use of spiritual disciplines in clinical practice. *Journal of Psychology and Christianity, 21*, 266–280.

Elias, M. (2007). Mentally ill die 25 years earlier on average. *USA Today,* 5/3/2007, retrieved July 15, 2008 from http://www.usatoday.com/news/health/2007-05-03-mental-illness_N.htm.

Ellis, A. (2000). Can rational emotive behavior therapy (REBT) be effectively used with people who have devout beliefs in God and religion? *Professional Psychology: Research and Practice, 31*(1), 29–33.

Fayard, C., Harding, G., Murdoch, W., & Brunt, J. (2007). Clinical implications for psychotherapy from the Seventh-day Adventist tradition. *Journal of Psychology and Christianity, 26*(3), 207–217.

Frame, M. W. (2000). The spiritual genogram in family therapy. *Journal of Marital & Family Therapy, 26*(2), 211–216.

Friedman, E. H. (1985). *From generation to generation: Family process in church and synagogue.* New York: Guilford Press.

Gingrich, F., & Worthington, E. L. (2007). Supervision and the integration of faith into practice: Research considerations. *Journal of Psychology and Christianity, 26*(4), 342–355.

Hardy, K. V., & Laszloffy, T. A. (1995). The cultural genogram: Key to training culturally competent family therapists. *Journal of Marital and Family Therapy, 21*(3), 227–237.

Helmeke, K. B. (2006). "My spiritual life": Conducting a spiritual life review with the elderly. In K. B. Helmeke, C. Ford Sori (eds.), *The therapist's notebook for integrating spirituality in counseling, II*, pp. 115–126. New York: Haworth Press.

Helmeke, K. B., & Sori, C. Ford (eds.). (2006). *The therapist's notebook for integrating spirituality in counseling II.* New York: Haworth Press.

Hernandez, B. C., & Wilson, C. M. (2007). Another kind of ambiguous loss:

Seventh-day Adventist women in mixed orientation marriages. *Family Relations, 56*(2), 184–195.

Hill, P. C., & Hood, R. W. (1999). *Measures of religiosity.* Birmingham, AL: Religious Education Press.

Hodge, D. R. (2005). Spiritual assessment in marital and family therapy: A methodological framework for selecting among six qualitative assessment tools. *Journal of Marital and Family Therapy, 31*(4), 341–356.

Hubble, M. A., Duncan, B. L., & Miller, S. L. (eds.) (1999). *The heart and soul of change: What works in therapy.* Washington, D.C.: American Psychological Association.

Jankowski, P. J. (2003). Integrating postmodern therapies and spirituality: A solution to the contemporary crisis of the self. *Journal of Psychology and Christianity, 22*(3), 241–249.

Jones, J. W. (2007). Training supervisors to integrate psychology and Christianity. *Journal of Psychology and Christianity, 26*(4), 336–341.

Kaiser, T. L. (1997). *Supervisory relationships: Exploring the human element.* Belmont, CA: Thomson Brooks/Cole Publishing Co.

Kass, J. D., Friedman, R., & Lesserman, J. (1991). Health outcomes and a new index of spiritual experience. *Journal for the Scientific Study of Religion, 30*(2), 203–211.

Lee, C. (2007). Patterns of stress and support among Adventist clergy: Do pastors and their spouses differ? *Pastoral Psychology, 55*(6), 761–771.

MacDonald, S. V. (2006). Spiritual journey mapping with lesbian, gay, and bisexual clients. In K. B. Helmeke & C. Ford Sori (eds.), *The therapist's notebook for integrating spirituality in counseling, II,* 177–188. New York: Haworth Press.

McMinn, M. R., Chaddock, T. P., & Edwards, L. C. (1998). Psychologists collaborating with clergy. *Professional Psychology: Research and Practice, 29*(6), 564–570.

NASW (2006). *Code of ethics of the National Association of Social Workers.* Washington, D.C.: National Association of Social Workers.

O'Leary, E. (1997). Confluence versus empathy. *Gestalt Journal, 20*(1), 137–154.

Onedera, J. D. (2007). *The role of religion in marriage and family counseling.* New York: Routledge.

Pargament, K. I., Murray-Swank, N. A., & Tarakeshwar, N. (2005). An empirically based rationale for a spiritually-integrated psychotherapy. *Mental Health, Religion, and Culture, 8*(3), 155–165.

Parmer, T., & Rogers, T. (1997). Religion and health: Holistic wellness from the perspective of two African American church denominations. *Counseling and Values, 42*(1), 55–67.

Patzer, N. L., & Helm, H. W. (2007). Categories of success endorsed among religiously identified Seventh-day Adventist students. *Psychological Reports, 88*(3, Pt. 2), 1121–1128.

Phrenology: Fad and Science—A Nineteenth Century American Crusade, (1971). New Haven, CT: Yale University Press, pp. x, xi., as cited in H. E. Douglass, *Messenger of the Lord* (n.d.), accessed July 13, 2008 at http://www.whiteestate.org /books/mol/Chapt43.html#Phrenology.

Poling, J. N. (2006). Preventing family violence: An educational model. *Pastoral Psychology, Special Issue: Asian-American Reflections, 54*(4), 377–391.

Protinsky, H., & Coward, H. (2001). Developmental lessons of seasoned marital and family therapists: A qualitative investigation. *Journal of Marital and Family Therapy, 27*(3), 375–384.

Prouty, A. M., Helmeke, K. B., & Lyness, K. P. (2002). Opportunities for mentorship in supervision. *Family Therapy Magazine, 1*(1), 44–46.

Rayburn, C. (2004). Assessing students for morality education: A new role for school counselors. *Professional School Counseling, 7*(5), 356–362.

Richards, P. S., & Bergin, A. E. (1997). *A spiritual strategy for counseling and psychotherapy.* Washington, D.C.: American Psychological Association.

Richards, P. S., & Bergin, A. E. (2005). Religious and spiritual assessment. In P. S. Richards & A. E. Bergin, *A spiritual strategy for counseling and psychotherapy* (2nd ed.). Washington, D.C.: American Psychological Association.

Shafranske, E. P. (Ed.) (1996). Religion and the clinical practice of psychology. Washington, D.C.: American Psychological Association.

Shafranske, E. P., & Malony, H. N. (1990). Clinical psychologists' religious and spiritual orientations and their practice of psychotherapy. *Psychotherapy: Theory, Research, Practice, Training, 27*(1), 72–78.

Shulman, L. (2005). The clinical supervisor-practitioner working alliance: A parallel process. *Clinical Supervisor, 24*(1–2), 23–47.

Sorenson, R. (2004). *Minding spirituality.* Hillsdale, NJ: The Analytic Press.

Stoltenberg, C. D., & Delworth, U. (1987). *Supervising counselors and therapists.* San Francisco: Jossey-Bass.

Walsh, F. (2003). *Spiritual resources in family therapy.* New York: Guilford Press.

Weiss-Rosmarin, T. (1990). Adler's psychology and the Jewish tradition. *Individual Psychology: Journal of Adlerian Theory, Research, and Practice, 46*(1), 108–118.

White, E. G. (1862). Phrenology, psychology, mesmerism, and spiritualism. *Review & Herald*, February 18, quoted in H. E. Douglass (1998), *Messenger of the Lord: The prophetic ministry of Ellen G. White*. Nampa, ID: Pacific Press.

White, E. G. (1884). Science falsely so called. *Signs of the Times,* November 6.

White, E. G. (1888). *The great controversy*. Mountain View, CA: Pacific Press.

White, E. G. (1904). The day of the Lord is near and hasteth greatly. *Review and Herald,* November 24.

White, E. G. (1909). *Ministry of healing*. Mountain View, CA: Pacific Press.

White, E. G. (1940). *The Desire of Ages*. Mountain View, CA: Pacific Press.

White, E. G. (1973). *Evangelism*. Washington, D.C.: Review and Herald.

White, E. G. (1990). Manuscript Releases, volume 6. The complete Ellen G. White writings, retrieved March 14, 2009 from http://egwdatabase.whiteestate.org/nxt/gateway.dll?f=templates$fn=default.htm$vid=default

White, M. B., & Russell, C. S. (1997). Examining the multifaceted notion of isomorphism in marriage and family therapy supervision: A quest for conceptual clarity. *Journal of Marital and Family Therapy, 23*(3), 315–333.

Worthington, E. L., Wade, N. G., & Hight, T. L. (2003). *Journal of Counseling Psychology, 50*(1), 84–96.

Zarski, J. J., Sand-Pringle, C., Greenbank, M., & Cibik, P. (1991). The invisible mirror: In-home family therapy and supervision. *Journal of Marital and Family Therapy, 17*(2), 133–143.

Psychiatry and the Spiritual Life: Loma Linda University's Curriculum for Psychiatry Residency Training

William Murdoch, Antonia Ciovica, and Carlos Fayard

Religion plays a central role in the lives of the general North American population, and religious beliefs often permeate the innermost aspects of one's life, shaping identity and life course and providing the framework for one's sense of hope, meaning, and suffering. In 1994, over 96% of North Americans endorsed a belief in God or a transcendent power, and 88% reported that religion is important in their lives (Gallup, 1994). Close to nine out of ten (86.7%) Americans identify with an organized religion, while only one in ten (10.8%) claims no religious affiliation (Dougherty, Johnson, & Polson, 2007); 65% pray between "a few times a week" and "several times a day," and 51% attend church between "once a month" and "several times a week" (Bader, Mencken, & Froese, 2007). Given the religiosity of the general population, of which 72% agreed with the statement, "My whole approach to life is based on my religion," it is interesting to note that only 46% of psychotherapists endorsed the same statement (although, with great variability among different mental health professions: from 62% of marriage and family therapists to 46% of clinical social workers, 39% of psychiatrists, and 33% of clinical psychologists endorsing the same statement; Bergin & Jensen, 1990). Further, while 46% of mental health professionals affirm that their personal life approach is based on their religion, only 29% feel that religious content is important in the treatment of "all or many of their clients" (Bergin & Jensen, 1990, p. 6). Bergin and Jensen conclude that the discrepancy between psychotherapists' personal religious involvement in their lives "may be due to the fact that training, education, and practice currently provide little place for such considerations" (p. 6). Further, a growing trend has been noted for mental health practitioners to embrace spirituality (Curlin, Lawrence, Odell, Chin, Lantos, Koenig, & Meador, 2007); however, this is not necessarily true for religion (Zinnbauer & Pargament, 2005). With this disconnect between the belief system and private lives of the general population and the delivery of mental health services, psychiatric practice continued to occur in the context of what has been termed a "religiosity gap" (Lukoff, Lu, & Turner, 1992; Sansome, Khatain, & Rodenhauser, 1990).

While historically religious adherence and beliefs have been considered pathological, essentially a "psychological crutch," inherent positive aspects and protective factors have more recently been identified. Religion and spirituality have been associated with better health, lower levels of pain, increased longevity, decreased depression and anxiety, and a number of other physical and psychological benefits (Ellison & Levin, 1998; Harrison, Edwards, Koenig, Bosworth, Decastro, & Wood, 2005; Koenig, 2007; Matthews, McCullough, Larson, Koening, Swyers, & Milano, 1998; Mueller, Plevak, & Rummans, 2001).

Further, research has highlighted considerable benefits of including issues related to religion and spirituality into psychiatric treatment (Bergin, 1988, 1991; Fleischman, 1990; Fukuyama & Sevig, 1999; Koening, 1998; Lovinger, 1984, 1990; Miller, 1988, 1999; Propst, 1988, 1996; Shafranske, 1996; Shafranske & Malony, 1996). Noteworthy findings point out that psychiatric practice that includes religion and spirituality leads to better clinical outcomes (Payne, Bergin, Bielema, & Jenkins, 1991; Pollner, 1989; Powell, Shahabi, & Thoresen, 2003; Propst, 1988); that religious patients prefer psychiatric treatment that cannot only accommodate, but also competently incorporate, issues related to their religious beliefs, values, and practices (Quackenbos, Pribette, & Klentz, 1985); and that religiously committed patients view clinicians who integrate religion into therapy more optimistically and as more competent than clinicians who do not (Keating & Fretz, 1990; McCullough & Worthington, 1995).

The "religiosity gap" between practitioners and recipients of psychiatric treatment, the identification of aspects of religion and spirituality as protective factors, and the evident benefits of addressing issues related to religion and spirituality as part of proficient treatment lead to an increasing awareness of an unmet necessity in psychiatric practice. As a result, a significant change occurred in 1994 when the Accreditation Council for Graduate Medical Education (ACGME) acknowledged the importance of spirituality and religion (S/R), and mandated residency programs to include these issues in psychiatric training, particularly as they relate to competent patient care in a multicultural setting (Puchalski, Larson, & Lu, 2001). The aim of this mandate was that psychiatry residents become conversant in the S/R factors "that significantly influence physical and psychological development" (ACGME, 1994), cultural issues, diversity, and issues of sensitivity to patients' background and values (ACGME, 2001).

The inclusion of spirituality and religion among other diversity factors is a necessary and long awaited recognition in psychiatric practice. However, we would like to further propose that issues related to religion and spirituality encompass more than the crucial aspect of honoring patients' cultural diversity and heritage, or the much needed emphasis on strength-based treatment. Each theory of psychotherapy was developed from within a specific understanding of human nature, with its own implications for personhood, suffering, and growth. These embedded philosophical assumptions are greatly reflected in the various treatment approaches and hold a powerful sway in each therapeutic encounter, affecting treatment process and outcome. The relationship between psychiatric practice and religion has historically been characterized by significant tension, and some philosophical assumptions hold direct dissonance to religious views. A commitment to involving issues of religion and spirituality in psychiatric practice calls for grappling with these dissonant views, and engaging our examined and, at times, unexamined assumptions regarding human nature, personality and development, models of health and illness, motivation, and change. More basic than acknowledging the importance of patients' religious diversity and right to psychiatric treatment that competently addresses their beliefs and culture are the foundational worldviews that we implicitly or explicitly employ when arriving at conclusions regarding persons, psychopathology, health, change, well-being, suffering, and ultimate meaning in life. These worldviews are most often intertwined, whether in harmony or disagreement, with religious and spiritual principles. Psychiatric treatment can be either greatly restricted or enhanced by these underlying suppositions on human nature.

One considerable way of closing the "religiosity gap" that still exists in psychiatric practice is addressing matters of religion and spirituality early on in psychiatrists' careers, particularly during their psychiatric residency training, arguably the most formative years of professional development. The current chapter provides an overview of current training practices in North American psychiatric residency programs, specifically as they relate to issues of religion and spirituality. Such established training practices and guidelines served as a model for the development of the Religion and Spirituality in Clinical Practice curriculum at Loma Linda University, School of Medicine, Department of Psychiatry. Further, because psychiatric practice can hardly be conceptualized and implemented outside a specific worldview and set of assumptions regarding human nature, we will illustrate a training curriculum which was explicitly developed from within a Christian worldview, more specifically, the Adventist tradition. Psychiatric practice from within an Adventist worldview takes into account a holistic concept of the person, views spirituality as a core component of being, and advocates a respectful stance towards the patient's values while at the same time encouraging the clinician to maintain the courage of his or her convictions (Fayard, Harding, Murdoch, & Brunt, 2007).

Loma Linda University is uniquely prepared to attend to issues of faith and spirituality while addressing the various needs of the patient. As an institution we have long acknowledged the role of religion and spirituality as a basic aspect of human beings' function and purpose.

Health and wellness principles that are now recognized and widely accepted by health professionals everywhere have long been practiced and advocated in the Adventist tradition.

One of these main principles is the focus on the "whole person," as opposed to simply addressing physical, mental, or spiritual aspects, each taken in isolation. "In the Adventist synthesis human beings have no real, even spiritual, existence apart from the body....Mind affects body, body affects mind, and both interact with the surrounding environment. A whole healing ministry has been integrated around this understanding" (Provonsha, 1994, p. 14). We are strongly rooted in the belief that Christ "came to give [men and women] health and peace and perfection of character" (White, 1905, p. 17), and help them to follow in His example by promoting *physical*, *emotional*, and *spiritual* restoration. Ellen White, the founder of Loma Linda University, articulated Jesus' lifelong ministry as bringing "*complete restoration*" to humanity. It is a sacred undertaking to "further the healing ministry of Jesus Christ," and we seek to fulfill it by what Jones and Butman (1991) called integrating "head, heart and hands."

CURRENT SPIRITUALITY AND RELIGION (S/R) TRAINING PRACTICES IN NORTH AMERICAN PSYCHIATRIC RESIDENCY PROGRAMS

Given the historical antagonism between religion and psychiatry, and the overwhelmingly irreligious context in which psychiatric training has taken place for so long, the relatively new task of training psychiatrists to effectively address their patients' religious/spiritual lives is not an easy one. An initial important step was taken in 1994 when the Accreditation Council for Graduate Medical Education stated that all psychiatry residencies must include didactic training in religion and spirituality as far as these matters pertain to psychiatric treatment (AGME, 1994). Another important advance was the development of a "model curriculum" by Larson, Lu, and Swyers (1996).

THE MODEL CURRICULUM

To aid psychiatry training programs with the inclusion of S/R in didactic sessions and clinical practice, Larson, Lu, and Swyers (1996) developed a "model curriculum." This model curriculum is organized into eleven modules (two core modules, and nine optional modules to be used depending on the time available for each program); a module is defined as "organized learning experiences in a topical area" (p. 6). Each module is structured and provides a sequence of possible learning objectives (in the three areas of knowledge, skills, and attitudes), didactic content, references and further reading, suggested applications, and anticipated problems and barriers. Residency programs are encouraged to "design their own 'tailor-made' course" by following the suggested training priorities (p. 6).

The two core modules, intended to provide basic knowledge regarding religious/spiritual issues, present an introductory overview of religion and spirituality in mental health (Module 1) and teach interviewing and assessment skills with regards to the patient's religious/spiritual practices, beliefs, and attitudes (Module 2). Accessory modules focus on topics such as S/R and human development, consultation-liaison, collaborating with clergy, S/R and substance abuse, S/R and treatment of women, S/R and treatment of abused persons, God images, and various religious experiences as they relate to mental health.

LEARNING FORMATS

Following the ACGME (1994) standards for the inclusion of S/R in psychiatric training, the learning objectives for curricular development are divided into knowledge, skills, and attitudes. Didactic training, the most frequently encountered teaching method, best addresses knowledge and skills objectives. Skills objectives can further be attained and honed through case conferences, resident presentations, supervision, and rotations in inpatient, outpatient, and consultation-liaison settings. Attitudinal objectives can be fulfilled through small-group discussions, role-playing exercises, and mentoring relationships with supervisors.

Didactic training. The most common form of teaching religion and spirituality as it relates to psychiatric practice is through deductive methodologies, such that clinicians in training are exposed to various classroom lectures, books, and articles, and then tested on the information they assimilated (Sorenson, 1997). Indeed, such coursework and didactic teaching is not only essential, but also developmentally appropriate for beginning clinicians, who need specific guidance in their advance of knowledge and skill acquisition through a directive and structured training experience and supervision. This teaching method lends itself well to specific issues such as the assessment and understanding of various belief systems, theoretical orientations (particularly in regards to the main assumptions and teachings of various theories of psychotherapy as they relate to religion), selection of treatment plans and goals compatible with a particular set of religious beliefs and values, awareness of professional ethics codes, models for assessing the functionality of a patient's spiritual path, and models of spiritual development through the life cycle (Aten & Hernandez, 2004; Berkel, Constantine, & Olson, 2007; Blass, 2001; Butman & Kruse, 2007; Ingersoll, 1997).

Experiential training. A number of psychiatry residency programs have augmented the didactic coursework with more experiential components, such as encouraging authentic role modeling through the supervisory relationship, participation in workshops, open dialogues, and experiential exercises. Thus, Butman and Kruse (2007) argue for a supervisory relationship characterized by authentic role-modeling, believing that helping trainees learn has a greater impact than "telling" them ("what we do is far more important than what we say," p. 308). Ingersoll (1997) supports the use of role-plays to highlight S/R issues. Blass (2001) advocates for a bi-directional dialogue between psychiatry and religion, in which "a psychiatrist, working together with a member of the clergy, could assess whether a patient's belief is idiosyncratic, possibly rendering it delusional, or if it is a part of the group's shared beliefs" (p. 80). Berkel, Constantine, and Olson (2007) also encourage the utilization of community resources, such as sponsoring open dialogues between trainees and ministers in which clergy members are invited to present their denomination's beliefs, rituals, practices, the types of mental health issues with which their communities struggle, and their opinion on how best to incorporate S/R issues within the context of mental health interventions.

Self-exploration. An additional area of focus in training is that of encouraging the resident's self-exploration. Hage (2006) emphasizes the necessity for training programs to allow "opportunities for self-exploration and reflection related to the potential impact of [residents'] spiritual values and biases on others…for example, [residents] should be encouraged to explore spiritual or religious practices and messages in their families and how these practices and messages may impact the way that they relate to their clients. Similar efforts at self-exploration across diversity areas have been shown to increase [residents'] overall sense of therapeutic competence and self-awareness (e.g., D'Andrea, Daniels, & Heck, 1991)" (p. 306). Aten & Hernandez (2004) encourage residents to not only know themselves, but also to know themselves in relationship; this includes examining their own beliefs and values, reflecting on their own experiences with religion, exploring differing religious issues and traditions, recognizing the unique epistemological assumptions of the clients' religious system, as well as differentiating between self and patient, being aware of the countertransference, and gaining an increasing ability to shift their perspective.

Supervision. Finally, above and beyond providing didactics and coursework, experiential learning opportunities, and an environment propitious for self-exploration, Sorenson (1997) challenges Christian training programs to offer more than competent education, to do "more than merely replicate what is already available from a secular equivalent" (p. 531). What he is referring to is cultivating moral virtues and character qualities. Butman and Kruse (2007) argue that a "supervision framework that builds competencies and then moves on to also focus on character formation through mentoring relationships, is greatly needed" (p. 309). According to Butman and Kruse, this model of supervision is characterized by "a developmental relationship... [where] supervisors see themselves as deliberately partnering with supervisees to shepherd them safely through vulnerable transitions... work[ing] to hone clinical competencies while showing concern for the supervisee's broader welfare and professional development..." (Johnson, 2007, p. 262, as cited by Butman & Kruse, 2007). Sorenson, Derflinger, Bufford, and McMinn (2004) also discuss a relational supervision model that "emphasizes process as much as content" (p. 355). In a national collaborative research studying how students learn the integration of psychotherapy and religion, Sorenson and colleagues (2004) found that students learn through "relational attachments with mentors who model that integration for students personally" (p. 363). "Students want broad and candid access to integrators so they can see how their mentors think, weigh choices, make clinical judgments, pursue courses of research, and most importantly, how they interact with themselves and others, including God" (Sorenson et al., 2004, p. 364). Palmer (1993) likens the educational journey with a "spiritual journey." Sorenson (1997) proposed that students "use faculty as subsidiary attachment figures or transitional objects, particularly the professors' own ongoing life of faith, to facilitate students' integrative pilgrimage" (p. 530). Thus, the importance of "secure attachment" within the context of supervisory relationships "lies not only in the feeling of well-being and security it provides but also in its facilitation of exploration of the world and of oneself" (Eagle, 1995, p. 128).

APPLICATIONS OF THE MODEL CURRICULUM

There now exists a wide variety of practical applications of this curriculum, from programs offering the bare minimum of one to six sessions integrated into already existing residency courses (incorporating information from the two core modules described above), to those with more specialized interests offering a thorough and comprehensive focus on S/R and clinical practice spanning the full four-year residency training (including, but not limited to, those described in the accessory modules). The vast majority of psychiatry residency programs view spirituality and religion as diversity factors and design their training to focus on gaining multicultural competencies when working with religious patients. Starting in 1997, outstanding psychiatry residency curricula addressing issues of spirituality and religion and mental health have been recognized by the John Templeton award program. Twenty-four residency programs have received this award so far. In 2006, the following programs were awarded:

- ◊ Baylor College of Medicine, Menninger Department of Psychiatry and Behavioral Sciences
- ◊ George Washington University Medical Center, Psychiatry and Behavioral Sciences
- ◊ Texas Tech University, Health Sciences Center, School of Medicine, Department of Neuropsychiatry and Behavioral Sciences
- ◊ University of California, Irvine, Department of Psychiatry and Human Behavior

The 2005 awards include:

- ◊ Rush University Medical Center, Department of Religion, Health & Human Values
- ◊ University of British Columbia, Vancouver General Hospital, Department of Psychiatry
- ◊ University of Kansas Medical Center, Department of Psychiatry and Behavioral Sciences
- ◊ University of South Carolina, School of Medicine, Department of Neuropsychiatry and Behavioral Science

Sample course assimilating spirituality and religion in psychiatric training. McCarthy and Peteet (2003) describe the "Mental Health, Religion, and Culture" course they co-directed at Harvard Longwood

Psychiatry Residency Training Program. This course included both didactic and experiential components. Training activities included residents pairing up and taking a religious/spiritual history of one another, participation in meditation and prayer exercises, and presentation of cases that have a religious aspect. Outside speakers were invited (for example, psychoanalyst Ana-Maria Rizzuto) to discuss research about internal God representation, and a faculty member presented a long-term psychotherapy case, followed by an opportunity for the residents to interview the patient, and later discuss issues regarding boundaries and the use of religion ideation as a defense as well as source of comfort/strength and countertransference.

THE RELIGION AND SPIRITUALITY IN CLINICAL PRACTICE CURRICULUM AT LOMA LINDA UNIVERSITY

The LLU, Department of Psychiatry, Religion and Spirituality in Clinical Practice curriculum consists of specialized training in the incorporation of religion, spirituality, and faith-based experiences into psychiatric practice. The goal of the Religion and Spirituality in Clinical Practice curriculum is to promote complete (physical, emotional, social, and spiritual) restoration through compassionate acceptance, dedicated care, and without discrimination. The process of educating psychiatry residents at LLU fully incorporates an Adventist worldview, throughout the didactic coursework and supervisory relationships, and also in order to develop character values in the personal lives of the residents. The importance of incorporating the supervisors' and supervisees' worldviews as a foundation for clinical practice cannot be overstated. Worldviews involve a set of beliefs about humans and the world. Worldviews answer basic questions about what exists, how we know it, how things work, what is good and bad or right and wrong, and who we are (or what it means to be human). In the words of Bevan and Kessel (1994), "worldviews are like sand at a picnic; they get into everything: (p. 506)" (Bufford, 2007, p. 293). Meador (2006) argues that spiritually sensitive psychiatric practice cannot exist outside a religious worldview. He makes a clear distinction between spiritually informed therapeutic techniques (such as meditation or mindfulness) and spirituality. Accordingly, the goal of the Religion and Spirituality in Clinical Practice curriculum is to not only provide the required skills and competencies (i.e., spiritually informed techniques), but also to foster the residents' spiritual development, who will then be better prepared to attend to the needs of their patients and to provide "whole person" care. The faculty at LLU are particularly well suited to prepare and guide residents in this model; while being exceptional professionals in their fields, they are also committed to acknowledging and embodying a particular religious worldview (a Christian, more specifically Seventh-day Adventist, worldview) in their teaching and clinical practice, and to continually extend the boundaries of their instruction above and beyond simply teaching how to skillfully apply a set of techniques. Residents have the unique opportunity to develop as clinicians from the "inside" of a particular religious tradition, as they are mentored by faculty members who aim "to cultivate clinicians who are able to be deeply engaged and present with matters of the soul, and who do not shrink away from grappling with suffering, sin and injustice" (Butman & Kruse, 2007, p. 310).

Within this framework, the Religion and Spirituality in Clinical Practice curriculum is designed as a two-step process: a core curriculum (spanning the first three years of psychiatric residency) and an advanced certificate program (fourth-year elective which provides the option for advanced training in S/R issues). Every psychiatry resident is expected to complete the *core curriculum*, while fourth-year residents can elect to obtain an *advanced certificate* in Religion and Psychiatry. The three main goals the curriculum sets out to achieve focus on helping residents gain knowledge and understanding of major factors related to religion/spirituality and mental health, attain necessary competencies and skills, and develop personal attitudes congruent with Adventist values and convictions. Following we will present a brief summary of the curriculum (see Appendix A for a detailed description).

Religion and spirituality in clinical practice: Core curriculum. In terms of knowledge objectives, graduating psychiatry residents are expected to demonstrate understanding of the theoretical and philosophical environment surrounding religion/spirituality and mental health, the empirical foundations of psychiatry and religion/spirituality, and the practical applications of religion/spirituality and clinical practice. The skills to be attained include assessment and interviewing skills, interventional skills, and engagement of other disciplines. Finally, residents should demonstrate in their behavior and demeanor values that regulate interpersonal transactions (respect, compassion, and teamwork) as well as values that point to ideals of emotional maturity.

These objectives are to be achieved through didactic teaching, clinical training opportunities, and an experiential component. The didactic teaching will take place in Grand Rounds as well as the seminar series (e.g., the Mental health and religion seminar: Theoretical, theological and philosophical background; Psychiatry and religion seminar: Empirical foundations; and the Psychotherapy and religion seminar: Practical applications). Clinical training opportunities include rotations through the outpatient psychiatry department, inpatient units, chemical dependency unit, and consultation liaison. The experiential component consists of individual focused supervision on spiritual/religious issues and case conferences.

Religion and spirituality in clinical practice: Advanced certificate program. The advanced integration certificate program is designed as an elective year-long specialty course for psychiatry residents in the final year of their residency. It is designed to further promote reflection on, and application of, the integration of religion/spirituality and psychiatry and to cultivate opportunities for residents to demonstrate their grasp of key concepts and techniques presented in the didactic, clinical, and experiential modules in earlier years of the program. Fourth-year psychiatry residents electing to participate in this certificate program will pursue a deeper understanding and application within a specific area of psychiatry as it relates to spirituality and religion. Potential areas of concentration include, but are not limited to, a focus on spirituality and severe mental illness, religion and psychotherapy, spiritual issues and the treatment of chemical dependency, psychiatry and spirituality in the care of terminally ill medical patients, spiritual aspects of child and adolescent psychiatry, the interface of forensic psychiatry and religion, trauma and religion, international missions and psychiatry, or a research focus on psychiatry, religion, and spirituality.

Above and beyond the core curriculum objectives presented for the core curriculum, the advanced certificate program allows residents to contribute to the development of knowledge as it relates to the interface of religious, spiritual, and psychological functioning; to further develop their skills in the integration of religion/spirituality in clinical practice with both individuals and communities; and to embody values necessary to serve effectively in diverse communities locally and/or globally. Successful candidates in this program will be able to demonstrate competency in addressing spiritual and religious issues within their traditional psychiatric practice, and will also be able to provide preventative and transformational mental health services to churches or other faith communities. The goal of this program is to prepare psychiatry residents to embody values necessary to serve effectively in diverse communities, both locally and globally, by providing services for underserved populations and integrating, both in practice and personal life, the disciplines of compassion and charity.

Didactic training at the advanced level includes a more personalized and profound exploration of a subject of interest to the resident culminating in the development of a research project and opportunities for teaching junior residents. Under the mentorship of a faculty member, the resident pursues a particular topic of interest within the area of psychiatry and spiritual life, and designs the specific focus of his or her didactic, clinical, and experiential training for the year; faculty members review and guide the resident's proposal, supervising the implementation of the didactic, clinical, and experiential modules of training. The clinical training will focus on providing spiritually sensitive services in both individual and community settings, culminating with a case presentation of a long-term psychotherapy patient and the development of a program or consultation services to local or overseas churches or communities. The experiential component will include participation in supervised experience as well as the provision of supervision to junior residents; the completion of the advanced program in the integration of S/R into clinical practice will conclude with a personal wholistic worldview thesis paper focusing on the relationship between psychiatry and spiritual life and demonstrating the personal reflection and application of psychiatric practice and religious/spiritual factors.

Evaluating the outcome and impact of training. Program evaluation and outcome measures will be incorporated into the course from its beginning, allowing for extensive research regarding the efficacy and impact of the training. Throughout each training year, residents' reactions to training will be assessed through course evaluations. Knowledge gains will be assessed through small quizzes and end-of-the-year examinations. Psychotherapy supervisors will evaluate whether the learning has been translated into behavior change in a patient care setting at mid-point and conclusion of each rotation. At the end of the three years of core training, supervisors and faculty will review videotapes of residents' psychotherapy sessions, both from initial patient encounters (in the resident's first year of training) as well as sessions at the end of the course. The focus of the review of videotaped sessions will be the residents' willingness and development of their ability to include communication about the spiritual dimension in their treatment process. An anticipated barrier to the implementation of this course includes the possible unwillingness of residents to engage with religious and spiritual material. To address this issue, Loma Linda Medical School faculty and literature clearly identify the program's dedication to religious and spiritual integration in clinical practice. Residents applying to the program will be fully educated regarding the required participation in the course, and ongoing supervision will provide the opportunity to discuss any concerns of residents in the program.

CONCLUSION

As an institution, LLU has been entrusted with the responsibility of educating competent health professionals and encouraging the pursuit of their personal and professional growth, as well as providing proficient and compassionate services to our patients. For the psychiatry residents we aim to provide more than an intellectual endeavor alone; it is our hope to create an environment that leads to transformation, an atmosphere that leads to the development of character, in which compassion and convictions flourish. In turn, we trust our graduating residents will not only learn to provide excellent mental health services, but also bring wholeness, healing, and hope to the individuals and communities they serve.

REFERENCES

Accreditation Council for Graduate Medical Education (1994). *Special requirements for residency training in psychiatry.* Chicago, IL: Accreditation Council for Graduate Medical Education.

Accreditation Council for Graduate Medical Education (2001). *Program requirements for residency training in psychiatry on cultural issues.* Chicago, IL: Accreditation Council for Graduate Medical Education.

Aten, J., & Hernandez, B. C. (2004). Addressing religion in clinical supervision: A model. *Psychotherapy: Theory, Research, Practice, Training, 41,* 152–160.

Bader, C. D., Mencken, F. C., & Froese, P. (2007). American piety 2005: Content and methods of the Baylor Religion Survey. *Journal for the Scientific Study of Religion, 46,* 447–463.

Bergin, A. E. (1988). Three contributions of a spiritual perspective to counseling, psychotherapy, and behavior change. *Counseling and Values, 32,* 21–31.

Bergin, A. E. (1991). Values and religious issues in psychotherapy and mental health. *American Psychologist, 46,* 394–403.

Bergin, A. E., & Jensen, J. P. (1990). Religiosity of psychotherapists: A national survey. *Psychotherapy, 27,* 3–7.

Berkel, L. A., Constantine, M. G., & Olson, E. A. (2007). Supervisor multicultural competence: Adressing religious and spiritual issues with counseling students in supervision. *Clinical Supervisor, 26,* 3–15.

Bevan, W., & Kessel, F. (1994). Plain truths and home cooking: Thoughts on the making and remaking of psychology. *American Psychologist, 49,* 505–509.

Blass, D. M. (2001). A conceptual framework for the interactions between psychiatry and religion. *International Review of Psychiatry, 13,* 79–85.

Bufford, R. K. (2007). Philosophical foundations for clinical supervision within a Christian worldview. *Journal of Psychology and Christianity, 26,* 293–297.

Butman, R. E., & Kruse, S. J. (2007). On creating a healthy supervisory environment: A Christian relational and developmental perspective. *Journal of Psychology and Christianity, 26,* 307–312.

Curlin, F., Lawrence, R., Odell, S., Chin, M., Lantos, J., Koenig, H., & Meador, K. (2007). Religion, spirituality, and medicine: Psychiatrists' and other physicians' differing observations, interpretations, and clinical approaches. *American Journal of Psychiatry, 164,* 1825–1831.

D'Andrea, M., Daniels, J., & Heck, R. (1991). Evaluating the impact of multicultural counseling training. *Journal of Counseling & Development. Special issue: Multiculturalism as a fourth force in counseling, 70,* 143–150.

Dougherty, K. D., Johnson, B. R., & Polson, E. C. (2007). Recovering the lost: Remeasuring U.S. religious affiliation. *Journal for the Scientific Study of Religion, 46,* 483–499.

Eagle, M. (1995). The developmental perspectives of attachment and psychoanalytic theory. In Goldberg, S., Muir, R., & Kerr, J. (Eds.), *Attachment theory: Social, developmental, and clinical perspectives* (pp. 123–150). Hillsdale, NJ: Analytic Press, Inc.

Ellison, C. G., & Levin, J. S. (1998). The religion-health connection: Evidence, theory, and future directions. *Heath Education Behavior, 25,* 700–720.

Farr, C., Lawrence, R., Odell, S., Chin, M., Lantons, L., Koenig, H., & Meador, K. (2007). Religion, spirituality, and medicine: Psychiatrists' and other physicians' differing observations, interpretations, and clinical approaches. *American Journal of Psychiatry, 164,* 1825–1831.

Fayard, C., Harding, G., Murdoch, W., & Brunt, J. (2007). Clinical implications for psychotherapy from the Seventh-day Adventist Tradition. *Journal of Psychology and Chirsitianity, 26,* 207–217.

Fleischman, P. R. (1990). *The healing spirit: Explorations in psychotherapy and spirituality.* New York: Paragon Press.

Fukuyama, M. A., & Sevig, T. D. (1999). *Integrating spirituality into multicultural counseling.* Thousand Oaks, CA: Sage.

Gallup, G. (1994). The Gallup poll: Public opinion 1993. Wilmington, DE: Scholarly Resources.

Gingrich, F., & Worthington, E. L. (2007). Supervision and the integration of faith into clinical practice: Research considerations. *Journal of Psychology and Christianity. Special Issue: Clinical supervision, 26*, 342–355.

Harrison, M. O., Edwards, C. L., Koenig, H. G., Bosworth, H. B., Decastro, L., & Wood, M. (2005). Religiosity/spirituality and pain in patients with sickle cell disease. *Journal of Nervous and Mental Disease, 193*, 250–257.

Hage, S. M. (2006). A closer look at the role of spirituality in psychology training programs. *Professional Psychology: Research and Practice, 37*, 303–310.

Ingersoll, R. E. (1997). Teaching a course on counseling and spirituality. *Counselor Education and Supervision, 36*, 224–233.

Johnson, W. B. (2007). Transformational supervision: When supervisors mentor. *Professional Psychology: Research and Practice, 38*, 259–267.

Jones, S., & Butman, R. (1991). *Modern Psychotherapies: A comprehensive Christian appraisal.* Downers Grove, IL: InterVarsity Press.

Keating, A. M., & Fretz, B. R. (1990). Christians' anticipations about counselors in response to counselor descriptions. *Journal of Counseling Psychology, 37*, 293–296.

Koenig, H. G. (Ed.) (1998). *Handbook of religion and mental health.* New York: Academic Press.

Koenig, H. G. (2007). Religion and remission of depression in medical inpatients with heart failure/pulmonary disease. *Journal of Nervous and Mental Disease, 195*, 389–395.

Larson, D. B., Lu, F. G., & Swyers, J. P. (Eds.) (1996). *Model curriculum for psychiatry residency training programs: Religion and spirituality in clinical practice.* Rockville, MD: National Institute for Health Care Research.

Loma Linda University (2011). School of Medicine: Mission. Retrieved from Loma Linda University (2011). School of Medicine: Mission. Retrieved from http://www.llu.edu/medicine/mission.page?

Lovinger, R. J. (1984). *Working with religious issues in therapy.* Northwale, NJ: Jason Aronson.

Lovinger, R. J. (1990). *Religion and counseling: The psychological impact of religious belief.* New York: Continuum.

Lukoff, D., Lu, F., & Turner, R. (1992). Toward a more culturally sensitive DSM-IV: Psychoreligious and psychospiritual problems. *Journal of Nervous Mental Dissorders, 180*, 673–682.

Matthews, D. A., McCullough M. E., Larson, D. B., Koening, H. G., Swyers, J. P., & Milano, M. G. (1998). Religious commitment and health status: A review of the research and implications for family medicine. *Archives of Family Medicine, 7,* 118–124.

McCarthy, M. K., & Peteet, J. R. (2003). Teaching residents about religion and spirituality. *Harvard Review of Psychiatry, 11,* 225–228.

McCullough, M. E., & Worthington, E. L. (1995). College students' perceptions of a psychotherapist's treatment of a religious issue: Partial replication and extension. *Journal of Counseling and Development, 73,* 626–634.

Meador, K. (2006). An illusion of the future: Temptations and possibilities. In P. McNamara (Ed.), *Where God and science meet: How brain and evolutionary studies alter our understanding of religion—The psychology of religious experience* (pp. 269–282). Westport, CT: Praeger.

Miller, W. R. (1988). Including client's spiritual perspectives in cognitive behavior therapy. In W. R. Miller & J. E. Martin (Eds.), *Behavior therapy and religion: Integrating spiritual and behavioral approaches to change* (pp. 43–55). Newbury Park, CA: Sage.

Miller, W. R. (1999). Integrating spirituality into treatment. Washington, D.C.: American Psychological Association.

Mueller, P. S., Plevak, D. J., & Rummans, T. A. (2001). Religious involvement, spirituality, and medicine: Implications for clinical practice. *Mayo Clinic Proceedings, 76,* 1225–1235.

Palmer, P. (1993). *To know as we are known: Education as a spiritual journey.* San Francisco: Harper San Francisco.

Payne, I. R., Bergin, A. E., Bielema, K. A., & Jenkins, P. H. (1991). Review of religion and mental health: Prevention and the enhancement of psychosocial functioning. *Prevention in Human Services, 9,* 11–40.

Polling Report (2002). CNN/USA Today/Gallup Poll, December 9–10, 2002. Retrieved June 8, 2008 from http://www.pollingreport.com/religion.htm.

Pollner, M. (1989). Divine relations, social relations, and well-being. *Journal of Health and Social Behavior, 30,* 92–104.

Powell, L., Shahabi, L., & Thoresen, C. (2003). Religion and spirituality: Linkages to physical health. *American Psychologist, 58,* 36–52.

Propst, L. R. (1988). *Psychotherapy within a religious framework: Spirituality in the emotional healing process.* New York: Human Sciences Press.

Propst, L. R. (1996). Cognitive-behavioral therapy and the religious person. In E. P. Shafranske (Ed.), *Religion and the clinical practice of psychology* (pp. 391–407). Washington, D.C.: American Psychological Association.

Provonsha, J. (1994). Conceptual foundations of our health message. In A. Whiting (Ed.), *Health 2000 and beyond: A study conference of Adventist theology, philosophy, and practice of health and healing* (pp. 9–16). Silver Spring, MD: General Conference of Seventh-day Adventist Health and Temperance Department.

Puchalski, C. M., Larson, D. B., & Lu, F. G. (2001). Spirituality in psychiatry residency programs. *International Review of Psychiatry. Special Issue: Religion and Psychiatry, 13*, 131–138.

Quackenbos, S., Pribette, G., & Klentz, B. (1985). Psychotherapy and religion: Rapprochement or antithesis? *Journal of Counseling and Development, 65*, 82–85.

Sansome, R. A., Khatain, K., & Rodenhauser, P. (1990). The role of religion in psychiatric education: A national survey. *Academic Psychiatry, 14*, 34–38.

Shafranske, E. P. (Ed.) (1996). *Religion and the clinical practice of psychology.* Washington, D.C.: American Psychological Association.

Shafranske, E. P., & Malony, H. N. (1996). Religion and the clinical practice of psychology: A case for inclusion. In E. P. Shafranske (Ed.), *Religion and the clinical practice of psychology* (pp. 561–586). Washington, D.C.: American Psychological Association.

Sorenson, R. L. (1997). Doctoral students' integration of psychology and Christianity: Perspectives via attachment theory and multidimensional scaling. *Journal for the Scientific Study of Religion, 36*, 530–548.

Sorenson, R. L., Derflinger, K. R., Bufford, R. K., & McMinn, M. R. (2004). National collaborative research on how students learn integration: Final report. *Journal of Psychology and Christianity, 23*, 355–365.

Stoltenberg, C. D. (2005). Enhancing professional competence through developmental approaches to supervision. *American Psychologist, 60*, 857–864.

White, E. G. (1905). *Ministry of healing.* Mountain View, CA: Pacific Press.

Zinnbauer, B., & Pargament, K. (2005) Religiousness and spirituality. In R. Paloutzian & C. Park (Eds.), *Handbook of the Psychology of Religion and Spirituality.* New York: The Guilford Press.

APPENDIX A

CONTENTS

RELIGION AND SPIRITUALITY IN CLINICAL PRACTICE CURRICULUM: DEPARTMENT OF PSYCHIATRY LOMA LINDA UNIVERSITY SCHOOL OF MEDICINE

BACKGROUND

Loma Linda University was founded with the purpose of "furthering the healing ministry of Jesus Christ." Ellen White, its founder, articulated the meaning of attending to the faith experience of those served in medical settings in her book, *Ministry of Healing* (1905) in this way:

◊ "Our Lord Jesus Christ came to this world as the unwearied servant of man's necessity.…It was His mission to bring men to complete restoration; He came to give them health and peace and perfection of character" (p. 17).

◊ "During His ministry, Jesus devoted more time to healing the sick than to preaching" (p. 19).

◊ "The Saviour made each work of healing an occasion for implanting divine principles in the mind and soul. This was the purpose of His work. He imparted earthly blessings, that He might incline the hearts of men to receive the gospel of His grace" (p. 20).
◊ "Gracious, tenderhearted, pitiful, He went about lifting up the bowed-down and comforting the sorrowful. Wherever He went, He carried blessing" (p. 24).
◊ "Christ recognized no distinction of nationality or rank or creed.…He passed by no human being as worthless, but sought to apply the healing remedy to every soul" (p. 25).

In summary, the goal is to promote complete (physical, emotional, social, and spiritual) restoration through compassionate acceptance, dedicated care, and without discrimination.

MISSION

The Religion and Spirituality in Clinical Practice curriculum consists of specialized training of psychiatry residents in the incorporation of religion, spirituality, and faith-based experiences into clinical practice. The Loma Linda University School of Medicine Psychiatry Residency Program seeks to further the healing and teaching ministry of Jesus Christ, "to make man whole," bringing health, healing, wholeness, and hope to humanity as informed by a Christian worldview particularly framed by the teaching and experience of the Seventh-day Adventist community. It seeks to fulfill its mission by:

◊ Educating ethical and proficient health professionals
◊ Promoting healing in a competent and compassionate manner reflecting a unique sensitivity to the biological, psychological, social, and spiritual dimensions of patient care
◊ Delivering comprehensive care that is patient-centered
◊ Advancing research in the area of mental health and spiritual practices and beliefs

- ◊ Encouraging the pursuit of personal and professional growth through effectively integrating knowledge, experience, and research

VALUES

The Religion and Spirituality in Clinical Practice curriculum seeks to provide a stimulating clinical and research environment for the education of psychiatry residents. The curriculum is informed by the following set of guiding values and principles:

Compassion. *Reflecting the love of God through compassionate, empathetic, and respectful personal and professional behavior.*

- ◊ Seek to reflect the character of Jesus, who met people in their need and was moved into action by compassion.
- ◊ Seek to follow Jesus' example "as the unwearied servant of [humanity's] necessity…to bring [people] complete restoration… to give them health, and peace, and perfection of character" (White, 1905, p. 7). That is, wholistic care.
- ◊ Seek to understand the emotional state of another as well as oneself, in order to alleviate pain and show compassion to those who suffer.
- ◊ Consistently treat others with courtesy, respect, and kindness; demonstrate empathy, humility, and patience; and promote forgiveness and hope.
- ◊ Exceed expectations when responding to needs in an effective and timely manner.
- ◊ Anticipate the needs of patients, family members, and co-workers, and respond in the spirit of a servant-leader.

Integrity. *Ensuring that all actions are consistent with Christian virtues by seeking to embody the example of Jesus in the interactions with the various communities served. Integrity is shown by:*

- ◊ Affirming our own identity in humility
- ◊ Honoring the sacred trust of those we serve

- ◊ Honoring, respecting, and affirming the values and worldviews that differ from our own
- ◊ Building trust by giving open and honest feedback
- ◊ Actively soliciting feedback and willingly accepting responsibility for actions
- ◊ Respecting personal dignity and privacy
- ◊ Following through with commitments and keeping promises
- ◊ Holding self and others accountable for actions and outcomes

Excellence. *Providing care that is safe, reliable, efficient, and patient centered. Every physician should realize that poor-quality work not only does injury to the sick, but is also injustice to fellow physicians as well as dishonor to Christ.*

- ◊ Constantly endeavor to reach a higher standard, seeking for increased knowledge, greater skill, and deeper discernment
- ◊ Take all necessary measures to ensure safe and respectful patient care
- ◊ Challenge the status quo to ensure an exceptional experience for patients and their family members
- ◊ Set high standards to achieve and support world-class excellence in education and research
- ◊ Partner with physicians and caregivers to ensure accurate, honest communication with patients and family members

Teamwork. *Collaborating to achieve a shared purpose.*

- ◊ Seek to restore health through the cooperation of the human and the Divine, draw together resources in order to minister to every aspect of human need, and bring about spiritual life and physical restoration
- ◊ Share information and create opportunities for increasing knowledge

- ◊ Recognize the contributions of others (patients, families, colleagues in the various health-care professions) and affirm and celebrate their successes
- ◊ Respect and encourage differing opinions
- ◊ Clearly communicate ideas and collaborate to break down barriers to safe patient-centered care
- ◊ Commit to continuous learning to ensure team strength and retention of the best talent

Wholeness. *Embracing a balanced life that integrates mind, body, and spirit.*

- ◊ Support the spiritual mission of Loma Linda's faith-based health ministry
- ◊ Demonstrate a positive, peaceful, and hopeful attitude
- ◊ Incorporate daily choices that promote physical and spiritual well-being
- ◊ Use appropriate humor in interactions with others
- ◊ Demonstrate caring to promote a compassionate healing environment for patients, families, and caregivers
- ◊ Practice faith-affirming activities

Relational Restoration. *As Christ came to this earth to restore the relationship between God and humankind, so the healer is in a privileged position to facilitate in turning the "heart of the fathers to the children, and the heart of the children to their fathers" (Mal. 4:6, KJV).*

- ◊ Initiate a corrective emotional experience between the physician and the patient(s)
- ◊ Demonstrate the appropriate inclusion of family members in treatment
- ◊ Facilitate relationship-enhancing activities between the patient and significant others

◊ Identify the influence of family relationships on spiritual/religious experience
◊ Empower patient and family members to resolve or address issues that contribute to spiritual disorientation
◊ Promote spiritual understanding and support within relationships
◊ Assist patients to resolve spiritual or relational issues with their faith community

RELIGION AND SPIRITUALITY IN CLINICAL PRACTICE: CORE CURRICULUM

OBJECTIVES

Knowledge

The resident should be able to demonstrate understanding of the following:

◊ Theoretical and philosophical background of religion/spirituality and mental health
- Define spirituality in its various aspects
- Understand the history of the tension between religion and psychiatry
- Understand the philosophical and theoretical underpinnings of wholeness—the integration of mind, body, and spirit—in relation to mental health
- Understand the role of culture-congruent healers and healing experiences
- Understand various major world religions and spiritual experiences (including beliefs, practices, and role in shaping health belief systems)
- Understand and articulate clearly the role of worldviews in theoretical areas in religion/spirituality and mental health
- Understand Loma Linda University's philosophy of wholeness

in the care of mental health patients

- ◊ Empirical foundations of psychiatry and religion/spirituality
    - Understand the research data on spiritual practices and health
    - Understand current research literature on the neurobiology of spiritual experience
    - Understand the unique impact of religious/spiritual/cultural experiences on human development
    - Understand how spiritual/cultural values can be effectively incorporated into treatment planning
    - Understand the role of religion in life-threatening conditions
    - Understand the contributions of spirituality and religion to mental health and psychopathology (e.g., depression, suicide, anxiety, trauma reactions, and additions)
- ◊ Practical applications of religion/spirituality and psychotherapy
    - Understand the differential diagnosis appropriate to an individual's religious/spiritual/cultural presentation
    - Understand transferential and countertransferential aspects of therapeutic work with religious populations
    - Understand the cultural and spiritual issues in treatment
    - Understand how spiritual/cultural values can be a hindrance to therapeutic gain
    - Understand the ethical aspects of including or failing to include cultural/spiritual issues in treatment planning
    - Understand the potential impact of the power difference between the physician and the patient

Skills

The resident should demonstrate competence in the following:

- ◊ Assessment and interviewing skills
    - Assess and interview religiously committed patients with sensitivity to their unique worldview
    - Recognize the potentially harmful aspects of a patient's

religious belief
- Recognize the differential diagnosis in regards to spiritual issues
- Recognize implicit spirituality as relevant to assessment and treatment planning

◊ Interventional skills
- Recognize one's own countertransferential bias in working with spiritually diverse populations
- Work with issues of transference in religious and non-religious patients
- Incorporate relevant spiritual issues into the patient's overall treatment plan
- Utilize appropriate culture-congruent strategies in treatment
- Utilize psychotherapeutic interventions informed by spiritual practices (i.e., prayer, meditation) congruent with the patient's worldview and institutional values
- Appropriately manage the potentially harmful aspects of a patient's religious belief
- Develop a respectful and compassionate approach for diversity in cultural and religious beliefs
- Develop an awareness regarding evidence-based practices in religion/spirituality and mental health

◊ Engagement of other disciplines
- Work cooperatively with clergy or other faith-based agents and communities

Personal Attitudes

Residents should demonstrate the following in their behavior and demeanor:

◊ Values that regulate interpersonal transactions
- Demonstrate respect and compassion for others
- Demonstrate dedication to teamwork
- Demonstrate the ability to relate to patients and co-workers as

equal human beings, recognizing and fostering others' ability to make valuable contributions within their own environment

◊ Values that point to ideals of personal emotional maturity
  - Demonstrate integrity, excellence, and personal wholeness
  - Develop an awareness of one's own cultural experience and history, and likely impact on patient care
  - Show sensitivity to the diversity of spiritual experiences
  - Demonstrate a non-judgmental attitude when working with a variety of religiously committed patients, clergy, or other faith-based agents
  - Demonstrate appreciation for the expressed goals of family members and patients in regards to therapeutic interventions that include culture-congruent approaches

TRAINING ACTIVITIES

Didactic Training Module

◊ Grand Rounds: Psychiatry and Spiritual Life Grand Rounds

◊ Mental health and religion seminar: Theoretical, theological and philosophical background
  - Relevant religious/spiritual definitions
  - Introduction to spirituality and mental health
  - Beliefs and practices of the world's major religions
  - Worldviews and values in spirituality and religion
  - Christianity and mental health
  - Understandings of human nature and implications for mental health
  - Theories of psychotherapy: A cultural, philosophical, and theological critique
  - Relational aspects of human nature and mental health
  - The psychology and neurobiology of religion and spirituality
  - History of the psychiatry-religion interface: Implications for current theory and practice

- Importance of spirituality in major life transitions
- Gender and diversity considerations in the study of religion/spirituality

◊ Psychiatry and religion seminar: Empirical foundations

- Overview of research findings in religion, spirituality, and medicine
- Religious/spiritual development throughout the lifespan
- Overview of research findings in psychotherapy and religion: Review of protocols and clinical implications
- Religion, spirituality, and chronic or life-threatening conditions: Oncology and cardiovascular disease; clinical implications for consultation liaison
- Religion, spirituality, and psychopathology: Review of research findings and clinical implications (with particular attention to depression, anxiety, suicide, trauma reactions, and addictions)

◊ Psychotherapy and religion seminar: Practical applications

- The assessment process: A patient-centered, culture-congruent approach
- Models of integration of spirituality and religion in therapy
- Differential diagnosis of religious experience
- Religious manifestations of psychopathology
- Transference and countertransference issues in working with religiosity and spirituality
- Incorporating issues of religion and spirituality in case formulation and treatment planning
- Psychotherapeutic interventions informed by Western spiritual practices: Prayer, meditation, collaboration with ministers
- Cognitive behavioral therapy interventions for religious populations
- Forgiveness as a psychotherapeutic intervention: Promise and limitations
- Psychotherapeutic interventions informed by Eastern spiritual practices

- Group psychotherapy interventions and research findings: Oncology and addictions
- Values and ethics in the treatment of religious and non-religious patients
- Spirituality and self-care for psychotherapists

Clinical Training Module

◊ Outpatient psychiatry

- Develop the ability to provide spiritually sensitive services for religiously committed individuals
- Develop the ability to take a comprehensive admissions history including religious/spiritual history
- Gain case conceptualization skills, including formulating the role of a patient's religion or faith in his/her functioning and difficulties
- Develop appropriate treatment plans, addressing, when appropriate, issues concerning faith and religion
- Develop proficiency in the differential diagnosis of spiritual and psychological conditions
- Provide individual, family, and group psychotherapy that is spiritually sensitive
- Offer referrals to and intensive case management with pastoral care services in the community

◊ Inpatient psychiatry

- Train in taking a comprehensive admissions history including religious/spiritual history
- Develop proficiency in the differential diagnosis of spiritual and psychological conditions
- Train on how to address issues of severe and chronic loss of hope, meaning, and purpose
- Consult with chaplains and pastoral care services
- Facilitate of psychotherapy groups addressing spiritual needs of various populations (i.e., geriatric, children, etc.)

- ◊ Chemical Dependency
  - Participate in spiritual model 12 Step recovery groups
  - Participate in pastoral care facilitated groups
- ◊ Consultation Liaison
  - Develop ability to provide spiritually sensitive consultation
  - Address trauma issues (i.e., suddenly becoming paralyzed after an accident)

Experiential Module

- ◊ Individual focused supervision on spiritual/religious issues
  - Observation of interviewing/therapy session (live or video tape)
- ◊ Case conference
  - Spiritual interventions in psychotherapy: Case examples
  - Presentation and discussion of specific cases involving:
    - ▫ Forgiveness as psychotherapeutic intervention
    - ▫ Spiritual disciplines as psychotherapeutic intervention
    - ▫ The use of prayer, meditation, and consultation with clergy

RELIGION AND SPIRITUALITY IN CLINICAL PRACTICE: ADVANCED CERTIFICATE PROGRAM

OBJECTIVES

This advanced integration certificate program is designed as an elective year-long specialty course for psychiatry residents in the final year of their residency. It is designed to further promote reflection on, and application of, the integration of religion/spirituality and psychiatry and to cultivate opportunities for residents to demonstrate their grasp of key concepts and techniques presented in the didactic, clinical, and experiential modules in earlier years of the program.

Knowledge

- ◊ Develop a deeper understanding of a specific area of psychiatry, religion, and spirituality. Potential areas of concentration include:

- Spirituality and severe mental illness—it may be connected with BMC, VA, and/or PSH
- Religion and psychotherapy
- Spiritual issues in chemical dependency—it may be connected with BMC, VA, and/or PSH
- Psychiatry and spirituality in palliative care, cancer, cardiomyopathy, or other chronic/life-threatening medical conditions—connected to the C & L rotation
- Spiritual aspects of child and adolescent psychiatry—it may be connected with BMC
- The interface of forensic psychiatry and religion—it may be connected with PSH
- Trauma and religion/spirituality—it may be connected with BMC and/or VA
- International missions and psychiatry
- Research elective with a focus on psychiatry, religion, and spirituality

Skills

◊ Demonstrate competency in the integration of religion/spirituality in clinical practice

◊ Demonstrate competency in addressing spiritual/religious issues within the context of patient relationships

◊ Demonstrate the ability to provide excellent preventative and/or transformational mental health services to churches and/or communities

Personal Attitudes

◊ Embody values necessary to serve effectively in diverse communities locally and/or globally by providing services for underserved populations and integrating, both in practice and personal life, the disciplines of compassion and charity

TRAINING ACTIVITIES

Didactic Module

- ◊ Under the mentorship of a faculty member, the resident identifies topic of interest within the area of psychiatry and spiritual life, and then designs the specific focus of his or her didactic, clinical, and experiential training for the year based on personal interest and unmet need within the department. The resident submits a proposal with the topic, training experiences, and a list of relevant literature to be read throughout the year and receives feedback from faculty members.
- ◊ Attend meetings twice a month with faculty mentors and/or peer group to discuss progress of individual readings and focused clinical experience
- ◊ Identify and attend relevant national conferences and training seminars

Didactic Module Outcome *(choose two of the following three options)*

- ◊ Design and complete original research project or comprehensive literature review on the topic of interest. Resulting paper to be presented at a conference or published in a peer reviewed journal
- ◊ Prepare and deliver a lecture on the topic of interest in the area of psychiatry and religion/spirituality
- ◊ Participate in co-teaching seminar(s) for other residents

Clinical Training Module

- ◊ Gain experience in providing psychiatric care with a spiritual focus in the specialty area selected
- ◊ Engage in community outreach
- ◊ Participate in the clinical training for other psychiatry residents integrated into their rotation and selected area of specialty (e.g.,

the resident selects to focus on addictions; during a rotation in the chemical dependency unit, the resident provides guidance to other residents on the topic of chemical dependency and spirituality)

Clinical Training Module Outcomes

- ◊ Prepare an Integrative Case Conference for a Grand Round on the specialty area selected. The focus of the presentation is on articulating religion and spiritual issues into clinical care.
- ◊ Participate in a community-based short-term intervention (e.g., prepare and deliver relevant mental health seminars to local churches, or participate in an overseas mission, or develop and help community-based interventions). The possible focus of these short-term community-based interventions includes disaster intervention, after-school programs, geriatric issues, whole person care, etc.
- ◊ Demonstrate competency in training junior psychiatry residents on the selected specialty focus related to psychiatry and spiritual life

Experiential Module

- ◊ Individual supervision
- ◊ Provide peer supervision to junior psychiatry residents during the specialty clinical rotation

Experiential Module Outcomes

- ◊ Obtain satisfactory evaluations from patients, peers, and faculty as already prescribed by residency standards
- ◊ Write a personal integration paper demonstrating the personal reflection and application of psychiatric practice and religious/ spiritual factors

CONTRIBUTORS

Bruce Anderson, M.D.: President, Adventist Health California Medical Group, St. Helena, California; Silverado Psychiatric Center, Calistoga, California.

Jamie D. Aten, Ph.D: Dr. Arthur P. Rech and Mrs. Jean May Rech Associate Professor of Psychology; Director, Catastrophe, Spirituality, and Trauma Laboratory, Wheaton College, Illinois.

Jana K. Boyd, Ph.D: Christian Counseling Service, Redlands, California.

Kendal C. Boyd, Ph.D: Assistant Professor, Department of Psychology, Loma Linda University.

Merlin D. Burt, Ph.D: Assistant Professor of Church History; Director, Center for Adventist Research; Seventh-day Adventist Theological Seminary, Andrews University.

Antonia Ciovica, Ph.D: Postdoctoral Fellow; Department of Psychiatry, Loma Linda University.

Carlos Fayard, Ph.D: Associate Professor, Department of Psychiatry; Director, Clinical Psychology Internship, Loma Linda University School of Medicine.

George T. Harding, IV, M.D.: Former Chair and Professor of Psychiatry, Loma Linda University; Clinical Professor, Department of Psychiatry, Ohio State University; Former Chair, Section on Religion and Psychiatry, American Psychiatric Association.

Barbara Couden Hernandez, Ph.D: Associate Professor; Director of Doctoral Clinical Training; Medical Family Therapy Program Director; Department of Counseling and Family Science, Loma Linda University.

Miroslav Kiš, Ph.D: Chair, Department of Theology and Christian Philosophy; Professor of Ethics; Seventh-day Adventist Theological Seminary, Andrews University.

Henry H. Lamberton, Psy.D, M.Div: Associate Dean for Student Affairs, School of Medicine; Associate Professor of Psychiatry; Associate Professor, School of Religion; Loma Linda University.

David Mee-Lee, M.D.: Training and Consulting, Davis, California;

Former Clinical Assistant Professor of Psychiatry, University of Hawaii, Harvard University.

William Murdoch, M.D.: Chair, Department of Psychiatry, School of Medicine; Acting Director, Student Counseling Services, Loma Linda University; Medical Director, Loma Linda University Behavioral Medicine Center.

Richard Rice, Ph.D: Professor of Theology, Philosophy, and Religion; School of Religion, Loma Linda University.

David R. Williams, Ph.D, MPH, M.Div: Professor of African and African American Studies and of Sociology; Florence & Laura Norman Professor of Public Health; Harvard School of Public Health.

Gerald R. Winslow, Ph.D: Vice President for Mission and Culture, Loma Linda University Medical Center; Professor, School of Religion, Loma Linda University; Vice President for Spiritual Life, Loma Linda University Adventist Health Sciences Center.

Deane L. Wolcott, M.D.: Vice President, Clinical Program Development, Aptium Oncology, Los Angeles; Department of Psychiatry and Behavioral Neurosciences, Cedars-Sinai Medical Center, Los Angeles; Associate Clinical Professor, Department of Psychiatry and Bio-Behavioral Sciences, David Geffen School of Medicine at UCLA; Associate Clinical Professor, Department of Psychiatry, Loma Linda University School of Medicine.

E. Edward Zinke, M.Div: Treasurer, Adventist Theological Society; President, Foundation for Adventist Education, Silver Spring, Maryland.

INDEX

Note: Page references followed by f refer to figures; t, tables.

A

C

D

E

F

G

H

J

M

N

S

U

V

W

Y

Z